The
WELFARE
of
NATIONS

The
WELFARE
of
NATIONS

James Bartholomew

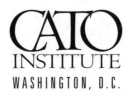

CATO
INSTITUTE
WASHINGTON, D.C.

This edition of *The Welfare of Nations* is published by arrangement with Biteback Publishing. Originally published in Great Britain by Biteback Publishing Ltd.
© James Bartholomew 2015.

ISBN: 978-1-939709-91-2
eBook ISBN: 978-1-939709-92-9

Library of Congress Cataloging-in-Publication Data available.

Printed in the United States of America.

CATO INSTITUTE
1000 Massachusetts Ave., N.W.
Washington, D.C. 20001
www.cato.org

Dedication

To the people who really went out of their way to help me with
the research for this book: Jeremy Hosking played the key role
of giving me some funding. Meir Kohn, economics professor at
Dartmouth College, regularly sent me links to articles that could
be of use, provided contacts, and—just as important—gave me
encouragement. Christian Wignall chauffeured me from one appointment to another in San Francisco and Oakland, patiently waiting for me to emerge after each one. He also helped with contacts
and kindly did restlessly intelligent research for me on various
subjects. J. P. Floru of the Adam Smith Institute and Philip Booth of
the Institute of Economic Affairs both repeatedly suggested and introduced me to contacts around the world. As well as granting me
a couple of interviews, Leszek Balcerowicz, former deputy prime
minister of Poland, opened doors for me in Warsaw that otherwise
would have remained shut. Eva Cooper helped me with contacts in
various parts of the world and answered questions about Sweden.
Pedro Schwartz arranged interviews for me in Spain. Janadas
Devan, director of the Institute of Policy Studies in Singapore, set
up several days' worth of meetings. To my surprise, I found one
of them was with the deputy prime minister. Lindsay Mitchell,
in New Zealand, organized an extraordinary day for me in and
around Wellington, meeting one interesting person after another;
and Greg Lindsay, founder and executive director of the Centre for
Independent Studies in Sydney, set up a program of meetings for
me, gave me a bed for the night, and made the supreme sacrifice of
letting me play bad golf at his club.

Contents

CONTENTS

The World Quiz

How much do you know about the way the world works? Is Sweden really socialist to the core? Which country is the single-parenting capital of the world? Is America a free-market, capitalist nation with barely any social provision? How does Britain fare in treating breast cancer compared with other countries that do not have a national health service? Which country has the lowest unemployment?

Take the quiz. Write down your answers and see how you score:

1. **What is the average rate of "functional illiteracy" in the advanced world?**

   (a) 2 percent
   (b) 5 percent
   (c) 11 percent
   (d) 18 percent

2. **Which of these countries has the highest proportion of people living alone?**

   (a) United States
   (b) Italy
   (c) Australia
   (d) Sweden

3. **In early 2014, one of these countries had an unemployment rate of 25.6 percent and another only 2.8 percent. Which was which?**

   (a) Spain
   (b) Singapore
   (c) France
   (d) Poland
   (e) Japan
   (f) Switzerland

4. **Which of these countries has the worst five-year survival rate for breast cancer?**

   (a) United States
   (b) United Kingdom
   (c) Netherlands
   (d) Australia

5. **What is the percentage of elderly living in residential care in England and Wales that say that they wish that they were dead?**

(a) 3 percent
(b) 8 percent
(c) 12 percent
(d) 21 percent

6. **At what age are Polish soldiers and policemen eligible to retire on a pension?**

(a) 35
(b) 45
(c) 55
(d) 65

7. **Who said, "He who does not work shall not eat" (and that only those who work should be allowed access to consumer goods)?**

(a) Adam Smith
(b) Milton Friedman
(c) Margaret Thatcher
(d) Vladimir Lenin

8. **What is or was the "rubber room"?**

(a) A windowless room with rubber walls for uncontrollable students in a Bronx school
(b) A room in a French *mairie* to which records revealing the corruption of officials are taken to be destroyed
(c) A place in New York where teachers went during the long-winded process of firing them
(d) A rest and recreation room for union officials in Spanish companies

9. **What was the rate of youth unemployment in Spain in early 2014?**

(a) 17 percent
(b) 23 percent
(c) 34 percent
(d) 54 percent

10. **How many people in the United States received food stamps in 2013?**

    (a) 3 million
    (b) 12 million
    (c) 21 million
    (d) 48 million

11. **Which country has the highest proportion of "free" or "charter" schools?**

    (a) Australia
    (b) Sweden
    (c) United Kingdom
    (d) United States

12. **Which country has the lowest unemployment rate?**

    (a) Switzerland
    (b) Sweden
    (c) Singapore
    (d) United States

13. **Between 1987 and 2001, the proportion of social (public) housing in Germany changed. In which way?**

    (a) It more than doubled.
    (b) It increased by over a half.
    (c) It increased by a quarter.
    (d) It more than halved.

14. **Which country has the highest rate of criminal assaults and threats?**

    (a) Australia
    (b) England and Wales
    (c) United States
    (d) Sweden

15. **Which country has the highest number of angioplasty, hip replacement, and knee replacement operations per 100,000?**

    (a) France
    (b) United States
    (c) Germany
    (d) Sweden

16. Who said, "I propose to create a Civilian Conservation Corps to be used in simple work; more important, however, than the material gains will be the moral and spiritual value of such work"?

    (a) President Herbert Hoover
    (b) President Calvin Coolidge
    (c) President Franklin D. Roosevelt
    (d) President Ronald Reagan

17. Which country is the world capital of single parenting (has the highest rate)?

    (a) Sweden
    (b) Denmark
    (c) United States
    (d) United Kingdom

18. Which country spends a massive 29.4 percent of its government budget paying pensions?

    (a) Switzerland
    (b) United Kingdom
    (c) Italy
    (d) Netherlands

19. The proportion of women over 65 without partners who live with one of their children has declined to only 3 percent in one of these countries but has remained at 61 percent in another. Which is which?

    (a) Belgium
    (b) Portugal
    (c) France
    (d) Denmark
    (e) United Kingdom

20. Who suggested that law school training is excessively long and courses should last only two years instead of three?

    (a) Margaret Thatcher
    (b) Milton Friedman
    (c) President Barack Obama
    (d) Lee Kuan Yew

Answers: 1. d; 2. d;[1] 3. a and b, respectively[2] (Japan and Switzerland also had much lower than average unemployment rates); 4. b;[3] 5. d;[4] 6. a; 7. d; 8. c; 9. d;[5] 10. d; 11. b; 12. c; 13. d; 14. b;[6] 15. c[7] (in fact, Germany does the most in each of the three categories of operation); 16. c;[8] 17. c;[9] 18. c;[10] 19. d and b, respectively;[11] 20. c.[12] Give yourself a point for every correct answer.

How did you score?
1–7: You really need to read this book!
8–14: You are pretty well informed and obviously take an interest in the subject. For you, this book is like getting a free upgrade to first class.
15–22: Impressive. You are an expert. It would be an honor if you would read this book.

Preface

"No! No! No!" How Lady Thatcher Helped Prompt the Writing of This Book

In May 2006, I went to a lunchtime talk at the Institute of Economic Affairs, not far from the Houses of Parliament. After it finished, I was about to leave when, unexpectedly, John Blundell, who was then director general, invited me to join others at a reception in a room nearby. It was for Václav Klaus, president of the Czech Republic, who was visiting London at the time. Even more to my surprise, I saw that among the people who had come to see him was Baroness Margaret Thatcher.

Suddenly I found myself being introduced to her. John Blundell marched me up to her and instructed me to tell her about the book I had written. Startled, I said that the book—*The Welfare State We're In*—had argued that the modern British welfare state, despite its good intentions, had done a great deal of harm and we would be better off if it had not been created. Straight away she demanded to know what, if that were the case, should be done about it.

I had been asked this question repeatedly when I had given talks about the book. I gave my usual reply: "Unfortunately, I am very doubtful that a democracy would accept the changes that would make things really better. And I do not want to recommend something second best."

Baroness Thatcher was not having that. She said something like: "No! No! No! You can't say there is a problem and not come up with a solution! You must suggest an alternative! If you say the welfare state is no good, you must suggest an alternative!"

I resorted to another of my standard answers: "The research to arrive at any conclusion worth hearing would cost a great deal of time and money. And anyway, people find blueprints boring."

She was impatient with that, too, saying, "If you can't think of a good way of communicating it, you must *find* a way of communicating it!"—or words to that effect. I was like a junior minister getting his marching orders.

I am afraid I still believe that a democracy is unlikely to adapt and stick to an ideal solution. However, after the prompting I got from her and others and after years of a niggling sense that "surely at least something could be done," I came round to the concept of this book, which is, in part, an attempt to answer Baroness Thatcher's question.

I also wanted to try to assess how welfare states are changing world civilization. In my research, I have traveled to 11 countries and studied more. I have found that the bare statistics are often misleading. Talking to people on the spot can reveal this problem, and give rise to insights that no amount of deskbound study could reveal.

1. Why Are So Many Swedish People Disabled?

The World of Welfare from Opheltas to Bismarck to the Clever Research of Kathryn Edin

In the midst of the greatest economic depression the United States has ever known, 13 million people are unemployed.[1] More than 5,000 banks have folded. Hundreds of thousands of families have been made homeless after defaulting on loans. Many have gone to shantytowns. At this extraordinary time of national crisis in 1935, President Franklin D. Roosevelt introduces the New Deal—a collection of programs intended to end the crisis. His advisers have different ideas. They argue with each other. He himself has no great theory, but he is a confident man, willing to try things out and see how they go. One thing he is sure of is that he wants men to work. He does not want just to give them money. He is also concerned about overspending.

In June, he bypasses Congress and issues an executive order. He creates one of his lesser-known programs, the National Youth Administration. The goal is to find work for young people who have left school and cannot get a job. He does not want them to be idle at this formative age.

He signs the order on a Tuesday morning. That same day, an ambitious young man telephones key contacts to put himself forward for the job of administering the program in his home state of Texas. His speed of reaction and energy get him the job within a month. He becomes the youngest state director of the program in the country. He is only 27.

He finds sponsors to provide materials for each project. Housing has to be found for the young participants. Supervisors need to be hired. He brings astonishing energy and determination to the job. He builds a reputation for getting things done. He also creates a political base in his home state from which, as soon as possible, he will be able to run for national office. He travels by car and by plane.

He is on the phone. He starts work at 7 in the morning and goes on until 11 at night. "You would ask him about the weather, and he would start talking about projects," a friend remarks.

The young man swiftly signs up 350 sponsors. Within six months, he has 18,000 young people working on parks, constructing buildings, and so on. The national director of the program, Aubrey Williams, says the young man is the best administrator that he has. Eleanor Roosevelt, the First Lady, wants to meet the young man.

What is the name of this exceptional individual? Lyndon B. Johnson.

According to a biographer of Johnson, his successful experience as an administrator of the National Youth Administration "confirmed his belief that in order to meet public goals it was necessary only to pass a good bill and put a good man in charge."[2] Twenty-eight years later, Lyndon Johnson is U.S. president following the assassination of John F. Kennedy. Ambition still burns fiercely within him. Brought up as a supporter of Roosevelt and a successful administrator of a New Deal program, Johnson focuses his ambition on nothing less than "an unconditional war on poverty." Poverty has not been a major issue previously, but he makes many speeches in which he urges that the greatness of America is not compatible with the poverty that remains in it. He says this is "more than a beginning. It is a total commitment by this President and Congress and this nation to pursue victory over the most ancient of mankind's enemies."

When Johnson makes this speech to Congress in 1964, America has not long before been among the victors of the Second World War both in Europe and against Japan. It has enjoyed fast-growing prosperity. The can-do attitude of Americans is famous. Why should the American capacity for doing things not be applied to poverty, too? Johnson goes on, "If we can bring to the challenges of peace the same determination and strength which has brought us victory in war— then this day and this Congress will have won a more secure and honorable place in the history of the nation and the enduring gratitude of generations of Americans to come." He believes he is making history. In a speech on the campus of the University of Michigan, he refers to "the Great Society." He has used the phrase before, but in this speech it is central. It becomes the phrase by which his massive program of legislation becomes known.

We can see two things combining to produce Johnson's war on poverty: the powerful ambition of a man who wants to make his mark and widespread optimism that a government can achieve whatever it sets out to do. With Johnson's determination and experience at dealing with Congress, he pushes through a wide range of radical laws. Box 1.1 shows what followed 50 years later and just steps away.

Box 1.1
A CONTRAST IN WASHINGTON

The final country I visited for my research was the United States. One day, in Washington, D.C., I went to talk to an expert on care for the elderly who was based in one of the grand government buildings not far from the U.S. Capitol. After the meeting, I walked across the street toward the Capitol itself—a magnificent building designed in the neoclassical style and poised on top of a hill. It inspires a feeling of power and order.

Eventually, I turned away to set off back to my hotel. As I walked along a featureless, straight street, I saw some people ahead on both sides of the pavement. Some were standing. Others were sitting on a low wall. Some were in groups of two or three. Others were alone.

What were they doing?

As I got closer, I realized that most were black. I saw around the corner that still more were waiting—but waiting for what?

I looked at a building on the far side of the road and saw a sign saying John L. Young Center for the Homeless. Were they waiting for accommodations? It seemed strange. The journalist in me wanted to go up to them and ask. I also wanted to take photographs. But I felt I would be intruding on people in unfortunate circumstances. I said nothing and took no photographs. I just wrote down on my notepad: "very sad sight" and then "separate sadness." They were not chatting with each other. They were each in individual, separate experiences of misfortune.

Seeing them gave me a strong feeling of how important it is to get welfare as right as we can. None of us should insist on his or her political prejudices. We should look at the evidence and try to be honest about it. Too much is at stake to indulge barroom views.

Half a century ago, the president of this exceptionally rich country proudly decided to wage "an unconditional war on poverty." And yet only 500 yards away from the Capitol—grand symbol of democracy and power—more than 30 melancholy people are waiting for something in a public, humiliating way.

It so happens that nothing is new about the paradox of a wealthy country with a large number of welfare dependents. This is exactly what struck Alexis de Tocqueville when he visited England in 1833. He remarked how strange it was that while Britain was preeminently rich and successful, it had more paupers than other, poorer countries.

Lyndon Johnson is one of the founders of the American welfare state. At first sight, he seems a world away from the originator of another welfare state. But let's travel back in time to the late 19th century to meet this other one.

Otto von Bismarck is the most powerful man since Napoleon. In contrast to Johnson, he is a conservative and monarchist. He is politically brilliant, is dedicated to his cause, and has created modern Germany.

We know quite a lot about his thinking because of a strange circumstance. From time to time, he uses a friendly journalist, Moritz Busch, to plant stories in the newspapers. Unbeknownst to Bismarck, Busch keeps copious notes of his conversations with Bismarck, including the chancellor's off-the-record remarks.

On January 18, 1881, Busch writes to Bismarck "reminding him of my readiness to place myself at his disposal" in case he wishes "to have any matter of importance discussed in the German or English press."[3] Two days later, Busch receives a letter inviting him to call on Bismarck the following day. So on Friday, January 21, 1881, Busch goes to the chancellor's palace.

Bismarck starts their conversation by remarking to Busch, "So you have come for material, but there is not much to give you." Then he remembers something. "One thing occurs to me, however. I should be very thankful to you if you would discuss my working-class insurance scheme in a friendly spirit."[4]

Bismarck explains his motives with extraordinary frankness: "A beginning must be made with the task of reconciling the labouring classes with the state. Whoever has a pension assured to him for his old age is much more contented and easier to manage than the man who has no such prospect."[5] His idea is to make the working classes "easier to manage," thus enabling him to perpetuate the monarchical rule to which he is devoted. (But state welfare goes back much further than him, as can be seen in Box 1.2.)

Bismarck frankly admits that this social insurance may cost a lot of money. "Large sums of money would be required for carrying such schemes into execution, at least a hundred million marks, or more probably two hundred. But I should not be frightened by even three hundred millions. Means must be provided to enable the state to act generously towards the poor." He discusses how money might be raised through the tobacco monopoly. But he tells Busch he "need not emphasize this point." Presumably, he wants to present the advantages rather than the costs. But the money can be found,

Box 1.2
STATE WELFARE DID NOT BEGIN WITH BISMARCK

Government welfare programs date to the earliest records of western civilization. In part of ancient Greece, laws provided that those who were disabled fighting in war should be "maintained at the public charge." Peisistratus, who ruled in Athens most of the time between 561 and 527 BCE, so ordered, seemingly following a precedent set by Solon, who lived even earlier, from about 638 BCE to 558 BCE. Solon ordered that the sons of those killed in war should "be educated and bred up at the public expense." Polybius in his *Histories* reported that a politician called Opheltas, in the third century BCE in Boeotia, a region of Greece, "was always inventing some plan calculated to benefit the masses for the moment, while perfectly certain to ruin them in the future."[a]

Under the Romans, the "dole" of grain was first subsidized at the initiative of Gaius Gracchus in 123 BCE. After him, the generosity of the dole went further when Publius Clodius Pulcher, in 57 BCE, made it free. The dole was the ancient equivalent of food stamps. Those entitled to it had a ticket (*tessera*) that could be exchanged every month.

In medieval Europe, the church took the leading role in looking after the poor, aged, and disabled. Hospitals, almshouses, and schools were founded that received considerable donations from the devout. Some reminders of this system survive. In Siena, Italy, you can visit the hospital of Santa Maria della Scala, founded eight centuries ago, which stands opposite the famous cathedral. In Ghent, Belgium, you can visit some of the House of Alijn almshouses that were administered by the church.

But governments—particularly local governments—took an increasing role at the time of the Reformation. Leading intellectuals of the day considered how best to administer welfare. Martin Luther wrote that every town and village should make a register of poor people in need of aid—they were called "paupers"—because otherwise those who got the most money would be "vagabonds and desperate rogues." He admitted, "I have myself of late years been cheated and befooled by such tramps and liars more than I wish to confess."[b]

In 1525, the town of Ypres, Belgium, devised a system for the "relief" of paupers that had enormous influence. Under this system, begging was banned. Individual officials were meant to visit the poor in their homes and to act as their "common parents," making sure they had enough to eat and they went to school or got training for a job or, if they were workshy, that they were obliged to work. If they refused work, the officials would punish them. The money to pay for this assistance was to be obtained through house-to-house collection of alms as well as from boxes in churches and from bequests. With all this provision of relief in place, Ypres felt able to ban begging.

(continued on next page)

(continued)

The system was so controversial that it was brought to the Sorbonne for judgment as to whether or not it was in accordance with the Scriptures, the teaching of the Apostles, and the laws of the church. The Sorbonne decided, with provisos, that it was acceptable. The system was described as "hard but useful . . . pious and salutary."[c]

In the 19th century, rapid development of mutual aid organizations, provident societies, trade unions, friendly societies, and commercial insurance also took place to various extents in different countries. Finally, national governments took an increasing role—slowly in the 19th century but with increasing speed in the 20th.[d]

---

[a] Polybius, *Histories*, Book 20. The third century BCE seems implied, but it is not stated.
[b] Karl de Schweinitz, *England's Road to Social Security* (New York: A.S.Barnes & Co./Perpetua Books, 1961), p. 37.
[c] Paul Spicker, ed., *The Origins of Modern Welfare* (Oxford: Peter Lang, 2010), p. 142.
[d] Sources include *Plutarch's Lives*, trans. Bernadotte Perrin (London: Heinemann, 1914); Diogenes Laertius, *The Lives and Opinions of Eminent Philosophers*, trans. C. D. Yonge (London: Henry G. Bohn, 1853); H. H. Scullard, *From the Gracchi to Nero: A History of Rome from 133 BC to AD 68* (Abingdon, U.K.: Routledge, [1959] 2011); Schweinitz, *England's Road to Social Security*.

and he concludes, "If the sums thus acquired are used for securing the future of our working population, uncertainty as to which is the chief cause of their hatred to the state, we thereby at the same time secure our own future and that is a good investment for our money. We should thus avert a revolution, which might break out fifty or perhaps ten years hence."[6]

It could not be clearer. Bismarck is a conservative and monarchist. He is introducing social insurance largely for the purpose of foiling a socialist revolution that he believes would otherwise take place. The cunning chancellor is thinking long term, protecting his king and the society he cherishes.

He is soon criticized by some people for introducing what is sometimes called "state socialism." He replies, in the classic manner of a politician who is a realist, "It may be State Socialism, but it is necessary."[7]

And yet who can be sure what is going on in Bismarck's mind? A few months later, Bismarck invites Busch to visit him again. This time Bismarck refers to social insurance as "our practical Christianity."

Busch is surprised. He asks, "Practical Christianity? Did I right understand Your Serene Highness?"

Bismarck replies, "Certainly. Compassion, a helping hand in distress. The state, which can raise money with the least trouble, must take the matter in hand. Not as alms, but as a right to maintenance, where not the readiness but the power to work fails."[8]

So perhaps compassion is a part of his motivation. Or perhaps he is merely rehearsing arguments that will enable him to get the legislation passed without really believing in them.

Finally, we see his remorseless political intelligence, which is always looking well ahead. He declares, "This question will force its way; it has a future. It is possible that our policy may be reversed at some future time when I am dead; but State Socialism will make its way. Whoever takes up this idea again will come to power."[9]

Bismarck's prediction proves correct. All around the world in the following decades, politicians gain or keep power by espousing what he called "state socialism." It is what we now know as the "welfare state." It is hard to think of any politicians who did their careers anything but good in the hundred years after Bismarck's declaration by espousing the cause of social security.

Politicians like Lyndon Johnson and Otto von Bismarck who took part in creating modern welfare states may appear to have been very different characters with different agendas. But they all had some of the following motives in varying proportions:

- Compassion for the poor and afflicted
- Outrage at the perceived injustice of society
- A desire by conservatives or centrists to hold onto power by undercutting the appeal of socialism, which was seen as dangerously damaging
- Ambition to gain a prestigious place in history
- Belief that governments could completely eradicate poverty

The motives ranged from the cynical to the utopian, and—such is human nature—some politicians were motivated by both simultaneously.

So how did it all go? Did Lyndon Johnson win his war on poverty?

The United States has a bewildering array of welfare programs. So let's take just one: food stamps. The number of people in the United States deemed to need government help to get food on the table surpasses 46 million.[10] That is one in every seven Americans.[11] Given that America has been the outstandingly rich and successful large country of the past century, this figure is astonishing. But even this figure does not include every person in America currently described

7

as being in poverty. Lyndon Johnson's ambition to eradicate poverty appears to have failed—perhaps even to have backfired.

As the wealth of America has increased, so has the number of people apparently in need of help. The budget devoted to welfare has increased again and again. It now amounts to $523 billion a year.[12] Yet the numbers who need support still grow. What has gone wrong?

Some may be thinking, "Social welfare may have gone wrong in America, but America adopted a particularly bad kind of welfare." In France, more than anywhere perhaps, scorn exists for American economic and social policy. The "Anglo-Saxon" approach is seen as brutish, grudging, and damaging to the harmony of society. France has a great belief in "solidarity"—a binding together of the classes. In France, welfare is based on providing compulsory, universal social insurance, not on merely providing a safety net for the poor. Armed with this positive attitude and a different system, have the French succeeded in eliminating poverty and providing employment in a way that the Americans did not?

No. Unemployment in France has soared from an average of 1.5 percent in the 1950s to 9.0 percent in the 1980s and 10.4 percent in 2014.[13] If the country had decided to increase unemployment as a matter of policy, it could hardly have done better. It has been a major welfare failure. (See Box 1.3.) Social spending has correspondingly risen higher and higher as a proportion of gross domestic product, climbing from 12.5 percent in 1960 to 32.5 percent in 2010.[14] The official number of disabled rose by a quarter in the decade leading to 2007.[15]

"When one crosses the various countries of Europe, one is struck by a very extraordinary and apparently inexplicable sight.

"The countries appearing to be the most impoverished are those which in reality account for the fewest indigents, and among the peoples most admired for their opulence, one part of the population is obliged to rely on the gifts of the other in order to live.

"Cross the English countryside and you will think yourself transported into the Eden of modern civilization. . . .

"Now look more closely at the villages; examine the parish registers, and you will discover with indescribable astonishment that one-sixth of the inhabitants of this flourishing kingdom live at the expense of public charity."

SOURCE: Alexis de Tocqueville. *Memoir on Pauperism* (Chicago: Ivan R. Dee, 1997 [1835]), pp. 37–38.

Box 1.3
POVERTY IN FRANCE: A SNAPSHOT

In La Rochelle, France, Nicole Liguori started offering subsidized lunches once every two weeks. Diners had to pay €2.50 for the meal. Local supermarkets helped by providing food and donations. Liguori said, "I was aware of the condition of people I met and chatted to in the street. The retired, the homeless and the unemployed who, in addition to the material miseries, feel profoundly alone."

SOURCE: Isabelle Pouey-Sanchou, "Très populaire, la soupe," *Sud Ouest* (France), December 8, 2010, http://www.sudouest.fr/2010/12/08/tres-populaire-la-soupe-261516-1391.php?reagir=true.

What about other countries that have introduced welfare states?

In 1950, the unemployment rate in the member countries of the Organisation for Economic Co-operation and Development (OECD) was just under 4 percent. But if one goes back further still, to the beginning of the 20th century, before almost any country had created unemployment insurance benefits, the rate was lower still. No overall OECD figures exist for that time, but in Britain, the rate was a mere 2.5 percent in 1900. In Germany, it was 4.7 percent in 1903, falling to 2.7 percent in 1906.[16] Now, since welfare states have been introduced in full measure, average OECD unemployment has risen to 8.2 percent in 2011, moderating to 7.4 percent in mid-2014. In the European Union, where welfare states are most fully developed, the lowest rate in recent years was 7.0 percent (2008), and it has subsequently risen to a peak of 10.8 percent (2013).[17]

But the rise in the official number of people unemployed does not tell the whole story. In some ways, things are even worse. For many countries, "early retirement" has become a politically convenient disguise for further unemployment. France, Belgium, Austria, Greece, and Italy have this type of hidden unemployment. Belgium and Austria both have particularly large gaps between the official retirement age for men of 65 and the actual average retirement age of 59.[18]

One of the most remarkable statistics I came across in my research is that in Poland, in 2004, only 28 percent of people ages 55 to 64 were actually working.[19] In other words, the vast majority of people stopped working once they were past 55. Since 2004, the proportion working has crept up to 37 percent. But even now, huge numbers of men and women of working age in Poland are not working yet

9

are not officially classed as "unemployed." They are the hidden unemployed.

Hidden unemployment also exists among people on disability benefits. Of course, some are genuinely disabled. But many are not. Huge contrasts exist in the numbers who receive disability benefits in different countries. In Japan, 2 percent of working-age people are officially disabled. In Sweden, more than 10 percent are.[20] If these figures reflected reality, when walking through the streets of Stockholm, one would expect to see many people being pushed around in wheelchairs or struggling on crutches. Yet one does not.

It is astonishing and, frankly, hard to believe that the rate of disability in one advanced country is five times greater than that in another. Conceivably, Japan is refusing to recognize the true disabled condition of some people. But it seems more likely that the cause of the violent contrast is that many people in Sweden are not genuinely disabled but have found that welfare benefits for incapacity are well worth having and can be obtained without too much difficulty. In other words, they are unemployed.

The apparently disabled of Britain have historically been concentrated in areas of high unemployment, again suggesting that going onto disability benefits has been an alternative to going onto unemployment benefits. An analysis of the large numbers on the benefit by a Labour government in the 2000s suggested that a million people on the benefit were capable of work. Around the world, the proportion of people of working age who are apparently too ill to work has risen. In the United States, it doubled from 2.3 percent in 1989 to 4.6 percent in 2009.[21] (See also Box 1.4.) The rise in the numbers claiming a disability benefit took place in parallel with the fall in the numbers on the welfare rolls.[22] For many, disability has become an alternative way of obtaining payments without working.

"To provide for poor men is harder than men think, considering that it cannot be duly executed without great diligence, study and wisdom."

SOURCE: *Forma Subventionis Pauperum*, an evaluation of the Ypres system, published in 1531, as quoted by Karl de Schweinitz, *England's Road to Social Security* (New York: A.S. Barnes & Co./ Perpetua Books, 1961), p.30.

Box 1.4

RISE IN DISABILITY BENEFITS OUTPACES POPULATION GROWTH

The number of people of working age who receive disability benefits quadrupled in the United States over 30 years, even as the general health of Americans improved, as shown in the following figure.

FIGURE B1.4

WORKING-AGE RECIPIENTS OF DISABILITY BENEFITS IN THE UNITED STATES, 1970–2003

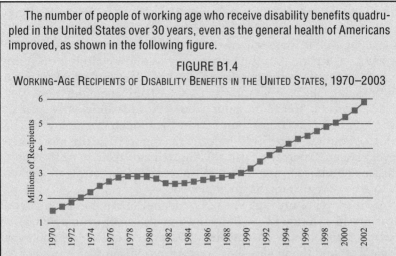

SOURCES: U.S. Social Security Administration, *Trends in the Social Security and Supplemental Security Income Disability Programs,* tables citing "Annual Statistical Supplement to the Social Security Bulletin," 2004, Table 4.C1; "Annual Statistical Report on the Social Security Disability Insurance Program," 2003, Table 1; Table equivalent for Chart 3, U.S. Social Security Administration Office of Policy website, http://www.socialsecurity.gov/policy/docs/chartbooks/disability_trends/sect01-text.html#chart3.

Disability benefits are distributed as Supplemental Security Income and Social Security Disability Income. The proportion of U.S. workers who receive disability benefits has risen from about 25 per 1,000 in 1970 to 73 in 2011. This is nearly a tripling in the proportion.[a] The number of recipients almost quadrupled over this period while the overall population of the United States rose by only 41 percent.[b] Since 2003, the number of disability benefits has continued upward and was approaching 7 million in 2012.[c]

The proportion of awards related to infections/parasites, injuries, respiratory ailments, endocrine/nutritional/metabolic problems, the nervous system, neoplasms, and circulatory problems has declined.[d] The awards related to mental and musculoskeletal problems proportionately increased. Those categories increased from 27.0 percent to 51.7 percent of all cases. The same trend has been seen in other countries. These two causes of disability have one thing in common with each other: it is not possible objectively to verify whether someone genuinely suffers from them or not.

---

[a] See Tad de Haven, "The Rising Cost of Social Security Disability Insurance," *Downsizing Government* blog, August 2013, Figure 3, http://www.downsizinggovernment.org/ssa/social-security-disability-insurance.
[b] From 205 million in 1970 to 290 million in 2003. See https://www.google.co.uk/publicdata/explore?ds=kf7tgg1uo9ude_&met_y=population&hl=en&dl=en&idim=country:US.
[c] Ben Gersten, "5 Charts Show Alarming Trend in Number of Americans Collecting Social Security," *Money Morning*, April 10, 2013, http://moneymorning.com/2013/04/10/5-charts-show-alarming-trend-in-number-of-americans-collecting-social-security/.
[d] "Trends in the Social Security and Supplemental Security Income Disability Programs," Table equivalent for Chart 27, Social Security Administration website, http://www.socialsecurity.gov/policy/docs/chartbooks/disability_trends/sect02-text.html#chart27.

The average proportion on disability benefits in OECD countries is 5 percent. Let us conservatively guess that the rate of genuine disability in an advanced country is, say, 3 percent, slightly above Japan's. If that estimate is right, then more than 2 percent of working-age people in the advanced world are claiming disability benefits without being genuinely disabled. If we add that figure to the official OECD unemployment rate, true unemployment rises to 10.2 percent. To this number should be added the early retirees, who are, in reality, other members of the hidden unemployed. That could amount to a further 2 percent, raising the true unemployment level to over 12 percent. Even this figure is unlikely to be the end of the story because it does not capture so-called discouraged workers who are not registered as unemployed.

Such a level of unemployment is unparalleled in human history. It amounts to a worldwide welfare disaster. Instead of winning a war on poverty, Lyndon Johnson—and other clever, generally well-intentioned leaders around the world—have created systems in which permanent mass unemployment has become normal. Although the wealth of the world has increased tremendously over the past 30 years, let alone the past 100 years, instead of achieving the economic well-being for all that our ancestors expected, we have mass dependency on handouts.

But the world has been even more reluctant to face another aspect of this situation. In Madrid, I talked to many people about the extraordinarily high unemployment there, which, at the time, had reached 23 percent of those of working age. One person I spoke to was the Madrid minister of health, Javier Fernández-Lasquetty. He stopped for a moment, midconversation, and remarked, "Actually, we don't know what is the level of unemployment. It is a mystery."

Fernández-Lasquetty meant that the government did not know the number of people who were working unofficially—without paying social insurance contributions or taxes. Spain undoubtedly has one of the biggest black economies in Europe. Many lower-paid immigrants—from Latin America and Romania especially—cannot get jobs at the minimum wage. But many get by on *chapuzas*—odd jobs for which they are paid in cash. And such hidden economies are not just in Spain. Hidden economies are part of many welfare states.

In America, Christopher Jenks, an academic, and his colleagues were puzzled that, in surveys, a lot of families on the lowest incomes said that they were not experiencing material difficulties. Most of these apparently very poor people said they were not going hungry or having their gas or electricity cut off. The academics hired a graduate student,

Kathryn Edin, to find out what was going on. She was to interview some of the people they had been questioning. She contacted them but found they were reluctant to talk openly. She realized they suspected she was working for the welfare department or some other government agency. So she decided to take a different approach. Instead of interviewing people who had no reason to trust her, she arranged to be introduced by people who already knew and were trusted by welfare recipients. Then, once she had the trust of the people she was studying, she interviewed them and asked them to introduce her to others.

By gaining their trust and interviewing people two or more times, Kathryn Edin—and Laura Lein, who joined her—discovered the answer to the mystery of how women with very low incomes were getting by: they had other sources of cash.[23] Edin and Lein and their colleagues talked to 379 women and found only one who did not have an extra source of income. Except in a minority of cases in which the income was officially recognized or declared, the women kept their income secret from government officials. Among those Edin and Lein interviewed who were unemployed and receiving welfare benefits, the average benefits were $565 per month, but average spending was 55 percent more: $876.

The women had two main sources of extra money (see Tables 1.1 and 1.2). One was people they knew: family, friends, and, more

Table 1.1

MONTHLY INCOME OF WELFARE-RELIANT MOTHERS

Type of income	Amount
Welfare benefits	$565
Earned income tax credits[a]	$3
Reported work	$19
Unreported and "underground" work	$109
Family, friends, boyfriends, and absent fathers	$151
Agency-based support	$37
Total income	**$883**

SOURCE: Kathryn Edin and Laura Lein, *Making Ends Meet: How Single Mothers Survive Welfare and Low-Wage Work* (New York: Russell Sage Foundation, 1997), Table 2-6.

[a] Earned income tax credits are for wages earned the previous year.

13

Table 1.2
WHAT PROPORTION OF WELFARE MOTHERS GETS INCOME FROM
OTHER SOURCES?

Source of income	Share
Reported work	5%
Unreported work	39%
"Underground" work	8%
Total from work[a]	**46%**
Family and friends	46%
Boyfriends	29%
Absent fathers formally	14%
Absent fathers covertly	23%
Total from people[a]	**77%**

SOURCE: Kathryn Edin and Laura Lein, *Making Ends Meet: How Single Mothers Survive Welfare and Low-Wage Work* (New York: Russell Sage Foundation, 1997), Table 2-6.

[a] Some mothers have more than one kind of extra income.

important, current boyfriends or absent fathers. Their second source of cash was work. A small amount was officially reported, but the vast majority was off the books. A minority of the earnings came from so-called underground work, such as prostitution and dealing in drugs or stolen goods. About 39 percent of the women were doing work not officially declared, even without including all those doing underground work.

Because of Edin's remarkable and well-respected investigation, we know that American single mothers have been keeping a great deal of work secret from the authorities. Other groups, such as men, are likely doing something similar. It also seems probable that something similar is taking place in other countries where no one has yet done such painstaking research. Box 1.5 discusses an example of another kind of unseen reality of welfare from Great Britain.

One point that Edin and Lein do not belabor—but which is implicit in their study—is that the mothers are making ends meet

Box 1.5
WHEN IT MIGHT PAY TO SPEND INSTEAD OF SAVE

Pauline Ford was a poor woman who lived in a mobile home and claimed welfare benefits. She lived frugally. She never went out and didn't smoke or drink. In 2011, she was convicted of fraud because she had not disclosed that she had built up savings of £22,000.

Of course, she should have disclosed her savings under the law. But it is also true that if she had drunk and smoked or if she had bought furniture and gold chains, she would not have had the savings and she would not have committed a crime.

Most people on means-tested benefits in Britain are aware that if they build up savings, they will cease to be entitled to certain benefits. The British welfare state thus discourages saving by the poor.

SOURCE: John Hutchinson, "Frugal Spinster, 58, Who Saved £22,000 Nest Egg from Her Benefits for Her Old Age Has to Pay It All Back, Plus Another £6,000," *Daily Mail* (London), http://www.dailymail.co.uk /news/article-2075861/Pauline-Ford-58-saved-22k-nest-egg-benefits-pay-back.html.

by cheating. The vast majority of the extra income they get should be declared to their welfare officer and result in lower benefits. So cheating is normal. You could even argue that it is part of the system. It is easy to imagine those involved feeling that they would be fools not to do what so many others are doing. They would also be in even greater financial difficulty. Edin and Lein make crystal clear that the lives of these women are difficult despite the extra money. Fifteen percent said they had gone hungry at some point during the previous 12 months despite receiving food stamps. Seventeen percent reported having had their electricity or gas cut off.

The research by Edin and Lein takes the lid off the world of welfare benefits. It is supported by research commissioned by Peter Lilley, British secretary of state for social security in the 1990s. His staff similarly found that the expenditure of the poorest 10 percent of people was considerably higher than their apparent income.

The implications of this hidden world of economic activity are strange. We previously found more unemployment than the official figures suggest, but Edin's research tells us that simultaneously hidden employment exists. Edin's work means, among other things, that less poverty exists than the official figures suggest—particularly for countries where benefits are means tested and a strong incentive exists to keep income secret. So the most quoted measure of inequality of income—the Gini coefficient—is unreliable. It exaggerates inequality of incomes, especially in those countries where benefits are mainly means tested.

Amid the confusion, one powerful truth emerges from the clouds bright and clear: many welfare systems around the world have been highly dysfunctional:

- The number of unemployed has dramatically increased.
- More people have become benefit dependent despite countries becoming much richer.
- A large proportion of people now dependent on welfare or other benefits are lying about their incomes. Lying has been made normal.
- The cost of welfare systems has grown enormously. Welfare expenditure is now larger than all other government expenditure put together in Denmark, Finland, France, Germany, Austria, Italy, New Zealand, Spain, and Sweden.[24] The average expenditure in advanced countries is 22 percent of gross domestic product.[25]

The situation of the poor has also become worse in other ways—ways less susceptible to being weighed by numbers.

The change in the lives of many of the poor is reflected eloquently by Barack Obama in his book *Dreams from My Father*.[26] Obama worked as a community organizer in Chicago in the late 1980s. Referring to the middle-aged, working-class, black Americans he met in Roseland, one of the less well-off suburbs, he wrote: "On the strength of two incomes, they had paid off house notes and car notes, maybe college educations for their sons or daughters whose graduation pictures filled every mantelpiece."[27] But he remarked that when his conversations with them turned to the future of the neighborhood, they "were marked by another more ominous strain."

People worried about "the decaying storefronts, the aging church rolls, kids from unknown families who swaggered down the streets—loud congregations of teenage boys, teenage girls feeding potato chips to crying toddlers, the discarded wrappers tumbling down the block—all of it whispered painful truths, told them the progress they'd found was ephemeral, rooted in thin soil; that it might not even last their lifetimes."

Obama came to think that much poorer people he had known earlier during his time in Indonesia had enjoyed better lives. "For all that

16

poverty, there remained in their lives a discernible order. The habits of a generation played out every day beneath the bargaining and the noise and the swirling dust. It was the absence of coherence that made a place like Altgeld [an area of public housing in Chicago] so desperate."

Obama felt that "something different" was also taking place on the South Side, another part of Chicago. There was "a change in atmosphere, like the electricity of an approaching storm." This brought the "sense shared by adults and youth alike, that some, if not most of our boys were slipping beyond rescue."

This evocation of how a culture and a way of life were changing before his eyes involves more than just unemployment. It brings in other aspects of the welfare state that are covered later in this book, such as parenting, housing, education, saving, and behavior. But the central thing that goes wrong in so many welfare states is that so many people are unemployed. Without jobs, they cannot pay off "house notes and car notes." They cannot enjoy normally functioning family structures. They cannot have order in their lives of the sort that even Indonesian slum dwellers have.

Why do so many welfare states have so much unemployment? The question needs answering.

2. Heart of the Darkness

Welfare States and Unemployment

Phil started working when he was 17. He got married and had children. It sounds like a pretty normal kind of life. But when he was 32, the business he was working for in Ireland went bust, and he lost his job. He thought he had managed to deal with the crisis when he got a job with another company. But his new employer failed to pay him. Naturally, he became extremely worried. He was not the only adult in his home who could earn. He had a wife. But he felt it was his job to bring in the money, to finance the home, and to provide for his children.

He kept pressing the company to pay him. Instead, it fired him. Naturally his financial worries increased. He tried to get another job, but he could not find one. "I had to pay rent, petrol, and get a new school uniform for one of the kids. . . . I had to go on the social [claim welfare benefits]." The welfare money was useful, but it was not enough to keep the family going in the way he was used to. Phil began to think of committing suicide. "You start thinking, 'Is it easier for them if I'm not here? . . . If I'm not here, she [his wife] would probably get more money for the kids, the bills would die with me, you wouldn't be driving the car and using petrol.'"

Phil's life hung in the balance. He had gotten to this stage because of losing his job. He felt he was not playing the role in life that he had before. He missed feeling he had a certain status in life and a purpose. His unemployment also led to money worries, which caused arguments with his wife. We know the outline of this true story because Phil was so close to suicide that he contacted the Samaritans, a charity that supports those considering suicide. The Samaritans published his story (obviously changing his name).[1]

Of course, not all people who lose their jobs contemplate suicide. But unemployment is far more depressing than most realize. Some large-scale surveys are conducted on happiness and unhappiness. In the United States, 11.6 percent of the population declared themselves "not too happy" in surveys between 1972 and 1994.[2]

But when it came to the unemployed, the figure more than doubled to 29.6 percent. In Europe, the rise was from 18.6 percent to 33.0 percent. In Europe, people were also asked about their "life satisfaction." Among the general population, 4.9 percent were "not at all satisfied," but more than two-and-a-half times as many of the unemployed—13.3 percent—felt the same way. Of course, this correlation is likely to be partly because the unemployed are poorer. But it goes beyond that. An academic study of the figures found that "being unemployed increases the chance that the respondent declares himself dissatisfied with life, even after holding other things constant that may be expected to be associated with unemployment (e.g., family income, marital separation)."[3] Moreover, "the size of the impact is large and similar across countries."

The unemployed have increased susceptibility to malnutrition, illness, and mental stress.[4] They are more likely to have poor self-esteem, leading to depression. Goldsmith, Veum, and Darity, using data from the U.S. national Longitudinal Study of Youth, found that being jobless injured self-esteem and fostered feelings of "externality" and helplessness among youths.[5] The unemployed have lower life expectancy and are indeed more likely to commit suicide.[6]

Why do I mention all this? Because there has been a tendency in recent times to treat mass unemployment as something that does not matter that much. People who, a few decades ago, would have been passionate about attaining "full employment" have given up the battle cry and now demand "equality" instead. It seems as though they have given up hope of returning to full employment so they have convinced themselves that it does not matter so much. But unemployment matters a great deal. It causes misery and, of course, it makes people poorer. The need for money to pay for unemployment and welfare benefits also means that others must bear higher taxes, so they are poorer too. We have become accustomed to permanent, mass unemployment and have lost sight of the fact that it is relatively new.

Britain had full employment—less than 4 percent unemployment—in at least 4 of the 10 years before the First World War[7] (Figure 2.1). Germany did slightly better, enjoying full employment for 7 of those years. France managed full employment all the way up until the depression of the 1930s.[8] In Germany, there was full employment for 27 years up to 1974.[9] In Australia, the average unemployment rate was a mere 2 percent between 1950 and 1974.[10]

Why has unemployment skyrocketed since those days? Various explanations have been put forward. They include globalization and

Figure 2.1
UNITED KINGDOM UNEMPLOYMENT BEFORE THE WELFARE STATE

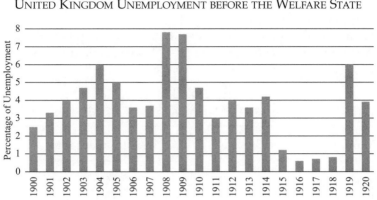

SOURCE: James Denman and Paul McDonald, "Unemployment Statistics from 1881 to the Present Day," *Labour Market Trends*, January 1996, http://www.ons.gov.uk /ons/rel/lms/labour-market-trends--discontinued-/january-1996/unemployment -since-1881.pdf.

NOTE: The U.K. government did not keep official figures until 1911, when employment exchanges were established. The figures before that are from the records kept by trade unions. In fact in most countries, it seems, it is quite difficult for statisticians to create a series of figures that is reliable and consistent. In Great Britain, the unemployment rate jumped to 16.9 percent in 1921 and stayed high until the outbreak of the Second World War. One possible reason is that unemployment benefits were made more generous at this time: see James Bartholomew, *The Welfare State We're In* (London: Politicos, 2004). It is extraordinary that unemployment remained so high through the 1920s as well as the 1930s. One reason it is extraordinary is that the same thing does not seem to have happened in France.

changes in the nature of work caused by such things as automation. The underlying idea in both cases is that, in rich countries, the cost of low-skilled people has become too high compared with the cost of labor from poor countries, when transferring the work to other countries is feasible, or compared with machines or computers such as automated checkout registers.

It is true that globalization has meant that much low-value work has been exported. It is also true that machines are doing many jobs that used to be done by people. But if either of those things were the real cause of overall unemployment, you would expect mass unemployment to have appeared in all rich countries. But it hasn't. Unemployment levels in such countries have varied dramatically.

21

(See Table 2.1). You would also expect the highest unemployment to be in the ri chest countries, where labor is most expensive. But that is not the case, either.

Switzerland is one of the richest countries per capita in the world apart from small tax havens and oil-rich states.[11] So unemployment

Table 2.1
UNEMPLOYMENT RATES OF COUNTRIES WITH NO MINIMUM WAGE

Country	Unemployment rate
Italy	12.6%
Finland	8.5%
Sweden	8.2%
OECD average	7.4%
Denmark	6.5%
Iceland	5.4%
Germany	5.2%
Switzerland	4.8%
Norway	3.3%
Singapore	2.0%

SOURCES: Organisation for Economic Co-operation and Development (OECD), OECD. StatExtracts for April 2014 or most recent available, http://stats.oecd.org/index .aspx?queryid=36324; Singapore government figure for Singapore. Countries with no minimum wages: various sources including OECD. Some articles refer to Austria as having no minimum wage, but it does appear to have one: see "Real minimum wages," OECD.StatExtracts, http://stats.oecd.org/Index.aspx?DataSetCode=RMW#. In Italy, although there is no national minimum wage, the unions negotiate minimum wages by sector. See Wageindicator.org, http://www.wageindicator.org/main/salary /minimum-wage/italy/minimum-wages-faq/minimum-wages-in-italy-frequently -asked-questions. The same is true in some of the other countries mentioned, but the impact and coverage of such agreements vary from country to country. For that reason, it is difficult or impossible to relate official statutory minimum wages to unemployment. In some countries, they are rendered irrelevant by union negotiated rates.

NOTE: Of advanced economies that have no national minimum wage, six of nine have unemployment rates below the average for the Organisation for Economic Co-operation and Development (OECD). The advanced country with the lowest unemployment rate in the world has no minimum wage. The country with the lowest unemployment rate in Europe—Norway—has no minimum wage. However, Italy, which also has no national minimum wage, has unemployment well above average. It may be that no national minimum wage (or a low one) is a necessary but not a sufficient condition for really low unemployment. Subsequent to this survey, Germany introduced a national minimum wage.

should be particularly bad here. But Switzerland has one of the lowest rates of unemployment in the advanced world. If Switzerland, of all countries, can manage relatively low unemployment in the face of globalization and the rest, something else must be going on. What? Does Switzerland have some special recipe for low unemployment?

I am in Zurich in the offices of the Schweizerische Arbeitgerberverband, an employers' organization. Everything is modern and practical. Behind a large desk sits Thomas Daum.

"Why has Switzerland got such low unemployment?" I ask him.

His answer is unexpected. "It is easy to fire people," he says.

It's a paradox but not a difficult one. His idea is that a company that knows it can fire people is more willing to hire them.

It is far easier to fire people in Switzerland than in France or Spain, Daum says. It is true that in Switzerland an employer has to give a reason for making someone redundant, but the explanation can be simply that the boss does not get along with him. A company also has to give some warnings, but the number is unspecified. Usually it is one, two, or three. If a company is found to have fired someone in a way that is not allowed—for being a member of a union, for example—then a fine is incurred. But even then the employer is not forced to take the worker back, unlike in France or Germany. The Swiss think that effective work depends on mutual trust and confidence, Daum says. When that is destroyed, continuing it is no use.[12]

The idea that being able to fire people matters is quite striking. But it seems unlikely that this could be the whole story. What other factors might enable Switzerland to have low unemployment?

During my time in Switzerland, I found that the country has no national minimum wage (Table 2.1). It does have minimum wages for workers from the European Union and in certain individual cantons (states), but there is no general minimum wage.[13]

What about welfare benefits? Could they be a factor? Switzerland, like many continental countries, has an unemployment insurance system. While you are working, you contribute. When you are fired, you get insurance benefits. The unemployment benefit in Switzerland is generous: single people get 70 percent of their previous salaries, while those who are married or who have children get 80 percent. These benefits last quite a long time too. If someone has worked for a company for 18 months, the unemployment benefit can last up to 400 days. That is the maximum for everyone. But throughout this time, recipients must prove every month that they are actively look-ing for a job. They must accept the offer of any suitable work.[14] And if the worker fails to get a new job, then, when the benefit runs out, he or she faces a major drop in income. Social assistance is assessed and paid for by the canton or commune—communes being the smallest and most local tier of government.[15] In some parts of Switzerland, local governments expect people to call on members of their fami-lies for support before claiming social assistance.[16]

Switzerland illustrates that it is possible to have relatively high benefits, at least for a while, yet still have low unemployment. But Switzerland is rigorous in demanding that the unemployed seek work. The OECD has said it "stands out as one of the [member] countries with the strongest search requirements."[17] Also significant is that, after the insurance runs out, the social assistance money is far less.

"In Switzerland, where unemployment has been around the 1 percent mark since the 1950s, each Canton is responsible for the welfare of its inhabitants. Workfare has been in force throughout this period."

SOURCE: Ralph Howell, *Why Unemployment?* (London: Adam Smith Institute, 1985), p. 9.

What about education? Is schooling a factor in Switzerland's low unemployment? The OECD's survey of educational attainment shows Switzerland is better than average in reading but not dramati-cally so. So that does not seem to explain it. However, one particular feature of education in Switzerland might be significant.

Still in Zurich, I walk from the city center across the long bridge that stretches above the river Limmat. I turn right alongside the river and then left up Ausstellungsstrasse. I come to an open patch of ground on the right with a modern building to one side. It is the entrance to the Technische Berufsschule (Technical Vocational School). I go in and am directed to an upper floor where the rector, Dr. Ernst Pfister, has his office. Pfister is correct, cordial, and a fount of knowledge.

He gives me a tour of the school. In the course of it, we come to two large rectangular rooms. They contain rows of engines and engine parts and four cars. At least one of the cars has wheels on rollers so that the engine can run with the car in gear. The exhaust pipes are connected to vents so that the gas emissions are safely removed. I am not a car enthusiast, but even I can't help finding it rather exciting to see real cars and working engines displayed and ready for use. It is easy to imagine a 16-year-old who has not been much interested in academic subjects such as algebra or languages suddenly discovering an enthusiasm for learning when brought into contact with these machines.

Every student at the school works for a company. They are all, effectively, apprentices. They are admitted to the school only after they have obtained a contract with an employer. In fact, most of their time is spent at work. Time at the school varies between one and two days a week.

The system is thus a combination of apprenticeship and vocational training. The schooling is intended to enrich the work and vice versa. The school also provides general education. The course lasts four years, and students must successfully reach one level before being allowed into the next. Companies take a leading role in this system. They hire the students and can request that schools come up with new courses as products and services change.

Is this form of education widespread? Yes. More students in Switzerland go to vocational schools than to universities. A purely academic education is reserved for a minority.

This system may make young people more "job ready" than other ones. Students who have been through one of these courses offer an employer a great deal of knowledge and experience. They can be productive immediately. That is quite a contrast with students who have graduated from a university in, say, media studies, philosophy, or history of art.

The rate of unemployment among younger people should give an indication of whether Swiss vocational training makes a difference. If so, the result is clear. Switzerland has half the youth unemployment rate of the rest of the advanced world.[18] More tellingly still, Switzerland is one of two countries with the lowest proportion of youth unemployment compared with adult unemployment.[19] In most countries, the youth unemployment rate is two to four times the adult rate. In Switzerland, it is only 70 percent higher. The other country with a similarly good ratio is Germany—which also has a strong emphasis on vocational education.

That is a flavor of how Switzerland, a rich country with low unemployment, manages things. Maybe we should now look at a country that is at the other end of the scale: a less-wealthy country that has had a real problem with mass unemployment.

I am in Madrid, climbing the stairs of an elegant but slightly creaky old building. I get to an antique wooden door and soon find myself in the tiny waiting area of a busy office. Felipe Navio González warmly greets me. He is a young entrepreneur who has created a new Internet-based business. To me, he looks so young he should still be in college.

He takes me out to a café, buzzing with enthusiasm. His head is full of the things he needs to focus on for his young business: getting customers, using technology, and so on. He has created a recruitment website using information from the "friends" that people have on Facebook. If someone applies through his website for a job at, say, L'Oréal, the company is automatically notified if any of the person's friends already work for the company. So L'Oréal can check out an applicant through someone it already employs. Navio González says this method increases the chances that an applicant will be hired.

Many young people are desperately eager to work for his young company. Interns work beyond normal working hours, hoping to impress him and to be hired full time. He has to tell them to go home in the evening. But he cannot take many of them into full-time work because when he does, he has to pay the industry-wide minimum wage established by the union.

The national minimum wage in Spain is low and irrelevant.[20] The important minimum wages are set by negotiation with unions across industries and regions. In Navio González's business, it is €15,000 (about $16,600)[21] a year, he says. There is no point trying to employ someone for less than that amount because even if a new employee agreed to work at a lower rate, once in the job, he or she could report Navio González to the union and get him into trouble.

"What would be the effect on your ability to grow if there were no minimum wage?" I ask.

"It would be transformational!" he exclaims excitedly. He could employ more people and grow faster. (See Box 2.1.)

This is the view of one young businessman. Does the experience of Spain provide any evidence to support it?

Let us look at how the economic crisis around the world in 2008 affected Spain. As it flared up, Spanish employers had no wage flexibility. Collective bargaining agreements there have a life of two to three years. At that moment of crisis, demand for labor was going down, but the price of labor could not fall. In fact, wage rates went

Box 2.1
MILTON FRIEDMAN ON THOSE WHO ADVOCATE A MINIMUM WAGE

"There are always . . . two groups of sponsors: there are the well-meaning sponsors and there are the special interests who are using the well-meaning sponsors as front men. . . . The special interests are, of course, the trade unions. . . . The do-gooders believe that by passing a law saying that nobody should get less than . . . whatever the minimum wage rate is you are helping poor people who need the money. You are doing nothing of the kind. What you are doing is to ensure that people whose skills are not sufficient to justify that kind of a wage will be unemployed.

"It is no accident that the teenage unemployment rate ... is over twice as high as the overall unemployment rate. It is no accident that that was not always the case until the 1950s when the minimum wage rate was raised very drastically, very quickly. Teenage unemployment was higher than ordinary unemployment because, of course, the teenagers are the ones who are just coming into the labor market. . . .

"The minimum wage law is most properly described as a law saying that employers must discriminate against people who have low skills.... The consequences of minimum wage rates have been almost wholly bad: to increase unemployment and to increase poverty. Moreover the effects have been concentrated on the groups that the do-gooders would most like to help. The people who have been hurt most by minimum wage laws are the blacks. I have often said that the most anti-negro law on the books of this land is the minimum wage rate."[a]

Otto von Bismarck, the 19th-century German statesman, also criticized minimum wages, saying, "Industry perishes, because it cannot bear the burden laid upon it of short work for high wages. Then the worker suffers from that as well as the entrepreneur."[b]

---

[a] Milton Friedman, interview posted on YouTube, https://www.youtube.com/watch?v=ca8Z__o52sk.
[b] Otto von Bismarck, speech in the Reichstag, March 20, 1884, quoted in *Bismarck,* ed. Frederic B. M. Hollyday (Englewood Cliffs, NJ: Prentice-Hall, 1970), p. 65.

on rising because of the minimum wage deals. It seems likely that the inflexibility of wages contributed to this situation: unemployment in Spain rose by more than seven percentage points in a single year. It was a disaster.

Could anything else in Spain be a factor? Here's another possibility: companies are required by law to pay some employees to work on trade union business once the companies have reached a certain size. One can imagine that this could discourage some companies from expanding. After all, the creation of jobs depends on two things: a willing and able employer and a willing and able employee.

What about the point that Thomas Daum made in Zurich? Employers are more likely to hire, he claimed, if they can fire employees without too much difficulty. How easy is it to fire employees in Spain? It depends. Long-term employees are extremely difficult to fire. Their removal has to be "justified," but the special labor courts set up to decide such matters have almost always decided that redundancy is *not* justified. Many judges in these courts are former active union members.

Until 2012, the cost of firing someone in an "unjustified" way was 45 days of redundancy pay for each year of service. So the longer someone had worked for a company, the more expensive it was to fire him. The maximum compensation was only reached after 28 years of service. The cost of firing someone then could amount to three and a half years' pay! This makes a huge contrast with Switzerland. Long-term employees of Spain have vastly superior rights. You could say that the unfortunate Swiss workers don't have rights. They only have jobs.[22]

What about the welfare benefits in Spain? Are they so generous that they discourage work? In fact, the benefits in Spain appear similar or perhaps even slightly less generous than those in Switzerland. After four years in a job, an employee builds up an entitlement to two years' unemployment benefit, which is worth 70 percent of the previous wages for 6 months, falling to 60 percent for the remaining 18 months. After that, the employee is entitled to social assistance, which, I am told, is very low and difficult to qualify for unless you are very poor. So far, there seems to be no great contrast.

In Spain, as in Switzerland, you are similarly required to seek work. But here we find a difference: in Spain, a public agency tries to find jobs for the unemployed. It appears to be spectacularly unsuccessful. Only a tiny fraction of hirings—less than 3 percent—have been made through this agency.[23] In theory, you are required to accept one of three jobs offered to you. But you do not have to accept a job over 30 kilometers away. And you do not have to accept it—at least for the first year—if it is not in your normal profession or line of work.[24]

In practice, the requirement to seek work does not seem strictly enforced anyway. Navio González tells me that some friends of his were fired and went off on a trip to Brazil for over three months. They continued to receive unemployment benefits. So, on the surface the unemployment benefits in Spain seem similar to those in

Switzerland, but in practice Switzerland seems far more rigorous in obliging people to seek work.

One other possible factor in Spain seems worth mentioning: the wedge. The "wedge" is the difference between what it costs a business to employ someone and what that person receives in cash after tax and social security contributions. Spain has a massive wedge. It is so big that Andalucía, a region of Spain, remarks on its website: "Social security payments can come as quite a shock to those new to the Spanish system."[25] The site gives an example of an employee whose salary is €1,500 a month. The employer has to pay €600 per month in social security contributions on the employee's behalf. So the total cost to the employer is actually €2,100 a month. As for the employee, about 6.4 percent is taken off his or her salary for unemployment insurance. Then income tax is deducted. After a tax-free personal allowance, the tax would be at a rate of 24.75 percent for this level of income.[26] The result is found in Table 2.2.

The employee receives €1,197 per month, but the cost to the employer is over 75 percent more: €2,100. When I bring the subject up with Navio González, he exclaims, "For every two people I hire, I

Table 2.2

THE TAX AND SOCIAL SECURITY WEDGE IN THE
ANDALUCÍA REGION, SPAIN

Cost of the employee for the employer	
Wage	€1,500
plus Social insurance	€600
Total cost	**€2,100**

Amount actually received by the employee	
Wage	€1,500
less Unemployment insurance	(€95)
less Income tax	(€208)
Cash received	**€1,197**

SOURCES: "Spanish Income Tax 2014," SpainAccountants website, http://www.spain accountants.com/it.html; "Rates and Allowances 2014," SpainAccountants website, http://www.spainaccountants.com/rates.html.

could hire a third if it were not for social security! And if I did that, it would cost the government less in unemployment benefit!"

How does the Spanish wedge compare with that of Switzerland? I calculate that in Geneva, the cost to an employer is about 37 percent more than what is received by the worker.[27] So the wedge is far smaller than in Spain.

These have been snapshots of how things work in Switzerland and in Spain. We have come across some possible causes of unemployment. But which one—or ones—are the real culprits, and which are mere distractions?

Here are the possible causes, one by one.

1. Regulations! Regulations! Regulations!

Thomas Daum in Zurich suggested that oppressive rules about firing people cause unemployment. Like other regulations, they increase the cost to a business of hiring someone (see Box 2.2). But in theory, this should not cause unemployment. Businesses should

Box 2.2
REGULATIONS VERSUS JOBS

Why does France have 2.4 times as many companies with 49 employees as with 50 employees? A company with 50 or more workers has to submit to a raft of rules and regulations that cost money and time. It must create three worker councils. If it wants to fire workers, it must submit restructuring plans to these councils. It must introduce profit sharing. And so on. Companies prefer to stop growing rather than to pay these extra costs. As a result, these companies produce fewer jobs than they would otherwise.[a]

Meanwhile, in the United States:

"Regulations sometimes overlooked in their impact on unemployment are those dealing with occupational licensing. If individuals cannot use their cars as cabs, sell homemade sandwiches on street corners, or move furniture without the appropriate licenses, then their job opportunities are limited. Licensing boards are typically controlled by practitioners in the relevant occupations, and these practitioners often use their licensing powers to restrict the number of entrants to their occupations."[b]

---

[a] Gregory Viscusi and Mark Deen, "Why France Has So Many 49-Employee Companies," *Bloomberg Businessweek*, May 3, 2012, http://www.businessweek.com/articles/2012-05-03/why-france-has-so-many-49-employee-companies.
[b] Farell E. Block, "Unemployment: Causes and Cures," Cato Institute Policy Analysis no. 4, October 10, 1981, p. 2.

simply pay lower wages to compensate. But if a high cost of regulations is combined with minimum wages—as in Spain—then lower wages are not allowed. So employing people becomes unprofitable. Businesses must close down or set up in another country.[28] It is a combination of the two factors—oppressive regulations and minimum wages—that damages employment.

2. The Wedge

Similarly, in theory, a big wedge should not cause unemployment. A company should simply pay a lower wage to compensate for the extra costs. But when a minimum wage has been set, the lower wage is forbidden. In that case, employing people may make no financial sense, leading to unemployment (see Figure 2.2).

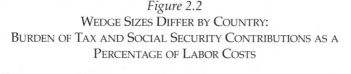

Figure 2.2
WEDGE SIZES DIFFER BY COUNTRY:
BURDEN OF TAX AND SOCIAL SECURITY CONTRIBUTIONS AS A
PERCENTAGE OF LABOR COSTS

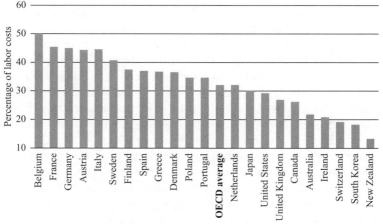

SOURCE: Organisation for Economic Co-operation and Development (OECD), "Taxing Wages 2014: Income Taxes, Social Security Contributions and Cash Benefits," http://www.keepeek.com/Digital-Asset-Management/oecd/taxation/taxing-wages-2014/income-taxes-social-security-contributions-and-cash-benefits_tax_wages-2014-9-en#page4.

NOTE: The wedge is income tax plus employee and employer contributions less cash benefits for single persons on 67 percent of average earnings as a percentage of labor costs, 2013, for selected countries. The numbers would be bigger if they were expressed as percentages of the net earnings of the employee. Note that continental European countries account for all of the nations with wedges above the OECD average.

3. Low-Quality Education

Wherever I have gone I have been told by those who try to find people jobs that illiteracy makes this task more difficult. But again, in theory, illiteracy should not of itself cause unemployment. Less-literate people should simply command lower wages. At the beginning of the 19th century, most people were illiterate, yet they worked. Switzerland suffers from a significant rate of functional illiteracy—13.7 percent. This rate is not much better than average, yet Switzerland has relatively low unemployment.[29] Illiteracy does not necessarily cause unemployment. But if a lower wage is ruled out by a minimum wage, then there will be unemployment.

4. A Minimum Wage

The three factors mentioned so far do not cause unemployment by themselves, but they lower the wages that an employer can afford to pay. People will probably reluctantly take lower pay unless something stops them. That something can be a minimum wage. It can also be welfare benefits that are more attractive than the lower wage. Welfare benefits can act as a proxy minimum wage. And welfare benefits can be combined with hidden employment to create an even better alternative.

In 2006, David Neumark and William Wascher reviewed more than 100 studies of the effect of minimum wages.[30] They concluded that "the preponderance of the evidence points to disemployment effects" and that 85 percent of the most credible studies pointed to negative effects. Most tellingly, they said that the studies that followed the least-skilled groups showed especially strong evidence that minimum wages cause unemployment.

I am suggesting that unemployment is not caused by a minimum wage alone nor by any other factor by itself but by the combination of a significant minimum wage (or easily obtained welfare benefits as a proxy minimum wage) with other factors.[31] The interplay of factors can be disastrous, as it has been in Spain. Unfortunately, many welfare states have gone ahead with this dangerous combination. They have increased the costs of employing people and reduced the cash benefit of working and then, on the other side, they have created high minimum wages or easily obtained welfare benefits. Politicians creating a high minimum wage or high benefits may have looked generous, but they have caused mass unemployment and, through this, they have created misery for millions of individuals (see Figure 2.3 and Box 2.3).

Figure 2.3
INCREASED UNEMPLOYMENT OF THE YOUNG UNSKILLED
IN THE UNITED KINGDOM FOLLOWING A
RISE IN THE MINIMUM WAGE

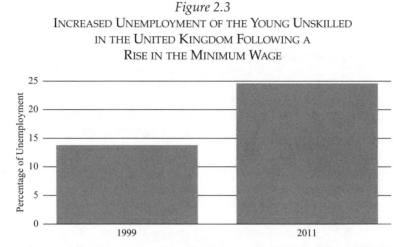

SOURCE: W. S. Siebert, "The U.K.'s Minimum Wage: A Bad Policy Implemented Well?," February 3, 2013. Paper obtained through the Institute of Economic Affairs, London.

NOTE: This big rise in the rate of unemployment for unskilled workers ages 16 to 24 in the United Kingdom took place when the minimum wage was increased by 13.4 percentage points more than average earnings and more than twice as much as consumer prices. The increase in the minimum wage took place over a slightly longer period (1999 to 2012). The slightly longer period is used because figures are available for that period from the Low Pay Commission's 2013 report. The national minimum wage rose by 71.9 percent, while average weekly earnings rose by 58.5 percent and the consumer price index by 34.4 percent. The retail price index rose by 48.7 percent, according to *National Minimum Wage: Low Pay Commission Report 2013*, Cm 8565, https://www.gov.uk/government/uploads/system/uploads/attachment _data/file/226822/National_minimum_wage_Low_Pay_Commission_report_2013. pdf, p. 26. Particularly big increases in the minimum wage occurred in 2001, 2003, and 2004. See *National Minimum Wage: Low Pay Commission Report 2012*, Cm 8302, https://www.gov.uk/government/uploads/system/uploads/attachment_data /file/32574/8302.pdf).

Unemployment jumped for low-skilled individuals not just because the economy was in a worse state in 2011. Over the same period, the rise in overall unemployment was far more modest, increasing from 6.3 percent to 8.1 percent. Meanwhile in France, youth unemployment went down.

Box. 2.3
THE MINIMUM WAGE AS A RACE ISSUE

"Before minimum wage laws were instituted in the 1930s, the black unem-ployment rate was slightly *lower* than the white unemployment rate in 1930. But then followed the Davis–Bacon Act of 1931, the National Industrial Recovery Act of 1933, and the Fair Labor Standards Act of 1938—all of which imposed government-mandated minimum wages, either on a particular sector or more broadly. . . . The inflation of the 1940s largely nullified the effect of the Fair Labor Standards Act, until it was amended in 1950 to raise minimum wages to a level that would actually have some effect on current wages. By 1954, black unemployment rates were double those of whites and have continued to be at that level or higher. Those particularly hard hit by the resulting unemployment have been black teenage males."[a]

More generally, Sowell stated,

"It would be comforting to believe that government can simply decree higher pay for low-wage workers, without having to worry about unfortunate repercus-sions, but the preponderance of evidence indicates that labor is not exempt from the basic economic principle that artificially high prices cause surpluses."[b]

[a] Thomas Sowell, *Basic Economics: A Common Sense Guide to the Economy*, 4th ed. (New York: Basic, 2011), p. 250.
[b] Ibid., p. 243.

Let's just stop for a moment and consider this: if all this informa-tion is correct, then the permanent mass unemployment we have seen in so many advanced countries is a result of their welfare states. The creation of a "welfare state" has brought about something wholly opposed to human welfare: unemployment. It is an irony—a tragic irony. (See Box 2.4.) The possibility that something as well intentioned, generally, as a welfare state should have caused such a tragedy should surely make us seek ways to make things better. Has any country ever found a way to improve matters when they have gone wrong?

After the Second World War, Germany was a star performer. Growth was faster and the people became richer than in nearby France and Britain. But gradually things began to go wrong. Each new high in unemployment was above the previous one. The unification of East and West Germany may have been a political triumph, but it increased unemployment still further.

Box 2.4
CAN UNEMPLOYMENT INSURANCE SURVIVE?

There are two basic kinds of welfare benefits: one based on insurance contributions paid by workers and the other based on people's needs. Continental Europe mostly has an insurance-based system. But the model has taken a battering. In some countries, such as Sweden and the Netherlands, the amount paid in insurance benefits has been reduced.[a] Also the period of time for which insurance is payable has been shortened in various countries, including Denmark, Sweden, France, and the Netherlands.[b]

When insurance benefits run out, individuals typically obtain means-tested benefits, which are lower and therefore cheaper for governments. But the trend is for more and more people to receive means-tested benefits rather than insurance-based benefits.

Will insurance benefits eventually become a mere facade for a benefits system that is predominantly based on means testing? That is what happened in Britain.[c]

Ian Sharp and Stephanie Fennessy of Kent illustrate one of the perils of a means-tested system. The couple lived together with their 10 children and received some £50,000 a year in welfare benefits. Fennessy remarked, "The benefits are being offered to me, so I'd be silly to turn them down." Benefits can prevent people from taking work.[d]

---

[a] Klara Stovicek and Alessandro Turrini, *Benchmarking Unemployment Benefit Systems* (Brussels: European Commission Directorate General for Economic and Financial Affairs, 2012), p. 17 footnote, http://ec.europa.eu/economy_finance/publications/economic_paper/2012/pdf/ecb454_en.pdf; Jelle Visser and Anton Hemerijck, *A Dutch Miracle: Job Growth, Welfare Reform, and Corporatism in the Netherlands* (Amsterdam: Amsterdam University Press, 1997).
[b] Stovicek and Turrini, *Benchmarking Unemployment Benefit Systems*.
[c] William Beveridge recommended an insurance-based system in which means testing would be a residual part. But the insurance element was reduced because it was more costly in the short term. The number of individuals receiving means-tested benefits grew enormously.
[d] "Parents of 10 Who Won't Get a Job . . . Because They're Better Off with £49,000 Benefits," *Daily Mail* (London), May 30, 2012, p. 25.

A great deal of significance can sometimes be attached to a particular number. In Germany, people were appalled that the number of unemployed people was approaching four million.[32] The level was first breached in 1996, but it soon fell back. Relief was only temporary, though, and in 2002 nearly 4.1 million people were unemployed—a number approaching 10 percent of the workforce.[33] The human and economic crisis became political.

A scandal in February 2002 added fuel to the fire. The government department responsible for finding jobs for the unemployed was revealed to have been fiddling the numbers. It had "extensively manipulated its job placement figures."[34] The department was exposed as untrustworthy and ineffective.

Gerhard Schröder, the German chancellor, had to act. He made a telephone call to a trusted friend, Peter Hartz, who was human resources director at Volkswagen. It was an unusual thing to do, and Hartz himself remarked later, "I was actually surprised when I got the call."[35] Schröder asked Hartz to head a commission to recommend what should be done about the unemployment crisis. The commission's recommendations resulted in four new laws that came into force between 2003 and 2005, known as Hartz I, II, III, and IV.

These reforms brought about a change in philosophy. Previously, welfare benefits were an entitlement. People were not under any strong pressure to take jobs that did not appeal to them. Hartz changed that. He put a clear and strong obligation on the unemployed to seek work. He introduced "Help and Hassle."[36] The government would help you if you were unemployed. But you had to seek work right away. In fact, you became obliged to notify the agency that you had been made redundant as soon as you were told—before your period of notice ran out.

If people did not seriously try to obtain a job or if they refused a job, their benefits could be temporarily suspended. The burden of proof was transferred to the claimants. If claimants dropped out of a training program, their benefits could be suspended. People were not allowed to be as choosy about what job they took. They had to take any reasonable job in relation to their qualifications, and they could be required to travel and even move.

Another change was that private companies were allowed to try to place people in jobs. Their payments were based on the results achieved. Training schemes were reformed, and people were required to go on them whether they were receiving unemployment insurance benefits or means-tested benefits.

The duration of some benefits was reduced and conditions tightened. Previously, an older worker who lost his job could live on benefits for at least two years and eight months. Older individuals used this concession as a form of government-financed early retirement. Hartz cut the entitlement period to 12 months or less for most people and 18 months for older people. It also became more difficult to qualify for unemployment insurance benefits. Employees had to have worked for 12 of the previous

Box 2.5
KEY ELEMENTS OF THE HARTZ REFORMS

1. Welfare recipients were required to seek work.
2. Private companies were used to find work for the unemployed.
3. Work was made to pay better than welfare benefits by removing tax and social insurance payments for mini-jobs and midi-jobs.
4. Restrictions on part-time work were relaxed.
5. It was made easier to fire employees.

24 months instead of 12 of the previous 36 months. And once the unemployment benefit ran out, individuals received a considerably larger drop in income when they moved to social assistance.

Two new legal categories of jobs were created: mini-jobs and midi-jobs. These were low-paid, temporary, and part-time jobs. A worker who took a mini-job was not taxed, did not have to pay social security contributions (nor did the employer), and could continue to receive benefits up to a point. In other words, mini-jobs scythed through possible financial disincentives to work. The maximum pay in these mini-jobs was only €400 (about $440) a month. But workers could take more than one. Hartz also loosened restrictions on temporary work. He also made it somewhat easier for employers to fire workers.[37] Box 2.5 lists highlights of the Hartz program.

The Hartz legislation amounted to a wide-ranging attack on possible discouragements to work both for employers and employees.

Did it work? Not immediately. In early 2006, unemployment was still high and Schröder was voted out of government. But by 2008, the number of unemployed had fallen all the way from over 5 million to 3.5 million. Even more impressive was Germany's performance after the financial crisis of that year. Most countries in the Eurozone suffered considerable increases in the number of unemployed lasting four or five years. But unemployment in Germany, after a brief rise, resumed its fall. From the peak of over 11 percent in 2004, unemployment fell to 5.5 percent in July 2012 (see Figure 2.4).

The improvement in youth unemployment was particularly good. While it rose dramatically following the financial crisis in the vast

Figure 2.4
The Turnaround in German Unemployment Ascribed to the Hartz Reforms, compared with France and the United Kingdom

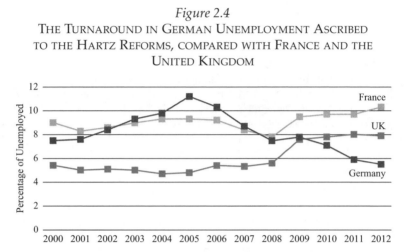

SOURCES: Eurostat. For the 2000–2011 figures, see http://epp.eurostat.ec.europa.eu /statistics_explained/index.php?title=File:Unemployment_rate,_2000-2011_(%25).png&file timestamp=20120502100338#filelinks; for the 2012 figures, see http://appsso.eurostat .ec.europa.eu/nui/show.do?dataset=une_rt_a&lang=en.

majority of countries, Germany was one of only four of the 34 OECD countries that managed to reduce youth unemployment between December 2007 and July 2012.[38] Germany achieved the lowest rate of them all: 8 percent. The average for the OECD was 16.1 percent. In Spain, youth unemployment was a horrendous 52.9 percent. Germany achieved this turnaround by increasing incentives for people to take jobs and by making it more cost-effective for businesses to employ people. (But see Box 2.6.) Put another way, Germany dismantled some of the disincentives it had previously created.

Box 2.6
Oh No! Not Speenhamland Again!

In the late 18th and early 19th century, in a Berkshire, England, village called Speenhamland, wages were subsidized according to people's perceived needs. Employers took advantage of the system and paid lower wages than they otherwise would have. The taxpayers picked up the bill. The same kind of thing was tried in Germany following the Hartz reforms. Government subsidies were paid to workers—partly to give them a better standard of living and partly to make sure they were better off working than not working. But employers took advantage by paying workers little, knowing that the government would supplement the wages.

The improvement in Germany is well known. But it was not the first time something like this has happened. The Netherlands previously had a similar turnaround. In that case, the improvement took longer because successive governments first tried remedies that made no effect. In the 1970s, they tried spending money on public works and subsidizing companies that were having difficulties. The unemployment problem got worse. Only after measures were taken that changed incentives—reducing the minimum wage, reducing welfare benefits, and increasing the requirement that people seek work—did the jobless rate fall. (See Box 2.7.)

But the fastest and most dramatic transfer of people from welfare benefits to work took place in the United States after President Bill Clinton signed the Personal Responsibility and Work Opportunity Act in 1996. The state that became perhaps the most famous for having success with the reform was Wisconsin. How did Wisconsin do it?

I am in Milwaukee, the biggest city in the state. I walk a few blocks from the faded grandeur of the Hilton Milwaukee City Center hotel to a modest office block. I am greeted by a slight, polite man named David Riemer, who leads me upstairs to his office. Riemer has a few mementos of President Franklin D. Roosevelt around the room because he is a fan and thinks the president has often been misunderstood.

Riemer is thoughtful and knowledgeable about the history of welfare in the United States. He is also part of it. He tells me how events developed from his point of view. In the early 1990s, the number of welfare dependents in Wisconsin was rising sharply. There was a growing feeling that something should be done. Wisconsin had long and proud traditions both of work and of caring for workers. It was one of the first states to introduce unemployment insurance.

Benefits in Wisconsin were higher than in the neighboring state of Illinois. It was discovered that people were taking the bus across the state boundary, traveling from Chicago to Milwaukee, just to get the higher benefits. Naturally, the people of Wisconsin did not want their taxes to be used to provide cash to nonresidents, some of whom had never even visited the state before.

Tommy Thompson, a Republican, was running for governor and proposed welfare reforms. He won the election and put forward his proposals. But David Riemer, who had thought about this issue more profoundly than most, believed they were just tinkering. The system needed more radical change. In 1993, he attended a picnic to celebrate the re-election of the mayor of Milwaukee, a Democrat.

Box 2.7
THE DUTCH MIRACLE

The Netherlands had a deliberately low-wage economy after the Second World War. The welfare system was cautious and there was full employment. In the early 1960s, the jobless rate fell to a mere 0.9 percent, a level that probably represented just people moving from one job to another.[a] But gradually the nation became "one of the most generous and extensive welfare states in the world," according to Jelle Visser and Anton Hemerijck.[b]

The proportion of gross domestic product raised in taxes and social security contributions jumped from 38.2 percent to 52.2 percent between 1968 and 1980. In 1977, the *Financial Times* declared that the Dutch had succeeded in establishing "one of the most prosperous and enlightened welfare states with minimum wages higher than in any other industrial society, high labour productivity, remarkably few strikes, and a widely developed social security network."[c]

Disaster followed. Nine years later, a sociologist working in the Netherlands referred to the country as "perhaps the most spectacular employment failure in the advanced world."[d] Two years before, unemployment had reached nearly 14 percent of the workforce.[e] Almost as many were on disability benefits or had taken early retirement. According to the OECD, broadly defined—or you might say "real"—unemployment had reached an astonishing 27 percent of the workforce.

The expression "the Dutch disease" began to be used in textbooks. The number of people receiving disability benefits multiplied from 200,000 to 700,000 between 1970 and 1985.[f] In 1990, the cost of paying disability benefits amounted to no less than 7.6 percent of all the nation's economic activity.[g] For those ages 55 to 64, the proportion claiming disability benefits in 1987 in the Netherlands was 980 per 10,000 workers—more than three times that of Germany, which had 262 per 10,000 workers, and more than twice that of Belgium, which had 434 per 10,000 workers.[h] In the Netherlands, the proportion of people working compared with those receiving benefits collapsed from 14.9:1 in 1970 to 2.9:1 in 1985.[i] (If you added in unpaid homemakers, a mere 1.2 people were working for each dependent in 1985. And that is leaving the retired and children out of the equation.)

Governments tried to combat the problem, of course. In the early 1970s, they tried public works programs focused on labor-intensive industries such as construction. That did not work. The government tried giving subsidies to struggling companies to keep them going. That did not work either.[j] Unions and employers agreed to restrain wages in 1982. But progress was minimal. Gradually the changes became more radical because the situation was so bad. But the process was still agonizingly slow. The minimum wage was steadily reduced from 80 percent of average wages in 1983 to 67 percent in 1994.[k]

In 1987, the unemployment benefit was cut from 80 percent to 70 percent of previous earnings.[l] Many younger people who in the past would have been

(continued on next page)

(continued)

entitled to full benefits got only "partial" benefits that did not last as long as before. The changes mostly affected the young. The value of disability benefits was significantly reduced for younger workers but not for older ones. The disability benefits fell from 70 percent of a worker's previous wage to 70 percent of the minimum wage. Disability recipients were required to have new, more objective medical examinations and greater obligations to seek work. The recipients had to accept all "normal" jobs instead of all "appropriate" jobs.

Finally, from the mid-1990s, the government embarked on "labor activation policies" that nudged people into work more firmly than before. Private companies were allowed to place people in jobs.[m] Job placement was something that the Netherlands had previously attempted only in a very minor way, with a bureaucratic and ineffective government-run employment service.[n] The government embarked on what looked very much like "workfare" programs for the long-term unemployed and for young people.[o] A program of retraining also was provided, followed by work experience and then job placement. The government also tried to reduce the size of the wedge for those who had been unemployed for a long time, provided the jobs paid low wages.

Eventually, these reforms had an impact. The rate of unemployment fell from 14 percent in 1983 to just over 6 percent in 1997. The Netherlands went from having one of the worst levels of unemployment in Europe to one of the best. But the process took a long time, and in the end, the Netherlands still had not fully managed to reverse the effect of having been "one of the most . . . enlightened welfare states."

---

[a] Stephen Nickell, Luca Nunziata, and Wolfgang Ochel, "Unemployment in the OECD since the 1960s. What Do We Know?," *Economic Journal* 115 (2005): 1–27, https://wwz.unibas.ch/fileadmin/wwz/redaktion/fai/EIB_Arbeitsmarkt_HS08/NickellNunziataOchel.pdf.

[b] Jelle Visser and Anton Hemerijck, *A Dutch Miracle: Job Growth, Welfare Reform, and Corporatism in the Netherlands* (Amsterdam: Amsterdam University Press, 1997), p. 119.

[c] Ibid., p. 120.

[d] Goran Therborn, *Why Some Peoples Are More Unemployed than Others*, cited in Visser and Hemerijck, *A Dutch Miracle*, p. 9.

[e] Visser and Hemerijck, *A Dutch Miracle*, p. 9.

[f] Ibid., p. 128.

[g] OECD, "Sickness, Disability and Work: Keeping on Track in the Economic Downturn," 2009, Table A2.1.

[h] Visser and Hemerijck, *A Dutch Miracle*, p. 138.

[i] Ibid., p. 128.

[j] Ibid., p. 159.

[k] Ibid, p. 135, Figure 10.

[l] Ibid., p. 136.

[m] Ibid., p. 184.

[n] Ibid., p. 161.

[o] Ibid., p. 173.

Over hors d'oeuvres, he started talking with Antonio Riley, a state legislator and also a Democrat. Riley agreed with Riemer that the changes being proposed were not sufficiently radical.[39] It was an unusual situation: two Democrats wanted more radical welfare reform than a Republican governor was proposing. Riley asked Riemer what he could do about the main legislation that was then up for debate, the AFDC (Aid to Families with Dependent Children) program, received mainly by unemployed single mothers.

"End it!" said Riemer.

Riley asked, "Can I do that?"

"You are a state legislator. You can introduce any law you want," Riemer recalls he responded. He argued that the state should not offer handouts for nothing. It should offer work.

Two weeks later, the two men sat down and drafted a bill. The Democrats controlled the state legislature, so the question was how Tommy Thompson, the governor, would respond.

Thompson then had two reform bills ready to go: the Republican one and the more radical Democratic one. He was lobbied by many people. One was Riemer himself, who urged the governor to accept the Democrats' bill, saying, "We will support you."

Thompson went with the Democratic proposal. He vetoed parts of it, but the essentials survived. And so, in this strange way, with elements of support from both sides of the American political divide, welfare reform in Wisconsin went through.

What were the key elements? Actually there was only one: work. That is why it was called "Wisconsin Works" or "W-2" for short. A vital part of the program was breaking down any barriers to work. The reforms went through several versions in the following years. But the original principles are worth recording partly because the publicity given to them helped make the changes effective. They were posted in welfare administration offices all over the state.[40]

1. For those who can work, only work should pay.
2. W-2 assumes everybody is able to work or, if not, is at least capable of making a contribution to society through work activity within their abilities.
3. Families are society's way of nurturing and protecting children, and all policies must be judged in light of how well these policies strengthen the responsibility of both parents to care for their children.

4. The benchmark for determining the new system's fairness is by comparison with low-income families who work for a living, not by comparison with those receiving various government benefit packages.
5. There is no entitlement. The W-2 reward system is designed to reinforce behavior that leads to independence and self-sufficiency.
6. Individuals are part of various communities of people and places. W-2 operates to enhance the way communities support individual efforts to achieve self-sufficiency.
7. The W-2 system provides only as much service as an eligible individual asks for or needs. Many individuals will do much better with just a light touch.
8. W-2's objectives are best achieved by working with the most effective providers and by relying on market and performance mechanisms.

"Activity conditions do succeed in getting people off benefits and into work, but they do it not by giving them the skills and opportunities they were previously lacking, but by making a life on benefits appear less desirable, relative to a life in employment, than it was before. This is the real (but often hidden) purpose of schemes like these and it works, for if you have to engage in 'work-like' activities to qualify for benefits, you might as well take a real job and get paid better for doing it."

Source: Peter Saunders, *Re-moralising the Welfare State* (St. Leonards, New South Wales, Australia: Centre for Independent Studies, 2013), p. 20 after citing OECD, British, and Australian research.

How did these principles work in practice? How do they work now? I am at the Dane County Job Center on the outskirts of Wisconsin's capital, Madison. I am in a meeting room with tables arranged in a square and myself in the middle of one side. About 14 administrators from the local office and the state face me from around the square. They range from front-line staff members to senior managers.

I put to them a practical problem: "Imagine a single mother gets off the bus and comes to this office. She has a baby with her. She says she needs money and somewhere to live. What do you say to her?"

One of the administrators immediately says that staff members ask her if she could not stay with her family.

"Imagine she says that her family members are 500 miles away in another state, and anyway they have rejected her. So where can she sleep tonight?"

They say they would suggest a shelter for the homeless such as one provided by the Salvation Army. But they add that the young woman will soon learn that this shelter is nothing she can settle into. She will be allowed to stay for only 90 days, and the shelter will be available to her only at night. The administrators don't flinch from saying that housing is hard to get. They tell me that a lot of people live doubled-up in apartments.

The young woman will probably be steered toward the Wisconsin Works program. On this first day or the next, she will attend a one-hour group class with 8 to 10 participants to introduce her to how the program operates. At the end of that class, she will have five minutes with an adviser and within three days she will have an "intake appointment," which could last between one hour and two and a half hours.

The aim is simple: to discover what barriers block the way of this person's standing on her own two feet and then to find a way to overcome them An individual employability plan is devised. Then the state official and the woman both sign the plan. It is like a contract.

I ask, "What are the top few obstacles to work that you come across?"

One of the administrators around the table says, "A criminal record." Another says, "Poor education." "Finding transportation to get to work," says a third. That sounds like a reasonable "top few." But then someone adds "housing," and others agree. Another common obstacle is mentioned and then another. In the end, I note down nine "top" obstacles to work:

1. A criminal record
2. Poor education
3. Difficulty getting transportation to a job
4. Lack of housing
5. Lack of support from family or friends
6. Mental health problems
7. Poor work history
8. Alcohol and drug use
9. Lack of a work ethic

One classic obstacle is not mentioned: the cost of childcare. That's because a key part of Wisconsin Works was always that the mother would have help with childcare. A center is available where children can be dropped off. The mother pays some of the cost so that she still has an incentive to save money by using a certified babysitter or family members.

If the young mother can't write a resume, she takes a course to help her to do that. If the problem is the cost of travel to work, she might be sent to a nonprofit organization that arranges shared travel to keep down the cost. The women take part in workshops for a week and get advice on dealing with the usual difficulties. There is a workshop on budgeting, for example. As soon as possible, the single mother is helped to find work or enrolled in training for a specific kind of job.

Various training programs are available. A common one leads to a qualification as a certified nursing assistant, but courses are also available in construction and clerical work.

"Men and women who have been unemployed for a certain period should be required as a condition of continued benefits to attend a work or training centre."

Source: Sir William Beveridge (later Lord Beveridge) in his influential report, *Social Insurance Allied Services* (1942). This part of his plan, however, was not implemented.

Once these training courses are completed, the search for a normal commercial job begins. That is the target they are working toward. But those who cannot get such jobs right away are allocated work provided by the state or by nonprofit organizations. The work could be in a charity shop or perhaps a warehouse at which the state has an arrangement with a commercial employer. In health care, jobs include acting as an attendant whose tasks involve taking people to appointments within a hospital.

If someone persistently fails to keep the jobs she takes, she has a "barrier screening" session. I am introduced to a woman who does this barrier screening. She says her job is to find out what the underlying problem is. Sometimes the single mother finds that just talking about her problems helps her to solve them. Sometimes a problem is not revealed at first because it is embarrassing. It might be the long-term impact of being abused as a child. Some are too ashamed to admit that they are unable to read and that illiteracy is what is causing the problem. The interview includes set questions designed to bring out hidden issues like that.

Three things are going on here: improving the employability of the woman, helping her overcome difficulties, and pressing and requiring her to seek work.

Wisconsin Works has been an astonishing success. It brought down the number of single parents on welfare from 55,000 to 10,000 between 1996 and 2004.[41] The result is all the more astonishing because the numbers had already been brought down from 90,000, probably because Governor Thompson tightened up conditions before Wisconsin Works came into effect. The reduction in numbers has been sustained too.[42] Some critics have objected that the improvement came about merely because people who were previously working in the shadow economy are now working on the books. They imply that the difference is insignificant. But, even if that were true to some extent, working "off the books" means getting welfare checks and not paying taxes. It amounts to defrauding taxpayers. The more people who do it, the greater the cost to taxpayers of financing this fraud. Taxes would have to be higher than they otherwise would be. And that, in turn, means that the incentive to cheat is all the greater.

It is a vicious circle that divides workers into those who commit fraud and those who are victims of fraud. Before the reforms, the long-term trend was of ever-rising numbers of single mothers on welfare. That trend has been stopped and reversed dramatically in Wisconsin but also in the United States generally. It is a decided improvement (Figure 2.5).

So the program has been a success, and yet there is a depressing aspect to reform in Wisconsin and elsewhere in the United States. During my visit, I gradually came to realize that the program for single mothers was only one part of a great web of welfare programs. Success has been achieved with single mothers—varying from state to state—but meanwhile the number of Americans receiving government handouts from another program, food stamps, has been soaring (Figure 2.6). The number of people claiming benefits on the basis that they are disabled has risen too (see Chapter 1).

What is the difference between what has been done with single mothers and, say, the food stamp program? There are many differences, no doubt. But one stands out. Food stamps can be obtained without having to turn up every day to do work or training.

Figure 2.5

THE U.S. TURNAROUND IN WELFARE DEPENDENCY OF SINGLE MOTHERS

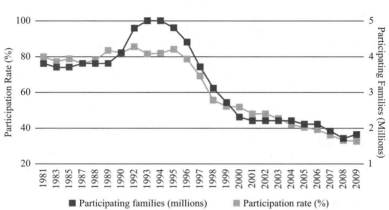

■ Participating families (millions)　　■ Participation rate (%)

SOURCE: U.S. Department of Health and Human Services, "Indicators of Welfare Dependence: Twelfth Report to Congress," Table IND 4a, http://aspe.hhs.gov/hsp/13/Indicators/rpt.pdf.

NOTE: Number and percentage of eligible families, mostly single mothers, participating in the Aid to Families with Dependent Children/Temporary Assistance for Needy Families cash assistance programs.

Figure 2.6

NUMBER OF AMERICANS WHO RECEIVE FOOD STAMPS, 1969–2013

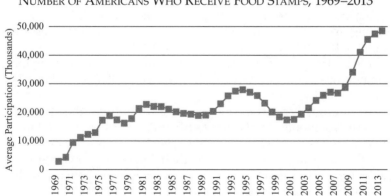

SOURCE: U.S. Department of Agriculture, Food and Nutrition Service, "National Level Annual Summary: Participation and Costs, 1969–2013," Supplementary Nutrition Assistance Program, http://www.fns.usda.gov/sites/default/files/pd/SNAPsummary.pdf.

NOTE: The program known as food stamps is now called the Supplementary Nutrition Assistance Program, or SNAP.

With some exceptions, the "workfare" idea has been applied only to single mothers. Otherwise, the American welfare juggernaut continues to thunder on its way.

The approach that Wisconsin took with single mothers has been radical and successful. But we should remember that America is not the place with the lowest unemployment in the advanced world. Nor is Switzerland, Germany, or the Netherlands. The country with the lowest unemployment rate in the advanced world—only 2 percent in early 2014—is Singapore.[43] What is that country's approach?

I am in a welfare benefits office in the South East region of Singapore near one of the mass rapid transit stations. The glass front is like that of any of the shops in the shopping center, and the front desk with a receptionist is like that of a hairdresser or clinic. Pamphlets are available from racks on the wall and seats are available for sitting while you wait. It is pleasant and unremarkable—a contrast to the bleak halls for benefit applicants I have seen in some countries.

Soon I meet Stanley Fong, the young general manager. We go to one of the four interview rooms at the rear. I ask him, "If I were a jobless man who came into this office saying I needed money, what would you say to me?"

He replies that sometimes people are seen immediately, but normally an appointment is made. The time set aside for the one-to-one interviews is 45 minutes to an hour. The meeting covers a lot of ground according to a plan, but it is still a conversation.

"Suppose that, at that meeting, I say I need money?"

Fong says right away I will be asked, "What are the resources available to you through family and friends?"

This is already different from most other countries. In Singapore, I am not meant to come to the welfare office at all if I can obtain help from my family.

The question is not some meaningless formality, either. If I persist in asking for money, I will have to fill out a form detailing all my income, expenses, and savings. I must also list all the members of my household, their occupations, and their incomes. I must agree that the welfare office may contact other government agencies to share information about my circumstances and those of all other members of my household. I will have to confirm that the other members of my household are aware of this requirement and have agreed to it. In other words, if I am living with my parents and one of them is earning a good wage, there is no way that I will get a cent from the government. The family is expected to provide.

Box 2.8
QUALITY OF ADMINISTRATION MATTERS

> In an online column, John Stossel recounted the difficulties his intern faced trying to find a job at a "job center":
>
> "There are no jobs!" That is what people told me outside a government "job center" in New York City.
>
> To check this out, I sent four researchers around the area. They quickly found 40 job openings. Twenty-four were entry-level positions. One restaurant owner told me he would hire 12 people if workers would just apply.
>
> It made me wonder what my government does in buildings called "job centers." So I asked a college intern, Zoelle Mallenbaum, to find out. Here's what she found.
>
> "First I went to the Manhattan Jobs Center and asked, 'Can I get help finding a job?' They told me they don't do that. 'We sign people up for food stamps.' I tried another job center. They told me to enroll for unemployment benefits."
>
> So the "jobs" centers help people get handouts. Neither center suggested people try the 40 job openings in the neighborhood.
>
> My intern persisted.
>
> "I explained that I didn't want handouts; I wanted a job. I was told to go to 'Workforce 1,' a New York City program. At Workforce 1, the receptionist told me that she couldn't help me since I didn't have a college degree. She directed me to another center in Harlem. In Harlem, I was told that before I could get help, I had to come back for an 8.30 a.m. 'training session.'"
>
> Our government helps you apply for handouts immediately, but forces you through a maze if you want to work.[a]

---

[a] John Stossel, "We Fund Dependency," townhall.com, October 3, 2012, http://townhall.com/columnists/johnstossel/2012/10/03/we_fund_dependency/page/full.

If that hurdle is crossed, I will probably still get no cash or other support unless I agree to conditions and sign up for a plan. The plan will be designed to get me into a job and into self-reliance. All help will be temporary. The welfare office's primary goal is to help me get a job. (For a different model, see Box 2.8.)

I will be tested to assess my abilities. If I am illiterate, I will get literacy lessons. I will get help with writing my curriculum vitae. On the basis of my qualifications and physical capabilities, we will agree what other training I might need. I might be sent to an education and training center to learn skills such as gardening or security. Or we might agree that I should train to work in the food or retail business.

As in Wisconsin, the office is trying to discover my barriers to work and to lower them. The idea is to make sure that people who get into the program get a job and become self-reliant. Although this is like Wisconsin, it is tougher and applies to all benefits, not just those for single mothers. As the conversation goes on, the phrase that keeps coming into my mind is "compulsory self-reliance."

Fong remarks, "Sometimes there is discomfort on the part of the resident. A lot would rather just have cash. We don't make it straight-forward and comfortable for them. We really want self-reliance."[44]

"We have arranged help but in such a way that only those who have no other choice will seek it. This is the opposite of attitudes in the West, where liberals actively encourage people to demand their entitlements with no sense of shame, causing an explosion of welfare costs."

SOURCE: Lee Kuan Yew, Prime Minister of Singapore, 1959–90, *From Third World to First: The Singapore Story, 1965–2000* (New York: HarperCollins, 2000).

Singapore takes a particularly robust attitude. But a further special and unusual aspect of Singapore may be significant. The tax wedge is much smaller than in other countries. Individuals on very low wages pay no tax at all. Even those earning well above the median wage have only 4.2 percent of their income taken in taxes.[45] Here is an even more remarkable fact: people make no social insurance contributions. They pay money into personal savings accounts instead.[46] It is a wholly different system.

So a person's money does not disappear into some government account from which benefits are paid out to others. Money is deducted from the worker's pay, but it is invested and attracts interest for that specific individual. The money can be used to provide a pension, to pay for health care, and to buy a home. People surely feel quite different about contributions to their own accounts than they would toward social insurance contributions. The more they put in, the wealthier they become. The problem of the wedge and the way it discourages the worker and the employer is largely removed.

Singapore appears like the ultimate welfare state for ensuring minimal unemployment. The regime would probably be too hard line for most democracies to accept. But some of its methods can certainly be copied.

Boxes 2.9 and 2.10 offer some conclusions about welfare and work.

Box 2.9
Two Different Kinds of Welfare: Each Has Its Merits

Why Social Insurance Is Better than Means Testing[a]

1. Social insurance encourages employment because people must work before they qualify for the benefit.
2. Means-tested benefits can discourage employment when large-scale benefits for people with substantial "needs" would be withdrawn if the person takes a job.
3. Under means testing, less money is paid when two parents live together but only one of them works. That policy can damage families.
4. Means testing results in more completely workless households.
5. Means testing tends to discourage saving.
6. Means testing incentivizes people to lie about their savings.
7. Means-tested benefits given to workers can encourage employers to pay lower wages. They know that the benefits will make up much of the shortfall.

Why Means Testing Is Better than Social Insurance

1. Means testing keeps the cost down in the short term—though not necessarily in the long term.
2. Means testing keeps social insurance contributions down, increasing net take-home pay and encouraging legitimate work.
3. Means testing can easily be framed to allow and encourage part-time work.
4. Means testing can leave those who don't need benefits free from state interference in their lives.

In purely economic terms, the arguments may seem fairly well balanced. But means-tested benefits have a much greater tendency to damage the behavior of recipients, discouraging saving, penalizing parents who stay together, and providing incentives to lie. So social insurance appears to be preferable. Singapore has succeeded with means-tested benefits only because those benefits have been minimal and have been rigorously policed.

There are other possibilities that have not been tried by modern governments. One could copy what has been done in Singapore with regard to pensions and health care and require workers to contribute savings to a designated account. The savings could be drawn on if the person becomes unemployed. Another possibility would be to require workers to take out unemployment and disability insurance with competing companies and mutual societies. Such a requirement would provide more choice, competition, and innovation. Mutual or friendly societies might also encourage mutual support.

---

[a] I am grateful to Peter Whiteford in Sydney for talking with me about this. He is knowledgeable on the subject, and I have benefited from some of his insights. However, the summary is my own, not his.

Box 2.10.
WHAT KIND OF GOVERNMENT PROGRAM BEST GETS THE UNEMPLOYED
INTO WORK?

Sometimes governments actively do try to get the unemployed into jobs. Efforts to do this are called "active labor market programs." Which kind works best?

Alessio Brown and Johannes Koettl looked at dozens of studies of the subject.[a] This is what they found:

Not-So-Good Programs

Subsidies to companies to retain employees despite a downturn were "very cost-ineffective." Money is wasted keeping people in jobs when many of them would have kept their jobs anyway. The money spent benefits those in jobs without helping the unemployed. The money encourages industries and individuals to delay adapting to changed circumstances.

In-work benefits for low-paid workers such as tax credits and reduced social security payments are "not cost-effective." A huge expense is incurred to subsidize employment that would have continued anyway. In some cases, employers rather than employees get the financial advantage.

Public works can crowd out private employment. They can "lock in" workers who consequently do not seek long-term employment elsewhere. Such programs are normally focused on low-skilled work and can remove the incentive for people to train and develop their skills. "The evidence on the ineffectiveness of public works has been widely documented,"[b] the authors note. However, one study has shown that the closer that public works are to regular work, the better the impact. Sometimes public works are combined with workfare (see the "best programs"). In those cases, they may be more useful.

Better Programs

Subsidies to companies to hire new employees can give the long-term unemployed experience in the workplace and help them become more employable. The subsidies give employers a chance to try out people they would not have tried otherwise. The subsidies can help the unemployed compete with the employed, making the market more competitive. But money also can be wasted on subsidizing people who would have gotten jobs anyway ("deadweight cost"). Companies might simply hire subsidized people rather than employing individuals without a subsidy. Overall, such subsidies can, with suitable targeting of beneficiaries, be cost-effective. "Self-employment subsidies are especially effective for the disadvantaged in the labor market, namely young, low-skilled, long-term unemployed and inactive workers."[c]

Training on the job or classroom training has achieved mixed results, even though governments spend more on this kind of program than on any other.

(continued on next page)

(continued)

On-the-job training is particularly effective compared with classroom training, according to the authors. One study found that combining on-the-job training with classroom sessions increased the impact by 30 percent compared with classroom sessions alone. Tightly targeted training in small programs has had better results. But people are less likely to get work while the training continues.

The Best Programs

Workfare and sanctions for not taking work—the threat of having benefits removed if a person does not seek work—have a "strong and significant" effect. One study found that the number of individuals taking jobs doubled after sanctions were imposed. Denmark had particular success by combining sanctions with tighter conditions for unemployment benefits.

Job search assistance also is "very cost-effective." Studies show the likelihood of getting a job increased between 10 and 30 percent with such programs. The assistance should be "targeted at workers with low employment probabilities at the beginning of the unemployment spell and at long-term unemployed workers,"[d] the authors say. If combined with the threat of sanctions, it can be more effective. The effectiveness may be lower during economic downturns.

What this report could not capture was the importance of the quality of the implementation of the programs. Job search assistance, for example, can vary from the extremely useful to a complete waste of time.

[a] Alessio J. G. Brown and Johannes Koettl, "Active Labor Market Programs: Employment Gain or Fiscal Drain?," Institute for the Study of Labor (IZA) Discussion Paper 6880, September 2012, http://ftp.iza.org/dp6880.pdf.
[b] Ibid., p. 27.
[c] Ibid., p. 22.
[d] Ibid., p. 34.

Seeing the experiences of Switzerland, Spain, Germany, Wisconsin, and Singapore makes the picture seem a lot clearer. For the most part, the permanent mass unemployment of modern times has been caused by welfare states. They have done it by increasing the costs of employing people for business and reducing the net cash benefit of working for employees. These factors have been particularly damaging when combined with a high minimum wage or proxy minimum wage in the form of easily obtained welfare benefits. Some welfare states have also contributed to unemployment through their housing, pension, labor market, and education policies, as we will see.

The permanently high unemployment that has been created has been highly damaging to the happiness of millions of people. It has been a scandal and a tragedy. It has also caused collateral damage, harming civility and honesty, weakening families, and, of course, enfeebling economic growth. We will come to those later in this book.

The remedies are of two sorts. The first is simply to minimize the obstacles to employment described previously: take away the extra costs imposed on businesses, reduce the tax and social insurance taken from employees, and lower or abolish minimum wages. There are precedents for all of these actions, including the reduction in the minimum wage in the Netherlands. The second kind of remedy that has been shown to be effective is "labor activation": requiring people to seek work, subsidizing training targeted at actual jobs, and removing barriers to work such as illiteracy.

Identifying such remedies is not difficult. The difficulty, in our representative democracies, has been for governments and people to face up to them and to implement them (See Box 2.11).

Box 2.11
A BETTER BENEFITS SYSTEM FOR FULL EMPLOYMENT

- Unemployment insurance as the main system, supplemented by much less attractive means-tested benefits
- The option of choosing from competing private unemployment insurance schemes
- No minimum wage or, failing that, regional minimum wages
- "Labor activation" policies for the unemployed that include work-seeking assistance, job-focused training, literacy courses, and workfare. Work is the priority.
- Private companies enlisted to help people get jobs and paid on the basis of results
- Elimination or reduction of conditions that deter companies from hiring, with policies that make firing employees easier, that minimize employment regulations, and that remove the requirement that companies pay for the staff of trade unions
- Clear and consistent financial advantages for low-paid workers to find and keep a job

---

3. In Search of the Best Health Care System in the World

Rather Like Looking for the Lost Ark of the Covenant

I am in the Zurich railway station with its magnificent, wide concourse and roof supported by soaring metal arches. Along the sides are some restaurants. At the far end are a newspaper stall and then the platforms. The concourse is bustling with people hurrying to catch their trains. I am going to catch a train, too, but on my way, a brightly lit temporary stall in the middle of the concourse catches my eye. Some young women are handing out leaflets. I wonder what they are advertising and I take one, but it is in German and I can't read it. Gradually I work it out, nonetheless. It is health insurance. Health insurance, I am discovering, is part of everyone's life in Switzerland.

I pass through this station several times during my stay in Zurich. On one occasion, I take a suburban train to Zug, a provincial town. It is a short journey, and I share it with commuters returning from their day's work. I am going to interview Konstantin Beck. I want to talk to him because I am trying to find a good health care system—in fact, the best health care system in the world. Various conversations I have had back in Britain have led me to think that Swiss health care is a candidate. Konstantin Beck knows it intimately because he works for one of the big Swiss health insurance companies.

As the train trundles along, I like to think I already have a moderately good grasp of Swiss health care. It is like this: Imagine you are a Swiss citizen. You are obliged to buy health insurance. That is the law. But you can choose between different health insurance groups that offer a range of policies. Whichever policy you buy will provide at least the minimum, government-specified coverage.

What about the poor who can't afford health insurance? They must buy it, too. They get help with the cost. True, they can't choose the most luxurious policies with private rooms and so on. But they are covered.

What about the elderly or people with major existing health problems, who, on average, have more medical expenses than the young and healthy do? Do they have to pay much more? No. Payments are "equalized." Insurers are obliged to accept customers regardless of their age or health history at the same price. The difference in risks is adjusted in a way that you, the buyer, do not see.

What if you, in a moment of rebellion or forgetfulness, fail to choose an insurer? You will be insured automatically anyway. There is no getting out of it.

So what is supposed to be good about this system? Those who like it admire the way that choice and competition run right through it. First, you choose your own insurance organization, so the insurers are competing for your business. They compete with each other partly on price and partly on extras. They need to offer an attractive deal or they will go out of business. Then the insurers, in turn, choose among competing hospitals, clinics, doctors, and so on. Some hospitals are private. Some are owned by one of the 26 cantons into which Switzerland is divided. All the hospitals need business, so they try to offer the best deals to the insurers. There are therefore two layers of competition: one among insurers and the other among health care providers such as hospitals. Some observers think this system encourages the best possible service at the lowest possible cost.

My train arrives at Zug. Konstantin Beck is on the platform waiting to greet me. We leave the station and walk to a café nearby.

Beck knows a lot about health care systems, not just the Swiss one. I ask whether he thinks the Swiss system is a good one.

"Yes," he replies.

It is an encouraging start.

He says it is true that newspapers complain that insurance premiums are expensive. But, in many cases, people themselves make the choice to buy the higher-priced policies. Premiums vary substantially. People can pay less if they choose a policy that has a "gatekeeper."

What is a "gatekeeper"?

A general practitioner. A policy with a gatekeeper is cheaper because you are not allowed to go straight to a specialist. You must first go to a general practitioner who will assess your condition and decide whether to send you on to a much more expensive specialist. The system saves money because, in many cases, general practitioners will decide that they can deal with your problem and you do not need to see a specialist at all.

You can also pay less for your policy if you choose "managed care." That means you can go to only a limited selection of doctors or hospitals. The most expensive policies allow you to go to any doctor or hospital in Switzerland.

The system as a whole has popular support, Beck says.

"How do you know?" I ask.

Because every now and then, he says, groups that do not like some aspect of the system challenge it, and the country holds a referendum. Consistently, the people vote to keep it.

As I come from Britain, with its history of people waiting a long time to be seen by specialists and waiting again to have tests and operations, I ask about waiting lists.

There are virtually none, Beck says. "If you want a hip replacement, you might possibly be asked to wait three months. But if it is urgent, it could happen more quickly."

"How long would you wait for an MRI [magnetic resonance imaging] scan?"

"No more than a few weeks."

It sounds good. Maybe this is indeed the best health care system in the world. But I am obliged to ask if there is anything wrong with it.

Beck admits that, yes, there are a few problems. A doctor can send excessively high bills to the insurance company. Or a doctor may refer patients to hospitals too readily. In both cases, the insurance companies have to pay up. I say nothing, but I am thinking that this defect does not sound too terrible.

Could the system be used in other countries, I ask. Does it depend on Swiss efficiency for it to work well? Beck does not comment except to say that the system does depend on the doctors to submit reliable claims. You have to be able to "believe the bills," he says.

One problem he notes is that the compensation that insurers receive for taking on customers with existing health problems is not as accurate as it should be. Insurers still have an incentive to sign up the young and healthy. Insurance companies have waged a 13-year battle to get extra compensation for taking on customers who have been in the hospital the previous year. The compensation would be a rough and ready adjustment, but it would help. As Beck talks, it becomes clear that the system is constantly being adjusted and refined. He says that, yes, Switzerland is improving, step by step. Eventually, he says, the Swiss system could become as good as the Dutch one.

It takes me a moment to digest what he has just said. I have come to Switzerland to hear about the much-praised Swiss system. Up until now, it has seemed that the news is good and that the system works well. But now Beck is saying that—in one respect, at least—the Dutch system is better. It is not often that a Swiss person tells you that another country does something better.

I can't remember whether I already intended to visit the Netherlands. But obviously now I have to.

A few months have passed and I am now in Rotterdam. Frankly, it is not the prettiest town in the Netherlands. It was severely bombed in the Second World War. But a major port and large areas of water give it a light, open feeling. I am visiting Erasmus Medical Center, the third or fourth largest hospital in Europe, serving 4.3 million people. It is a vast place and is being rebuilt. The press officer guides me through a labyrinth of corridors to get to the next person I am seeing. Finally, she knocks on a door and I am introduced to genial, smiling Dr. Eric Sijbrands.

Sijbrands specializes in diabetes. The hospital has a particularly difficult problem with this disease. Rotterdam is a multiethnic city. Among outpatients, 70 percent with diabetes do not speak Dutch, so communicating with them is difficult. What makes the situation worse is that many patients come from south Asia, Turkey, and Morocco, where people tend to have more problems with type 2 diabetes. Sijbrands tells me that those patients get diabetes when they are younger and thinner than when western Europeans develop it. The disease is "meaner" with them too.

He tries to get his patients to improve their diets. But that is difficult. He recalls that he once became very depressed about how things were going. In his experience, he would try for a year, then for a second year, and then a third year to persuade patients to change their diets. When he failed to persuade patients to make a significant change after three years, he admits he felt like giving up. He had a feeling that he had "achieved almost nothing." He had a few days off and gloomily sat at home wondering, "What am I doing here?" He wished he could help his patients more effectively.

Sijbrands wrestled with various ideas for what could be done to improve the situation. He gave up many of them, but he persisted with one: the notion of "diabetes stations." The stations would be rooms, not far from where patients live, where patients could go to administer tests on themselves. A computer would provide personalized guidance based on each test. It would communicate in each patient's own language. The patients would be able to see for themselves what sort of progress was being made. Any unexpected or worrying results could quickly be flagged automatically to their doctors.

Sijbrands went to the innovation department of the hospital and persuaded the staff members to support the idea. Now it is being tried out. These stations are being created around Rotterdam. One of the initial results has been a 70 percent reduction in patient visits to the hospital. It turns out that patients prefer visiting the machines to visiting the doctors. They are emailed recipe ideas written in their own language and in accordance with their traditional diets.

Sijbrands shows me one of the machines, and I do a few tests. I am impressed. This seems to be an innovation that might both save money and treat patients more successfully. It looks like public-spirited health care at its best.

From what sort of a system has it emerged? And, even more important, is this really a good system of health care?

I go on to see a clutch of doctors and academics in the Netherlands and try to discover the answers. But it is not easy. I gradually learn that the Dutch do not like to make dramatic statements. Everything is carefully expressed. Hardly anyone is frank and forthright. Gradually, though, I manage to work out that there has been a revolution in Dutch health care, but one that has taken place in slow motion.[1]

The health care system used to be very much government controlled. But in 1987 a leading businessman, Wisse Dekker, wrote a report that argued that it should be open to private competition.[2] This proposal provoked vehement opposition—by Dutch standards. It was blocked. Governments came and went. Some were in favor of the idea and some against. But over a long period of time filled with debate, argument, and consensus-building, the government-dominated system gradually allowed some private competition.

Planning and experimentation took place in the five years from 1995. In the five years after that, some hospitals began using parts of a new system. Different groups all had their say. It was long-winded and complex.

I am used to seeing governments make bold new changes decisively. In one interview in Amsterdam, I fail to hide my feeling that it sounds like a roundabout and irksome business. But Tom Groot of Vrije Universiteit replies, "If we hadn't done this, the current system would not have emerged." He and several others I talked to in the Netherlands believe the debate and consensus-building led to a better, more securely based system.

So what is it?

At first sight, it seems similar to the Swiss system. Everyone has to be insured, and everyone can choose among competing insurers.

But systems like this have tricky details to decide in two areas. One is the amount of compensation paid to the insurers for accepting high-risk patients. That is where Konstantin Beck seemed to think the Dutch were ahead of the Swiss. The other is the amount that the insurers pay to hospitals and clinics for treatments.

The Dutch have had problems with this second issue. Before the 1980s, the government doled out money to hospitals according to the number of beds they had and similar measures. The result was that the hospitals were not very productive and had waiting lists. They had no incentive to be productive. So the system was changed. Hospitals were paid according to their "production"—how many operations they did. This scheme encouraged hospitals to do more operations, and the hospitals had no incentive to innovate or keep costs down. So that became expensive.

Doctors were then asked to define typical conditions that patients suffer from and to specify normal procedures and how much they should cost. This was called a "diagnostic treatment combination." The hospitals or specialist clinics would be paid a fixed sum for each diagnostic treatment combination and so would have an incentive to come up with cheaper and better ways to treat patients. Increasingly, the insurers could also negotiate with hospitals and clinics over how much they paid for treating certain conditions. This situation led to an increase in specialist clinics, which make themselves very efficient in a particular treatment—laser eye surgery, for example. Waiting times decreased. But the trouble became that the huge number of diagnostic treatment combinations made the system cumbersome. The next move was drastically to reduce the combinations.[3]

The insurers are increasingly able to negotiate with hospitals and other providers on price and quality. In 2005, they could negotiate some of the terms on which they bought 10 percent of health care provision. In 2012, it was up to 70 percent.

It sounds to me as if the system is constantly being refined. It certainly seems much better than in the 1970s.

In the conversations I have, I get the impression that everyone thinks the Dutch system is pretty good. But no one is openly enthusiastic about it. So is it good or not?

I ask another academic, Erik Schut, a professor at Erasmus University in Rotterdam, which system he thinks is the best in the world. He is reluctant to make an outright judgment. He is only willing to indicate a relatively favorable view of the Dutch and German systems. That is it. It is a curious business. I came to the

Netherlands with the idea that it might have an even better system than the Swiss. Yet when I come here, many of the experts are surprisingly equivocal about it.

One evening near the end of my stay, I have supper with a personal contact, someone who has nothing to do with health care except, of course, for being a patient now and then. We meet in the Dauphine Café-Restaurant, a bustling place in Amsterdam, and I ask him almost incidentally what experience he has had with Dutch health care. He becomes quite agitated talking about it.

"You ring up the doctor and you can't speak to him! Instead, you speak to a receptionist who asks you lots of questions. But you might not want to discuss your case with a receptionist. To get to see the doctor soon, you have to be pushy. The pushy get through. The meek must wait." His description of general practitioners sounds as though the "gatekeepers"—through which patients normally go in the Netherlands—have gates with rusty old hinges that they are reluctant to open.

What about the hospitals? There are still waiting lists for operations, my contact exclaims. People go to Germany or Belgium if they want to get treated quickly. The French system, which he knows about because his wife is French, is much better because there are no gatekeepers and the general practitioners come to see you in your own home. They won't do that in Holland.

This is only anecdotal. Perhaps it is exaggerated or out of date. But the conversation reminds me of something a senior doctor said earlier in my visit. He was a German working in the Netherlands, obviously in a particularly good position to compare the two systems. What did he think?

At first he gave me what sounded like a balanced judgment in the Dutch style. He told me the Dutch system is structured, centralized, and evidence-based. There are gatekeepers, and the system is cheaper. The German system is good, but it is expensive.

Then he leaned forward confidentially: "Don't write this down," he smiled. "But I still have my German health insurance."

It was a telling moment. The Dutch system has its virtues, no doubt. It is fashioned and continually refined by highly intelligent, serious, public-spirited people. But when it comes to the crunch, some people, at least, prefer a less controlled system that costs more but offers faster service and more freedom for the individual. The German system is complex and varied. It has compulsory insurance, but a key element is that patients can choose whichever general practitioner or specialist they want to see. The physicians are in private practice and most hospitals are independent but not for profit.

It was confusing. Two systems that I had heard being touted as the best did not seem quite so good when I got a bit closer. Perhaps it was time to get a truly international assessment.

So, I am now in the headquarters of the Organisation for Economic Co-operation and Development (OECD) in Paris. The press officer takes to me to see a woman who, he says, has been much in demand to give presentations about health care systems. She has written an analysis that has caught many people's imagination. Along a corridor we come to a small room and I am introduced to a lively, charming woman, Isabelle Joumard.

I ask her to tell me about her research. She says that she analyzed the effectiveness of health care systems in relation to their costs. To put it another way, she looked at which health care systems produce the best results for the cash spent.

I am skeptical. I have previous experience with how difficult it is to measure how well a health care system performs. How did she measure performance? As part of her answer, she mentions life expectancy. I exclaim that I am astonished she should take life expectancy as a measure. It is extremely misleading! Life expectancy depends far more on lifestyle—especially diet—than on the quality of the medical system. She smiles indulgently and replies that her analysis included adjustments for lifestyle factors. It also excluded deaths by violence. She also used a measure of "avoidable deaths"—deaths from conditions such as asthma from which young people should not normally die.

Amused by my skepticism, Joumard tells me that what persuaded her that these measures were meaningful was that they were "highly correlated" with each other. The various measures she used produced similar results.

She suggests various papers I can read to get the full story. But it has been a long day and the thought of reading yet more OECD research papers fills me with dread. Yes, I will look at them, I assure her.[4] But in the meantime, could she tell me the answer, please?

She is reluctant to tell me the results of her extensive labors in a sentence. I cajole and encourage her, saying, "This is turning into a long journey. Please give me a little guidance!"

Finally, she relents. She offers me the result of her popular, learned study and her high correlations. What is the country with the most cost-effective health care system in the advanced world?

Australia.

Fine. I was not expecting that one. But Australia would be interesting. I was thinking of going there anyway.

I am now in lovely, spectacular Sydney. I am going to the Australian Club, which sounds charmingly old-fashioned. It turns out that the building I have been sent to does not look like a venerable gentlemen's club after all. I am going up in an elevator in an office building. However, when I arrive at the top, the club has evidently held onto relics of its past, including a certain formal manner. I am greeted by Dr. John Graham, an immaculately polite, retired doctor of the old school.

He takes me to a table for two by the window, which gives us a good view. I explain to him that I have been to the OECD headquarters in Paris, where I was told that Australia has the most productive health care system in the world. What does he think?

"They must be looking at it through funny-colored spectacles," he remarks. Graham strongly feels that the quality of health care in Australia has deteriorated. Consultations are too rushed. The general practitioner does not have time—and is not trained—to get to the bottom of what a person is suffering from. He just follows a quick routine. For example, he dishes out antibiotics, which will be the right treatment for only 1 in 10 of the patients he gives them to. For 8 of the patients, antibiotics will be unnecessary, and in 1 case he will have missed a completely different condition such as jaundice.

Waiting times have become long, Graham says. If you want a knee replacement, you can wait between 18 months and two years. The bureaucracy has mushroomed too. He is old enough to remember when health care in the state of New South Wales was administered by 65 bureaucrats. Now there are 15,000 of them. He has studied the proportion of people employed at the front line compared with managers, bureaucrats, and so on. In his research, he bent over backward to be fair, even including hospital gardeners as front-line staff because hospitals have gardens that need to be cared for and that are good for patients. Even after such a generous interpretation, he found that, for every four people delivering health care, another three were not on the front line.

So there is a huge waste of money. But there is a kind of "double whammy" of waste, too. First the administrators cost money. Then the inordinate amount of time that doctors and nurses must spend filling in the forms that the administrators create for them costs money, too. Graham expresses all this in a tone of regret rather than of anger, and I find that only makes his remarks all the more persuasive.

After lunch, he takes me along a busy street to Sydney Hospital. It was founded in the 19th century and still has remnants of the old colonial architecture. In one part, substantial, old stone arches run alongside a wide corridor open to the air at the first-floor level. Graham says he can remember patients being placed in beds out in the open there. He reminisces about the days when the hospital was bigger and a center of expertise where medical advances were made. Now politicians are trying to close it down. We go into various buildings. He retired only a year before, and all the staff members know and obviously respect him. They call him by his first name, and we are waved through wherever we go. He was probably working at the hospital before most of them were born.

In the emergency department, we talk to the senior nurse, who is exactly the sort of capable person you would want in that position. I ask her about waiting times for emergencies. She says that patients are put in one of five categories. Category One patients—the most serious—are seen right away. Category Four patients have relatively minor injuries. For example someone might have turned an ankle and still be in some pain. That person would be seen by a doctor within an hour. It all sounds pretty good. Then I mention to the nurse that Graham previously remarked that this emergency department is less busy than others. Ambulances are typically sent to a bigger hospital. She agrees. That is when she tells me about "ramping."

The nurse explains that sometimes hospitals, especially bigger ones, cannot accept all the emergency patients who arrive at busy times because they have insufficient capacity. So ambulances are told to wait on the ramp leading to the entrance. Or else the patients are allowed into the hospital but continue to be attended by the ambulance paramedics so that officially they have not been admitted. This procedure enables the hospitals to meet their target of seeing every patient within four hours of admission. Of course, ramping is a tacit acknowledgment that they are probably not going to be seen within four hours of arriving.

The nurse says she has a friend who was in serious condition and was kept on a stretcher waiting to be officially admitted for two hours. Once admitted, she had to begin another wait to see a doctor.

How often does this happen, I ask. "At the big hospitals, every week. The usual times are Monday afternoons and Friday evenings."

It sounds grim.

During my stay in Australia, I look into this issue more. Jeremy Sammut, a health care analyst, tells me that more than a third of emergency admissions to a public hospital have to wait more than eight hours for a bed.[5] That sounds positively frightening.

A few days later, I am having lunch with another doctor. We get onto the related subject of rationing of health care. Does rationing happen in Australia, I ask. He tells me I should talk to a specialist he knows. Without pausing, he makes a call on his cell phone. He quickly tells the person on the other end of the line who I am and passes over the phone. I find myself talking to a specialist who does bone marrow transplants. This can be a life-saving operation for a certain kind of cancer. I ask if there is rationing in his field.

There certainly is, he says. "We could do at least twice as many!"

So why doesn't he? Because the money made available by the government to pay for support staff and beds is restricted.

Does it matter? Does anyone suffer as a result? The specialist says that people who ought to have marrow transplants right away have to wait. The doctors naturally try to prioritize urgent cases, but some patients have relapses because they have to wait so long. They are often weakened so much by the relapses that they become unable to stand the strain of chemotherapy, which is part of the treatment. And because they cannot bear the chemotherapy, they die. The delay has caused their deaths. Medical rationing leads to deaths.

I ask whether he talks or writes articles about what is going on. He says it is against the terms of his employment. If it were revealed that he has said these things to me, he could be fired. He says no politician in Australia is telling the truth about health care rationing. No politician is willing to tell the truth, and no doctor is allowed to.

This is depressing. Yet it seems there are some good aspects of health care in Australia. People can see a general practitioner quickly and easily. If their own doctor is not available, it does not matter. They can see any general practitioner. Typically, the government pays for most of the cost of a treatment but not all, so the patient has to contribute. I am told the doctors may do too many procedures because they get paid according to what they do rather than how many patients they have. But seeing a general practitioner quickly is a good thing that does not happen everywhere.

Also the large minority of care in private hospitals seems to work well enough. The market in private health insurance is thriving. Private hospitals and other medical care are encouraged by the government in clever ways. For example, more affluent individuals have to pay an extra 1.0 to 1.5 percent of their income to help pay for the government's health insurance scheme, Medicare. But if they opt out and take private insurance, they do not have to pay this extra charge.

Private health care is big. One doctor tells me that 40 percent of hospital care is provided privately. Mostly this provision consists of planned operations, but having the critical mass of patients in private health care means that even some private hospitals with emergency departments are capable of handling major incidents. A friend living in a Sydney suburb tells me that if members of his family have an emergency, they go straight to the local private hospital.

How does such a large private sector continue to exist after a number of decidedly left-leaning governments in recent decades? A long-time resident tells me that the Labor Party has given up attacking private health care because private insurance is taken out by people fairly well down the income scale whose votes they need.

Overall, I am slightly disappointed. The numbers in Australia might look good from Paris, but if OECD staff members found themselves in an ambulance waiting on a ramp for a few hours before being admitted to the hospital, and then they had to wait some more, they would probably not be so impressed.

But one other advanced country might be worth looking at. The OECD tends not to examine it because it is not a member of the organization. It rarely appears in international comparisons of health care. This country is sometimes mentioned as having a good system, and it happens to be located on my way back to England.

My plane arrives in the early evening, and across the wide bay are dozens of massive merchant ships and tankers. In the dying sunlight, the view is a wonderful sight and a reflection of how far the country has come. Singapore is now the second busiest port in the world after Shanghai.[6] Singapore was once a British colony. It was much poorer than Britain, and its medical care was unsophisticated. But now babies born in Singapore are half as likely to die before their first birthday as those born in Britain. Life expectancy, for what it is worth, has surpassed that of the former mother country. It is age 82 compared with 80. I have heard no reports of "ramping" or long waiting lists there. Do these good results mean the system costs a fortune?

On the contrary, whereas Britain spends 9.4 percent of its national income on health care, Germany spends 11.3 percent, and the United States spends a staggering 17.9 percent, Singapore spends a mere 4.7 percent.[7] If Singapore had been included in the OECD comparison of cost-effectiveness, it would surely have come first. How does Singapore do it?

The most unusual aspect of the system is the way medical care is paid for. Money to pay the bills comes from a variety of sources. The system has been carefully assembled to try to reconcile competing goals.

One source of funds is the government. It provides a substantial subsidy to its own hospitals and clinics. The subsidy helps keep down the cost for patients of modest means. The government also provides further subsidies for the poor through some means testing. Next, a fund helps the poor who cannot manage any other way to pay for their health care. This is means tested too, to make sure that only the genuinely poor use it.

Then a government insurance scheme protects against the cost of an exceptional, extremely expensive stay in the hospital. Most people buy it because, again, it is subsidized.

Another source of payment is the patient's own pocket. The idea is that people will not waste their own money as they might waste government money. In particular, most people except the poorest are expected to pay for their general practitioner and normal prescriptions with their own cash. Some element of "co-payment" is fairly widespread in health care systems from Sweden to Australia. In systems in which practically everything is covered by insurance, as in France and in many American policies, the cost of health care is very high.

This brings us to the last big source of cash, which takes place on a national scale only in Singapore: all workers are required to pay between 7.0 and 9.5 percent of their income into a personal medical savings account called Medisave. Their employers pay slightly under half this amount. The money saved can be spent only on medical

---

"I was a student in Britain when the Labour government in 1947 implemented the National Health Service. Their belief that all people were equal and no one should be denied the best medical services was idealistic but impractical and led to ballooning costs. The British National Health Service was a failure. American-style medical insurance schemes are expensive, with high premiums because of wasteful and extravagant diagnostic tests paid for out of insurance. We had to find our own solution."

Source: Lee Kuan Yew, former prime minister of Singapore, from his book, *From Third World to First: The Singapore Story, 1965–2000* (New York: HarperCollins, 2000; New York: HarperBusiness, 2011), p. 100. All citations refer to the 2011 edition.

---

bills, but the key point is that it remains the property of the individual. When workers reach the age of 55, if the value of the Medisave account, combined with other savings accounts, is above a certain level, individuals can withdraw it. Moreover, when the individual dies, the saved money is distributed tax free to a recipient designated by the owner. The money in one's own personal Medisave account is used to pay for a great deal of that individual's health care. People can choose where they spend it. They have every reason not to waste it.

"We could spend our entire gross domestic product on healthcare in useful ways. In fact, we could probably spend the entire GDP on diagnostic tests alone—without ever treating a real disease."

SOURCE: John C. Goodman, *Priceless: Curing the Healthcare Crisis* (Oakland, CA: Independent Institute, 2012), p. 172.

The ingenious aspect of Singapore's system is the way it recognizes and addresses points that typically go wrong in health care systems around the world. On the one hand, everyone is covered. On the other hand, the system includes competition, choice, and the incentive not to waste money.

Even the government hospitals, which are semi-independent, compete with each other and with the private hospitals to attract patients. Patients can go to whichever hospital they prefer. Long waiting lists do not appear to be an issue, possibly because hospitals get cash for treating patients. Almost everybody has the money available to pay for treatment because of the savings accounts. Different levels of accommodation are available for different prices. The cheapest rooms are in open wards in government hospitals, which are 80 percent subsidized by the government.

I am keen to see one of the hospitals. Fortunately, a visit to Khoo Teck Puat Hospital in the northern suburbs has been arranged for me. When I arrive, I find large modern buildings with gardens like those of a top-class hotel. I meet the manager, Liak Teng Lit, a veteran government official who grew up alongside the tough, determined creators of modern Singapore.

Liak takes me around the different wards. The lowest C-class open ward we see is full of people and has no air-conditioning. I would find it oppressively hot, but perhaps local people are more acclimatized to the heat. The top A-class accommodations consist of private rooms that are quiet and cool. But I don't find them particularly welcoming.

These rooms have no government subsidy. I mention to Liak that someone told me that the people in the A-class rooms get better treatment. "That's rubbish," he replies. He says that, in fact, one of his biggest problems is keeping the patients in the A wards from being neglected. Doctors find it easier to do their rounds in the cheaper wards. They can move from one patient to another easily. Furthermore, the doctors have no reason to prefer the patients in the A-class rooms. Most doctors are on a fixed salary.

The Singapore system offers one further, subtle advantage. As a patient, you take responsibility for your own health care. You are not just told where to go by the government or an insurance company. You have your own resources and can make real choices. Yes, you have been compelled by the government to save. But you can use the money at any recognized hospital.

Are there any problems?

There is one thing that most advanced democracies would find shocking and unacceptable. Suppose a relative of yours—say, your sister—has a serious medical condition that requires repeated hospital stays and expensive drugs. Suppose, too, that the savings in her Medisave account have been exhausted. The government will come to you and your sister's other relatives and ask you to pay the bills from your own Medisave accounts. This is enforced family support. You might not even like your sister. You might not have seen her for 30 years. It does not matter. One person in Singapore tells me that this policy does not bring families together—it drives them apart. He adds that at times an elderly grandmother will not go for treatment because she does not want to drain the family finances. Most democracies would not accept such a policy.

Another possible issue is that some people may not like that the government hospitals are reluctant to use the latest, most expensive equipment. And, in some countries, it would be reasonable to worry whether the vast sums locked up in Medisave accounts might one day be raided by a government in financial difficulty.

The Singapore system probably cannot be simply copied. In fact, I meet several people in Singapore who would like it to be changed in one way or another. The government, too, feels obliged to make little changes now and then to fine-tune the program. Most people seem to want to increase the insurance element and reduce the amount of self-payment. But it must be admitted that the existing system appears to be the most cost-effective in the advanced world.

At this point, the reader might think I should finish the world tour and come to a conclusion. But please come with me on one final journey. At least it is to somewhere warm where the people are friendly and the wine is excellent.

I am in Valencia, Spain. This is the region that includes resorts such as Alicante. But I am not at any resort. I am in an inland town called Alzira. Not familiar with it? That's not surprising. This is a nondescript sort of place that no tourist would dream of visiting. Yet a new kind of health care system began here. It has become known as the "Alzira model," and it is studied and talked about far and wide. In fact, I first heard about it in Stockholm, of all places.

I am staying at a funny little hotel that is not exactly up to the highest international standards. My room is small and contains a refrigerator that is not plugged in. That does not matter because nothing is inside anyway. In the morning, I am collected by a public relations officer, who drives me the short distance to the hospital. The place seems normal enough, like hundreds of other hospitals. I am led to a meeting room where the manager and some senior staff are waiting for me.

The director general, Dr. Manuel Marín Ferrer, is a short man with an air of relaxed authority. He speaks some English, but when he needs help, Dr. Carlo Trescoli, a tall, urbane, and friendly man, steps in.

They give me a presentation. The hospital has so many visitors from around the world that they are well prepared. Afterward, I ask questions and am taken on a tour. Then I interview a variety of people through the day to try to understand as well as I can what is going on.

I discover that the Alzira model was created in a roundabout way. No one planned it at the outset. In 1982, the Socialist Party in Valencia promised that Ribera—the health department in which Alzira is situated—would get a hospital. Years rolled by and no hospital was built. Hospitals cost money, and there never seemed to be enough of it. While this was going on, it was becoming increasingly recognized in Spain that standards were low in many public hospitals. When I was in Madrid, before coming to Alzira, I asked someone how long you might have to wait to see a doctor in an emergency department. He told me it could be as long as seven days! I found that hard to believe. I had never heard of emergency wait times being measured in days.

So, in 1997, the national government passed a law decreeing that publicly financed health care did not have to be delivered by the government itself. The regional government in Valencia took advantage of this law to find a way to build the long-awaited new hospital in Alzira. The officials still had no money, but they had the idea of making a contract with a private company to design, build, and—crucially—pay for a new hospital. In recompense for this work, the company would run the hospital for 10 years and would then hand it back to the regional government. The private company would be paid a sum each year based on the number of people living in the Ribera area. The amount would be no higher than the sum spent per capita at hospitals elsewhere in the region.

For the regional government, the deal solved a political problem at no cost. In fact, the contract sounds so advantageous to the regional government and so tough on the private company that you might wonder why on earth the company would agree to it. How could the income over only 10 years ever cover the heavy cost of building a hospital and still produce a profit? I try all day to find the answer.

A cynic might think, "Oh, they could make money by having long waiting lists and not treating people properly while taking the government's money." But the contract was far too ingenious for that. Part of the deal was that if the people of Ribera voted with their feet and went to hospitals outside the department for their operations, the private company would have to pay the whole cost of their procedures. The contract was deliberately unequal. If the situation was reversed and people from outside Ribera came to the Alzira hospital, the company would receive only 80 percent of the officially determined value of the procedures. So the Alzira hospital had to attract local patients to avoid heavy penalties. And if people came to the hospital from elsewhere, the hospital managers had to find ways to treat them that were at least 20 percent less expensive than what other hospitals managed.

How could the private hospital hope to survive in these circumstances, let alone make a profit? The savings in cost per procedure would have to be enormous. It turned out that the contract was indeed so tough that the company could not make it work. A compromise was made. The deal was eased a little and, surprisingly, in the course of making this compromise, the negotiators created the new element that made the Alzira model special. The regional government agreed that the company would take over primary care—care provided by general practitioners or local clinics—in Ribera as well as hospital care. This change had remarkable consequences.

But first, before we get to those consequences, we need to get some idea of how the hospital was able to make major cost savings. Even after the original contract was made less tough, it was still very demanding. Throughout the day, I ask the people involved, "How can you make a success of the contract when you have to pay for building and equipping the hospital and then you have to hand it back?"

Marín Ferrer tells me some of the ways in which his hospital saves more money than public hospitals do. "We work the equipment from 8 a.m. to 8 p.m. instead of from 8 a.m. to 3 p.m.," he says. The staggering thing about this remark is the way it reflects on the public hospitals. MRI scanners and advanced computerized axial tomography (CT) scanners are extremely expensive. Operating theaters are the most expensive part of a hospital. It seems that the Spanish government-run hospitals allow this equipment to lie idle after 3 in the afternoon. Actually, that is scandalous. For any enterprise, public or private, the cost of financing expensive equipment continues without pause, day and night. Equipment needs to be used as much as possible to carry the burden. As a private company, the Ribera Hospital has to pay attention to this fact or lose money.

A similar difference involves the way the Ribera employs its staff. "Public hospitals contract, say, 60 cardiac specialists who are paid their salary regardless of their activity," Marín Ferrer says. But the Ribera Hospital adjusts the number of staff members on hand to the level of activity. Staff pay also is adjusted according to how well the hospital meets its targets. These targets include below-average inpatient mortality, a surgical waiting time of less than 90 days, and average stays of less than five days. Everyone in the hospital is on the same side, striving to achieve these goals.

Doctors at the Ribera work harder than in public hospitals, and they get paid more. Their time is more productive. The beds are used more efficiently. The shorter-than-usual waiting time for surgery brings in more patients—from outside the area as well as from Ribera itself.

Now we get to why it matters that the contract was changed to include primary care: one big fact about health care that most people do not think about is that hospital care is many times more expensive than primary care. When a patient has an operation in the hospital and stays for five days or more, the cost is measured in thousands of dollars. But when a general practitioner sees a patient, the cost is measured in tens. A health care system that can keep people out of the hospital saves vast amounts of money.

So once the company had responsibility for primary as well as hospital care, what did it do? It provided lots of active, preventive care to keep people from needing to go to the hospital. For example, during the winter, people typically go to the hospital with chronic bronchitis. When this happens at the Ribera, the hospital notes who the patients are. The following October, the company's primary care staff members contact the patients and offer to visit, to see how the patients are. If they are having problems, the patients receive preventive treatment. In many cases, monitoring and treatment in the fall keep the patients out of the hospital over the winter. The benefits are twofold: the health care system (paid for by taxpayers) saves money and the patient avoids a traumatic trip to the emergency room on a cold winter night.

People with known heart conditions are monitored, too. Many myocardial infarctions—heart attacks—can be avoided by monitoring the heart and offering early treatment. The Ribera now admits half as many myocardial infarctions as before—an astonishing result.

The company similarly goes to great lengths to encourage people over age 65 to have flu vaccinations each autumn. As well as sending out letters, it takes extra steps such as advertising on local radio. As a result, 95 percent of individuals over age 65 have the injections in Ribera compared with the national average of 70 percent.

In short, the company saves money by offering proactive primary care. It also has an incentive to keep the citizens of Ribera as healthy as possible. That, in brief, is why people from around the world make the pilgrimage to the modest little town of Alzira.[8] The introduction of this system has had the added benefit of encouraging the government hospitals in the region to improve their performance.[9]

So is the Alzira model the answer? Should health care be delivered by private companies working in the service of the public good? It seems like an improvement over relying on government services wholly provided by government hospitals. The idea of a government contracting out work to private companies has its echoes in some Swiss cantons, some Japanese regions, and the British National Health Service.

Unfortunately, the model has some drawbacks. There is a danger of corruption, of government officials taking bribes to give contracts. That sort of thing has happened in parts of Italy when health care contracts have been awarded. Then there is the lack of choice. A Ribera resident has to go to a general practitioner employed by the hospital. Some of us would like to be able to choose a doctor who is not employed by the same company as all the others. There is also the danger that, once a region has contracted out all of its care, it might reduce the funding and, when standards fall, put the blame on the private companies.

So which is the best system? Would you like to make a wholly logical decision on the basis of objective evidence? Wouldn't we all! Unfortunately, much of the "objective evidence" clearly does not lead to an ideal solution. The statistics suggested that Australia was particularly efficient, for example. But those waiting in an ambulance on a ramp outside a hospital would tell you that it is far from perfect.

"A healthy person is someone who has not been examined sufficiently well."

SOURCE: Tom Groot, Vrije Universiteit Amsterdam. The idea is well known among doctors that if you do enough diagnostic tests, you can find something wrong with everybody. Therefore, the potential cost of health care is virtually unlimited.

Again and again, I have looked at systems in different countries and found serious failings of one sort or another. Quite a few seem to have a strength that, unfortunately, is matched by a weakness. The Netherlands, for example, has a sophisticated method of paying hospitals, but its system makes seeing a local general practitioner difficult.

What should we do then? Having admitted that we have no wholly reliable way of reaching a conclusion, we might still find it worth looking at which countries produce the best and worst outcomes for patients according to international measures. None of these measures is perfect or wholly reliable, of course, and many cover only a limited number of countries. But by looking at a mix, we might detect a pattern.

For example, which countries do best when treating cancer? The greatest variety of cancers is covered only in purely European

Table 3.1
WHAT PROPORTION OF PEOPLE ARE STILL ALIVE IN DIFFERENT
COUNTRIES FIVE YEARS AFTER BEING DIAGNOSED WITH
BREAST CANCER?

Highest proportion of survivors	Lowest proportion of survivors
United States	Poland
Canada	Ireland
Australia	Czech Republic
Japan	United Kingdom
New Zealand	Denmark

SOURCE: Organisation for Economic Co-operation and Development, *Health at a Glance 2013* (Paris: OECD Publishing, 2013), p. 127, http://www.oecd.org/els/health-systems /Health-at-a-Glance-2013.pdf.

NOTE: The OECD table includes only advanced countries, although one could argue that economically some of the eastern European countries are much less advanced than the others. Smaller countries such as Slovakia and Slovenia are not listed in Table 3.1 and other tables in this chapter. Israel and Iceland also have been omitted in this table. They are advanced, but they are relatively small. This chapter does not mention them otherwise, so they do not help disentangle the relative merits of the others. The original study also does not include Switzerland or Singapore.

research, but for a few common cancers, more of the world is covered (see Tables 3.1 and 3.2).

Another measure of health care systems is the number of MRI scanners per capita (see Table 3.3). It is a rough and ready measure of the availability of advanced equipment.

One objection to the MRI figures could be that some countries prefer advanced CT scanners. So here are the figures for CT scanners as well (see Table 3.4).

How quickly are patients treated? Unfortunately, the figures are available only for a very limited number of countries. Still, it is an important measure and is worth including (see Table 3.5).

Another litmus test is how many operations of various sorts are performed. Take coronary angioplasty as an example. The obvious difficulty with this is that diets vary, so people who have more heart-friendly diets in the Mediterranean are less likely to need

Table 3.2
WHAT PROPORTION OF PEOPLE ARE STILL ALIVE IN DIFFERENT
COUNTRIES FIVE YEARS AFTER BEING DIAGNOSED WITH
COLORECTAL CANCER?

Highest proportion of survivors	Lowest proportion of survivors
South Korea	Poland
Japan	Czech Republic
Australia	Denmark
United States	United Kingdom
Germany	Portugal

SOURCE: Organisation for Economic Co-operation and Development, *Health at a Glance 2013* (Paris: OECD Publishing, 2013), p. 129, http://www.oecd.org/els/health-systems /Health-at-a-Glance-2013.pdf.

NOTE: The OECD table includes only advanced countries. The original study does not include Switzerland or Singapore.

Table 3.3
MRI SCANNERS PER CAPITA, 2011 OR NEAREST YEAR

Most MRI scanners per capita	Fewest MRI scanners per capita
Japan	Hungary
United States	Poland
Italy	Australia
Greece	United Kingdom
South Korea	Portugal
Finland	Czech Republic

SOURCE: Organisation for Economic Co-operation and Development, *Health at a Glance 2013* (Paris: OECD Publishing, 2013), p. 87, http://www.oecd.org/els/health-systems /Health-at-a-Glance-2013.pdf.

NOTE: The OECD table includes only advanced countries. The study also does not include Singapore. Table 3.3 omits Chile, Iceland, Israel, and Mexico, which are outside of this chapter's analysis. MRI = magnetic resonance imaging.

Table 3.4
CT SCANNERS PER CAPITA, 2011 OR NEAREST YEAR

Most CT scanners per capita	Fewest CT scanners per capita
Japan	Hungary
Australia	United Kingdom
United States	Netherlands
South Korea	France
Greece	Belgium
Switzerland	Poland

SOURCE: Organisation for Economic Co-operation and Development, *Health at a Glance 2013* (Paris: OECD Publishing, 2013), p. 87, http://www.oecd.org/els/health-systems/Health-at-a-Glance-2013.pdf.

NOTE: The table includes only advanced countries. The study also does not include Singapore. Table 3.4 omits Chile, Iceland, Israel, and Mexico, which are outside of this chapter's analysis. CT = computerized axial tomology.

Table 3.5
PERFORMANCE OF SELECTED COUNTRIES IN LENGTH OF PATIENT WAITING TIMES

Fewest patients waiting two months or longer to see a specialist	Most patients waiting two months or longer to see a specialist
United States	Canada
Germany	New Zealand
France	United Kingdom

SOURCE: Organisation for Economic Co-operation and Development, *Value for Money in Health Spending*, p. 130, citing 2008 Commonwealth Fund International Health Policy Survey of Sicker Adults.

NOTE: The patients concerned are adults with chronic conditions. Only eight countries were included in this survey. The others, in between, were the Netherlands and Australia.

Table 3.6
CORONARY ANGIOPLASTY OPERATIONS PER CAPITA, 2009

Most coronary angioplasty operations per capita	Fewest coronary angioplasty operations per capita
Germany	Ireland
Belgium	Canada
United States	New Zealand

SOURCE: "OECD Health Data 2011," cited in Organisation for Economic Co-operation and Development, *Health at a Glance 2011* (Paris: OECD Publishing, 2011), p. 91, http://www.oecd.org/els/health-systems/49105858.pdf.

angioplasty. Fortunately, no Mediterranean country is among the three best and worst anyway. (See Table 3.6.)

Similarly, the need for hip replacements is also affected by dietary factors. Arthritis is much less common in Japan and perhaps Korea than in the West. But we can bear that in mind when looking at the results (see Table 3.7).

Knee replacement is a less common operation, and the countries concerned are slightly different (see Table 3.8).

Table 3.7
HIP REPLACEMENTS PER CAPITA, 2009

Most hip replacements per capita	Fewest hip replacements per capita
Germany	South Korea
Switzerland	Poland
Belgium	Slovakia

SOURCE: "OECD Health Data 2011," cited in Organisation for Economic Co-operation and Development, *Health at a Glance 2011* (Paris: OECD Publishing, 2011), p. 93, http://www.oecd.org/els/health-systems/49105858.pdf

NOTE: Table 3.7 omits Chile, Israel, and Mexico, which are outside the study of this chapter. Singapore was not included in the study.

Table 3.8
KNEE REPLACEMENTS PER CAPITA, 2009

Most knee replacements per capita	Fewest knee replacements per capita
Germany	Ireland
United States	Hungary
Switzerland	Portugal

SOURCE: "OECD Health Data 2011," cited in Organisation for Economic Co-operation and Development, *Health at a Glance 2011* (Paris: OECD Publishing, 2011), p. 91, http://www.oecd.org/els/health-systems/49105858.pdf

NOTE: Table 3.8 omits Chile, Israel, and Mexico, which are outside the study of this chapter. Singapore was not included in the study.

As this is a mixture of measures, we might also include the results of the OECD analysis of what countries obtain the best results for the money spent (see Table 3.9).

Doubtless other people would have chosen other measures, but I chose these not knowing what results they would produce.

On looking at them, I am astonished by how well the United States ranks. It is among the best countries in seven of nine of these

Table 3.9
HEALTH OUTCOMES BY COST

Best health outcomes in relation to money spent	Worst health outcomes in relation to money spent
Switzerland	Ireland
Australia	Greece
South Korea	United Kingdom
Japan	Denmark

SOURCE: Isabelle Joumard, "Health Care Systems: Getting More Value for Money," Economics Department Policy Note no. 2, Organisation for Economic Co-operation and Development, Paris, 2010.

NOTE: Table 3.9 omits Mexico, which is outside the study of this chapter. Singapore was not included in the study.

Table 3.10
WORLD HEALTH CARE PIGGYBACKS ON U.S. INNOVATION

Share of pharmaceutical patents, selected countries (%)

United States	42.0
United Kingdom	6.0
France	4.0
Canada	3.0
Australia	1.5

SOURCE: OECD Science, Technology and Industry Scoreboard 2009, cited in Sally C. Pipes in *The Pipes Plan: The Top Ten Ways to Dismantle and Replace Obamacare* (Washington: Regnery, 2012).

measures (see also Table 3.10). Please note that these figures all relate to care before the implementation of Obamacare. One measure on which it most obviously does not excel is value for money. But even when cost is taken into account, it still is not among the worst—presumably because the results are so good.

One could doubtless find a string of measures on which the United States would rank lower. Life expectancy, perhaps. But, as I mentioned before, simple life expectancy reflects diet and lifestyle more than the effectiveness of a medical system.

Should we conclude that the U.S. system, currently undergoing huge changes, is a model for everyone? There are three reasons to hesitate. First is the extraordinary expense. (See Box 3.1.) The reasons for the amazing cost are a matter for a separate study all by itself. But whatever the reasons, the high price suggests something is not working well.

Second, many people are not covered by insurance. They are not the poor because the poor have Medicaid. They are not the old because the old have Medicare. They are the people not poor enough or old enough to have government-financed care and who have not bought insurance. Some argue that this circumstance is not as worrisome as it first appears. You might even argue that this drawback is worth having in exchange for the outstanding medical service available to the majority of Americans. But then we come to the third problem: the existence of the uninsured appears politically unsustainable in a modern democracy. In this system, there are certain

Box 3.1
TREATMENT FOR A SMALL CUT ON THE HEAD: US$2,300

Oscar, age 12, attended an American summer camp and slept on the top level of a bunk bed. When he got out of bed one morning, he bumped his head against a sprinkler in the ceiling. It was a small cut, but there was some bleeding. The camp called Oscar's father and suggested that the boy see a doctor. So Oscar was taken to the nearest hospital. After a three-hour wait, a doctor dabbed on some anesthetic liquid and "glued" the torn skin in place.[a]
The doctor's bill was $88.41.
The hospital's bill was $2,221.02.

[a] This story was told to the author by the father in 2012. He wishes to remain anonymous, and the boy's name has been changed because he has been in a dispute with the hospital.

to be cases of people who are financially ruined by an illness. Understandably, these cases cause outrage. (See Box 3.2.)

So if the United States does not have the answer, is there anything else we can learn from the medical outcomes?

One noticeable aspect is that better health care is closely correlated with wealth. Look at the countries that appear most frequently in this chapter's tables as being among the best: the United States (in seven of nine), Switzerland (in four of six), Japan (in five of eight), and (Germany in five out of nine).

It is striking that these countries are among the wealthiest countries per capita in the world. Wealth leads to better health care. Indeed, it is possible to argue that, if you want first-class health care, you should first get economic growth.

What else can we glean from the data? Let us look at the countries that come out worst in the tables: the United Kingdom (in six of nine), Ireland (in four of eight), and Denmark, Hungary, and the

"Why do doctors and hospitals deliver so much unnecessary care? There are many reasons. . . . Malpractice fears drive defensive medicine. . . . But the most powerful reason doctors and hospitals overtreat is that most of them are paid for how much care they deliver, not how well they care for their patients. They get paid more for doing more."

SOURCE: Shannon Brownlee, *Overtreated: Why Too Much Medicine Is Making Us Sicker and Poorer* (New York: Bloomsbury, 2007), p. 8.

Box 3.2
U.S. HEALTH CARE SYSTEM IS IN PIECES

There is no disputing that the U.S. health care system is a dysfunctional muddle. It can be roughly divided into five segments.

First, employer-sponsored health insurance. This became a major part of American health care because of a historical accident. During the Second World War, wage controls were introduced, but fringe benefits were not subject to the controls. So employers used health insurance to attract workers.[a] Additionally, the contributions of employers to such schemes were made tax free.[b] Employer-sponsored health insurance generally provides excellent health care.

The second segment consists of people who are not employed by a company but who pay for their own health insurance. Their premiums are much more expensive because they are not part of a mixture of low-risk and high-risk patients. Also, the rates are pushed up because some individuals who know they are going to need a great deal of health care buy insurance while others who are young and healthy do not buy it. Another feature that boosts the cost is that individual insurers get little or no tax relief.[c]

Because self-insurance is so expensive, millions of people do not take it out, and they are not only the young and healthy. These individuals are the third segment: the uninsured. They can be financially ruined if they suffer from an expensive illness.

The fourth segment consists of those at the poorest end of society. They are covered by Medicaid, a government program. The fifth segment is the elderly, who are covered by Medicare, another government program. These two programs pay limited amounts for procedures, and some doctors and hospitals refuse to treat patients who rely on them. An official from one independent, nonprofit hospital in the United States told me that the hospital lost money on Medicare patients. The hospital made up the shortfall by charging private patients more.

So the system is incoherent. It leaves a few to be ruined and many others to pay extraordinary amounts. Yet we have to acknowledge that, in terms of medical performance, it appears to have better outcomes than any other system.

The whole system has now been thrown into the air by the advent of Obamacare, formally known as the Affordable Care Act. This program does not, as casual observers might imagine, introduce clarity and coherence. In theory, everyone would be obliged to have insurance and pay the same rate. But, in fact, people can opt out by paying a penalty. Those who opt out might include the young who are earning little and not expecting to become ill. So the cost of the insurance may rise because the average risk will rise. Meanwhile, some of the people who opt out of the program will become seriously ill and be ruined, just as before.

Funding for Medicare is going to be reduced, so even more hospitals may find it uneconomical to treat Medicare patients. And as the government will effectively be establishing increased central control of medical care, it risks

(continued on next page)

(continued)

creating a greater bureaucratic burden that will increase the cost of treatment. Something will have to give. One senior person at a hospital told me that thinking about it kept her from sleeping at night.

For a while at least, the excellence that has been built up over the decades will probably persist. But in the longer term, the system could reach some kind of crisis.

---

[a] Thomas C. Buchmueller and Alan C. Monheit, "Employer-Sponsored Health Insurance and the Promise of Health Insurance Reform," National Bureau of Economic Research Working Paper 14839, April 2009, http://www.nber.org/papers/w14839.pdf?new_window=1.

[b] Ibid. This was confirmed in 1954. See also Alex Blumberg and Adam Davidson, "Accidents of History Created U.S. Health System," National Public Radio website, October 22, 2009, http://www.npr.org/templates/story/story.php?storyId=114045132 . The report says that corporate health insurance initially became tax free in 1943.

[c] If you have to pay your own insurance premiums and medical expenses, they are generally tax deductible only to the extent they exceed 10 percent of your adjusted gross income (roughly speaking, your annual income from all sources). So if you have income of $60,000 per year, you would have to pay the first $6,000 of premiums and medical expenses out of after-tax dollars. So the tax system favors being an employee over being independent. Information provided through an email from Christian Wignall in California. Also, see John Waggoner, "Tax Q&A: Are Health Insurance Premiums Deductible?," *USA Today*, March 26, 2014, http://www.usatoday.com/story/money/personalfinance/2014/03/26/tax-qa-health-insurance-deductible/6878171/.

Czech Republic (each in three of eight). The worst result of all is for Britain, which, exceptionally, is not one of the poorest countries. The distinguishing feature of the British health care system is that it is mostly a government monopoly. In recent years the government has been contracting out some health care to the private sector. But there is generally no mechanism for people to obtain private health care directly unless they pay twice: once for government care through taxes and a second time privately. Because of this system, most people obtain only government care. So the most monopolistic system also appears to be the least successful.

The Irish system is a close relative of the British one and also comes out badly. It has developed in different ways, but the 1953 Health Act essentially meant the government paid most of the bills and supplied the overwhelming majority of the doctors. One difference is that patients make some co-payments. In both Great Britain and Ireland, private provision has gradually increased, partly because waiting lists for treatment have become national scandals at various times.[10] (See Box 3.3.)

Box 3.3
HOW MANY HAVE TO WAIT FOR THEIR OPERATIONS?

The following rankings were based on the proportion of patients who waited four months or more for elective surgery,

Fewest	Most
Germany	Canada
Netherlands	Sweden
United States	Norway
Switzerland	United Kingdom
France	Australia

SOURCE: Organisation for Economic Co-operation and Development, *Health at a Glance 2011*, citing Commonwealth Fund International Health Policy surveys. Figures are for 2010.

NOTE: Survey of 11 countries. The other country was New Zealand.

The contrast between the groups that did best and least well was dramatic. In the best-performing countries, no more than 7 percent of patients wait more than four months. In all the relatively badly performing countries, at least 18 percent were waiting for more than four months. I would not want to place too much reliance on the figures because some have varied dramatically over relatively few years and because waiting times are notoriously prone to manipulation. However, I have included them because waiting times are very important, and this is the best comparative information available. As always with medical performance, no comparative figures are perfect.

After all that has been discussed, what should be the conclusion? What is the best system that a modern democracy might choose?

Clearly, it should not be monopoly government provision. Yes, it might be an improvement for a government to contract out hospitals and even to follow the Alzira model. But this also is not ideal because of the lack of competition and real choice for the individual. At the other end of the spectrum, a system that leaves some people wholly uncovered for their health care costs seems unlikely to be acceptable in a modern democracy.

A system is needed in which costs do not run out of control, as they have in many countries. Meanwhile, hospitals, doctors, and clinics need an incentive to come up with new drugs, devices, and ways of treating people. It seems undesirable that individuals who want private care should have to pay for it twice, because then private care becomes unaffordable for most people. It would be good for people to have free choice of hospitals and doctors. Everybody should be able to expect treatment. If we agree that we want all of these features, what system does it lead us to?

I suggest it might lead to a combination of the models found in Singapore and Switzerland/the Netherlands. The system could start with all of us having health savings accounts, as in Singapore—a personal account into which a percentage of our earnings is paid. We would use the money in this account to pay for most health care, such as seeing a general practitioner. This requirement would give us a reason not to waste money.[11] It would be vital to keep our health savings accounts out of the hands of the government by as powerful a constitutional lock as can be devised. And since much of the cost of health care would be paid out of our health accounts, our taxes could be reduced correspondingly.

What if the money in one's health savings account is not sufficient for a major medical bill? Then medical insurance would kick in. All of us would be obliged to take out medical insurance, as in the Netherlands and Switzerland. We would choose between companies that would compete to offer the best deals. We would pay premiums based on the coverage, not on our age and prior conditions.

As for general practitioners, they would all be private and independent. Our relationship with doctors would go back to being personal and direct because we would pay them from our personal health savings accounts or in cash.

The advantage of this system would go far beyond saving money from not having unnecessary treatments and tests. All sorts of suppliers would be inventive in creating medical services that are cheaper, faster, more convenient, and better. In the United States, patients can order their own blood tests from competing diagnostic testing facilities.[12] It is far cheaper than going through a hospital, and the results can be available online within 48 hours. Walmart, the large retail chain, offers hundreds of generic drugs at $10 for 90 days' coverage. Teladoc, a telephone doctor consultation service, provides advice from a qualified doctor at any time, day or night.

Hospitals could be both private and public. But perhaps they should be on a level playing field. The public ones should not be given subsidies or have losses guaranteed. It might be better to have

"The biggest change brought about by giving patients direct control over healthcare dollars is not on the demand side of the market. It's on the supply side."

Source: John C. Goodman, *Priceless: Curing the Healthcare Crisis* (Oakland, CA: Independent Institute, 2012), p. 160.

few or no public hospitals so that all hospitals can compete on an equal basis. Existing public hospitals could be made into charitable trusts or sold to private companies. In the Netherlands, many hospitals are independent trusts.

When framing the best possible system, it is important to think, "What could go wrong?" I can imagine a government fiddling with this system and undermining it. I would worry about excessive rules and regulations being imposed, increasing the costs. I would not be entirely happy that the health savings account and the insurance would be compulsory. But that compulsory element does seem necessary if we are to avoid cases in which people who are not covered incur hardships, causing outrage that leads to an abandonment of the whole system and replacement of it by something with even less freedom. In any case, at present, in countries that do not have a system like this, there is compulsory tax instead.

Some people have a strong aversion to private provision. To them, I would say that the evidence against government monopoly provision is overwhelming. If you want yourself and your loved ones to be seen reliably and quickly in an emergency and you want a better chance of surviving a heart condition or cancer, a public monopoly will not give you what you want.

The system suggested here would not be perfect. That's for sure. But my trip around some of the health care systems of the world leads me to believe that it would be better and more economical than most.

4. "Daisy, Cross Your Fingers"
The Scandal of State Education

In 1977, Marc Le Bris left teacher training school and went to work in the beautiful, rural region of Brittany in northwest France.[1] He had been taught at the school to scorn old-fashioned teaching methods. He believed that his predecessors were "teachers of a previous era" and "semi-incapable."

He began work and found that he had a colleague who was the epitome of an old-fashioned teacher, dictating to his class in a high-pitched voice and getting children to read aloud—something Le Bris had been taught to regard as an absolute heresy. But he came to notice a curious thing: the students who came from the class of this teaching dinosaur did better than the others.

As time went by, he came to believe that what he had been taught at his teacher training school was quite wrong. Worse than that, the kind of teaching it promoted had been a disaster for education in France—a disaster that still has not been corrected. He also found that the new, inadequate methods had affected members of his own family.

A few years ago, Le Bris's brother-in-law approached him. He and his wife were worried about their son, Martin. The boy was not doing as well as his older brother, and his parents were coming to think that he was less able. They were even worried that he might be rather dim. Le Bris replied that Martin might be a bit of a rascal, but he did not seem stupid, certainly not to the point of being unable to read.

The boy's parents explained that they spent one or two hours a day helping Martin with his school work, taking advantage of the way they had different shifts so that both could help him. But Martin's understanding was not getting better. It had reached the point where he did not like learning. There were sometimes screams and tears. Martin's teacher had talked about holding him back a year.

Le Bris looked at Martin's textbooks. He saw right away that the school was using the "whole word" method of teaching children to read, which was based on an educational theory that became fashionable in the latter part of the 20th century. According to this theory, children should learn how to read by recognizing words rather than letters. The teacher had even gone so far as to explain to the parents that they should not tell Martin the sounds of the letters. He should discover them for himself.

It was November. Le Bris suggested to the worried parents that they should try using the old-fashioned Boscher way of teaching, which dated to the 1950s and emphasized letters. He gave them some simple instructions about how to do it. So the father started to teach his son to read in this way.

The following June, seven months later, Martin's teacher reported on how he was doing. She said, "We don't know what happened but suddenly, over Christmas, Martin made great progress!" Martin's mother, normally a quiet, reserved person, remarked pointedly that it was over Christmas that they had started teaching Martin the sounds of letters. The teacher blushed. She said that, in any event, what mattered was that the boy could now read. Quite so.

Marc Le Bris, his words suffused with anger and outrage, comments: "In the end, it is the parents who teach the children to read. The teachers don't know how to."[2] He feels guilty about the children he thinks he failed when he started teaching and was using methods that did not work. But at least he eventually perceived something was wrong and changed his methods. He had the initiative and courage to change, but the teaching colleges and the authorities did not.

"This has been going on for more than 30 years," he wrote. "More than 80 percent of children are still subjected to dogmatic, stupid methods."

What becomes of the children whose parents, unlike Martin's parents, do not take it upon themselves to teach their children to read, Le Bris asks. They do not learn properly. But they are moved on to the next year anyway. Children are not held back for a year any more. Why? Because, he says, "It would look bad in the statistics." The title of the passionate book that Le Bris wrote is *Et vos enfants ne sauront pas lire, ni compter!—And Your Children Won't Know How to Read or Count*!

It might seem unlikely that more than one country would adopt and persist with a way of teaching that works so badly. But I have found that this has taken place in several countries at least.

We may have different ideas about the purpose of education. But most of us would agree that one thing that any schooling system

Box 4.1
STATE EDUCATION FOR EQUAL OPPORTUNITY?

State education ostensibly creates a level playing field for the children of the poor to compete with the children of the rich. But in many countries, public schools reinforce the difference instead because the rich get their children into the best public schools and the poor are left with the rest. This phenomenon certainly takes place in Germany, France, Britain, and the United States, among others. In Germany, children from a privileged background are four times more likely to attend a *Gymnasium*—the kind of school most likely to lead to university—than a child with similar grades from a working-class home.[a]

One way in which the rich get into the best public schools is by moving into the catchment area for those schools. This increases property values in the area, pricing out those who are poorer. In Britain, academic research has indicated that the best schools push housing prices in a particular area 12 percent higher than they would be if that area had the worst schools.[b] So there is a kind of auction for the advantage of the best government education. It is an auction that the rich tend to win, of course. As Becky Francis, professor at King's College, London, has observed, "Equality of opportunity is being undermined by the greater purchasing power of some parents."[c] It has even been found that one in 20 upper-middle-class parents buy a second home in the catchment area of a specific school so that their children can attend it.[d]

----

[a] Alexandra Topping, "Germany's Middle Class Happy with Rampant Inequality in Schools," *Guardian* (London), March 15, 2011, http://www.theguardian.com/world/2011/mar/15/germany -middle-class-inequality-schools.

[b] Steve Gibbons, "The Link between Schools and House Prices Is Now an Established Fact," London School of Economics blog, September 25, 2012, http://blogs.lse.ac.uk/politicsandpolicy /archives/27103. Gibbons notes, "A link between better schools and higher house prices has emerged as one of the most stable empirical regularities, with studies worldwide reporting effects of a similar order of magnitude."

[c] Quoted in Amanda Constance, "By Any Means...," *Absolutely Kensington*, February 2014, http://issuu .com/zestmedialondon/docs/abs_kensington_feb_2014/65. Professor Francis is one of the authors of a Sutton Trust report, "Parent Power."

[d] Ibid.

should do is teach children who have been in its care for 11 or more years how to read and write (see Box 4.1). How well do the schools of the advanced world succeed in this fundamental task?

As part of my visit to the Organisation for Economic Co-operation and Development (OECD) in Paris, I am on my way to see Andreas Schleicher. He is the man who established the OECD's Programme for International Student Assessment (PISA) studies of educational attainment around the world. All the OECD countries and a number of countries or cities that are not members of the OECD have taken part. Michael Gove, the former British secretary of state for education, has called Schleicher "the most important person in world education."[3]

The press officer who arranged my visit takes me along a maze of smart, light corridors. Everything is modern with lots of straight lines and glass. We find an office on an upper story with a large window overlooking an internal courtyard.

Schleicher gets up and greets me with a firm handshake. He looks like everyone's idea of a dynamic, intelligent German in his prime. He reminds me of Martin Kaymer, a golfer whose final putt enabled the European team to win the Ryder Cup in 2012. He and his staff have collected a great mass of information—the latest PISA report consists of six substantial volumes. So I ask him: what is his conclusion about literacy? How well do the schools of the world teach children to read?

Schleicher is a precise man and asks what level of literacy I mean. I specify "functional literacy." This is the literacy level that is good enough to be useful at work or in private life. A person is functionally literate, for example, if he or she can read a notice about donating blood and answer a fairly simple question about it (see Box 4.2). Answering the question does require a little intelligence but not much.

Six reading levels are defined in the PISA study. Schleicher tells me that individuals who manage to reach only level 1 are deemed to be functionally illiterate. He remarks that those who have not got further face a bleak outlook. If you have not learned to read by the age of 15, "nobody will teach you," he says. So what is the percentage of children among OECD countries, who, after many years of schooling, cannot read properly?

Schleicher picks out one of the PISA volumes and finds the page that shows the percentages of children who attain the various levels of literacy in each country and in the OECD as an average. Adding together percentages below level 1 and at levels 1A and 1B, we work out that the level of functional illiteracy among the children of the advanced world is 18.8 percent.[4]

I expected that the figure might be bad. But this statistic is truly appalling. I remark that it is a terrible indictment of the educational systems of the advanced world. Schleicher does not disagree and observes, "What is even more amazing is that they pass exams with this low level of literacy."

We see many statistics about education in newspapers, including tables of performance by schools and countries. But literacy figures

Box 4.2
SAMPLE QUESTION FROM THE PISA TEST

Blood donation notice from a French website:

Blood donation is essential.

There is no product that can fully substitute for human blood. Blood donation is therefore irreplaceable and essential to save lives.

In France, each year, 500,000 patients benefit from a blood transfusion.

The instruments for taking blood are sterile and single use (syringe, tubes, bags). There is no risk in giving blood.

Blood donation

It is the best-known kind of donation, and takes 45 minutes to 1 hour.

The 450-ml bag is taken as well as some samples on which tests and checks will be done.

A man can give his blood five times a year, a woman three times.

Donors can be from 18 to 65 years old.

An 8-week interval is compulsory between each donation.

The test asks various questions about this notice. This is the question at level 2—the level that indicates functional literacy:

An 18-year-old woman who has given her blood twice in the last 12 months wants to give blood again. According to "Blood donation notice," on what condition will she be allowed to give blood again?

A correct answer is one that identifies that enough time must have elapsed since the previous donation. The answer will be marked as correct even if the time of eight weeks is not mentioned.[a]

---

[a] Organisation for Economic Co-operation and Development, *PISA 2009 Results, vol. 1: What Students Know and Can Do* (Paris: OECD Publishing, 2010), p. 102.

rarely get any coverage. I suggest they are more important than any others. School systems that have not taught a large proportion of children to read have failed in their most basic task and have damaged the futures of millions of people.

Some countries do much better than others, and we will get to the possible reasons. But overall, it seems clear that the educational systems of most of the advanced world are failures, leaving an average of nearly one in five children functionally illiterate (Table 4.1 and see Box 4.3).

Table 4.1
HOW MANY CHILDREN ARE LEFT FUNCTIONALLY ILLITERATE?

Country or city	Percentage (%)[a]
Shanghai	2.9
Hong Kong	6.8
South Korea	7.6
Ireland	9.6
Japan	9.8
Singapore	9.9
Poland	10.6
Canada	10.9
Finland	11.3
Switzerland	13.7
Netherlands	14.0
Australia	14.2
Germany	14.5
Denmark	14.6
Belgium	16.1
Norway	16.2
New Zealand	16.3
United Kingdom	16.6
United States	16.6
OECD average	**18.0**
Spain	18.3
Portugal	18.8
France	18.9
Italy	19.5
Austria	19.5
Greece	22.6
Sweden	22.7

SOURCE: Organisation for Economic Co-operation and Development, *PISA 2012 Results, vol. 1: What Students Know and Can Do*, rev. ed., Table I.4.1b (Paris: OECD Publishing, 2014), http://dx.doi.org/10.1787/888932935705. The figure of 18.0 percent for the overall OECD average for functional literacy appears on page 196 in the text; see http://www.oecd.org/PISA/keyfindings/PISA-2012-results-volume-I.pdf. The OECD average of 18.8 percent referred to by Andreas Schleicher in our interview was from PISA 2009, the most recently published report at that time.

[a] Percentage of students below level 2 in reading, PISA study 2012, selected countries. The OECD figure Andreas Schleicher mentioned is slightly different because he was using the 2009 study.

Box 4.3
SCHOOLED BUT ILLITERATE

"How did I get through school when I couldn't read?"[a]

Professional football player Dexter Manley asked this powerful question during a hearing of the U.S. Senate Subcommittee on Education, Arts, and Humanities on May 18, 1989.

The obvious answer to Manley's question is that the tests applied by his school were not rigorous. The school system was graduating children who had not even learned to read. According to an account of the Senate hearing, "Dexter Manley, the All-Pro former defensive end for the Washington Redskins, offered a startling and embarrassing confession to Congress, saying he almost made it to the age of 30 without being able to read. Manley was embarrassed to say that he was illiterate and that he had memorized words and faked his way through life for years. 'I broke down and started crying,' Manley said in 1989. 'How did I get through school when I couldn't read?'

"Manley told Congress that at the age of 28, he entered The Lab School of Washington with a second grade reading level. He would eventually earn as much as $350,000 a year playing for the Redskins—and keeping his closely-guarded secret from his fellow players for years."[b]

Manley's experience growing up in Houston, Texas, is not isolated. Consider these observations from a 2011 report about Detroit, Michigan:[c]

- Of the 200,000 adults [in Detroit] who are functionally illiterate, approximately half have a high school diploma or GED.
- The National Institute for Literacy estimates that 47 percent of adults in the City of Detroit are functionally illiterate.

As we will see, the consequences of this education disaster are extremely serious. For example, as the U.S. Department of Justice reported, "The link between academic failure and delinquency, violence, and crime is welded to reading failure."[d]

---

[a] Michael H. Cottman, "Analysis: Illiteracy in Detroit a National Shame," New America Media website, May 11, 2011, http://newamericamedia.org/2011/05/analysis-illiteracy-in-detroit-a-national-shame.php.

[b] Ibid.

[c] Detroit Regional Workforce Fund, "Addressing Detroit's Basic Skills Crisis," http://cbsdetroit.files .wordpress.com/2011/05/basicskillsreport_final.pdf. GED (General Educational Development) tests are a group of five subject tests that, if passed, certify that someone has high school–level academic skills.

[d] Cited in "Literary Statistics," Begin to Read website, www.begintoread.com/research/literacystatistics .html.

It is an inescapable fact that all these systems are dominated by government schooling. Another question we will come to is whether private schooling would do better.

I can imagine some people reading this chapter and thinking, "Yes, well, the statistics might not look great, but there are plenty of schools doing a good job. Is there really a problem? Or is this a mere abstract thing without real consequences?" Let's see. What happens to people who cannot fully read and write?

Harriet Sergeant, a British journalist and author, wanted to understand why many white and Afro-Caribbean working-class boys were failing to go from school to normal jobs.[5] As part of her research, she went to West Norwood in south London to see if she could talk to the sort of youths who were dropping out of normal life. Accompanied by "Swagger," a worker from a local community center and former robber of security vans, she approached a small group of mostly black teenagers on the street. They were dressed in hoodies and low-slung baggy jeans, intimidating passers-by, glaring at shoppers, mooching cigarettes, shouting, and laughing. She thought they looked as though they could turn violent at any moment. She assumed they had knives—perhaps even a gun. She had not thought about the fact that she was wearing an expensive watch.

The short, young leader of the group gave his name as Tuggy Tug. In her book, *Among the Hoods*, Harriet wrote that Tuggy Tug was positively proud of his criminality. He showed her a red hoodie underneath his black one. He said he wore it in case he needed a quick change of identity. "I want no one recognisin' me when I about my business," he said.[6] He explained that he was looking for someone to mug and, as he spoke, he looked directly at Sergeant.

She asked why they were not at school. One of the group, who called himself Jiggers, was even smaller than Tuggy Tug and had scars on his little hands. He had a "pinched, watchful expression." Jiggers said he had problems with his English teacher. "Why did them teachers keep askin' me questions? They knew I couldn't read, but they kept on askin,'" he said. Jiggers and Tuggy Tug, along with Bulldog and Sunshine, all admitted having trouble with "them little words." That is why none of them was in school.[7]

Swagger, Sergeant's escort, later described how he himself had been affected by illiteracy: "I was embarrassed by my reading so I became the class clown," he said. By the age of 13, he had become bored, frustrated, and always in trouble. "I didn't feel good about myself. I got no pride in myself. I was angry over every little thing.

It did not take a lot to set me off." No teacher seemed to notice or address the problem. "So I think why not bunk school and go and do a bit of thieving?" he said.[8]

That is how he became a criminal. Eventually he was caught robbing a security van and went to prison. "We go from school to prison. I thought I would be dead by 40."

Swagger's parents—first-generation immigrants from Jamaica working in good jobs—had hoped their only son would become a lawyer or doctor. But he said, shaking his head sadly, "School shatters your dreams before you get anywhere."

Swagger was unusual in facing up to what had happened to him. It is human nature to try to make the best of one's situation and see it in as positive a light as possible.

Sergeant asked the gang members how they saw their future in the absence of education or jobs. "Tuggy Tug answered for them all. That did not seem a problem. His heroes were rap stars and the older drug dealers in the area. 'I know a man of 21 who owns five houses, and he never went to school,' he said."[9]

The gang gave another explanation for why they had left school, one which, coming from young, illiterate criminals, is all the more remarkable. They complained of a lack of discipline:

> "You can sit on the desk with your shoes off, your socks hanging out, on the phone, doing your ting [drug dealing], and the teachers won't give a toss," said Tuggy Tug.
>
> His friends all nodded, eager now to contribute. This was a subject that raised strong feelings. . . . "There's bare [lots of] people in your class just messin' around," said one mixed-race boy called Sunshine. "You don't feel like you're learnin' so what's the point of goin' to school?"[10]

These gang members felt that they were let down by their schools. And the failure of schools to teach them to read had, according to their own testimony, led them toward crime. In turning to crime, they were probably ruining their own lives as well as harming those whom they mugged or robbed. As Harriet Sergeant predicted at the time, some of the gang have since gone to prison. Of course, they are contributing nothing to the economy. They are costing money instead.

Their story suggests that a failed education, in general, and illiteracy, in particular, lead to crime. Is there evidence to support this idea? Here is some from the United States: only a minority of children are not taught to read proficiently, yet the overwhelming majority of those who get in trouble are from their ranks. Some 72 percent of prison inmates have a low level of literacy and 40 percent are at the lowest of five levels of literacy—almost twice the proportion in the general population.[11] These are remarkable statistics. It is as though literacy were a superb defense against criminal activity. As ever, correlation is not the same as causation. It is genuinely conceivable that some third factor contributes to a child's becoming both illiterate and criminal. Indeed in Chapter 6 we will consider the role of parenting.

Further support for the idea that illiteracy contributes to crime comes from the reoffending figures. Learning to read reduces the rate at which prisoners reoffend. The average effect is to reduce reoffending by 6 percent, and the best results can reach 14 percent.[12] These and other similar statistics are so powerful and make so much sense that it seems overwhelmingly likely that illiteracy makes people more likely to be criminal in the modern world.

Why is illiteracy so powerfully connected to crime? It surely goes back to the comment of Tuggy Tug and his gang: if you can't read, you have trouble getting a job. It is the same thing that officials in the Job Center in Madison, Wisconsin, said in Chapter 2. Most jobs require at least some ability to read. Even a driver needs to be able to read road signs. It is surprising how much even fairly low-wage jobs involve reading.

If a young man cannot get a job because he can't read, what is he to do? Live on welfare? Possibly. But the temptation to turn to crime is much greater than it would be if he could get a job. So we see two possible results of functional illiteracy: crime and unemployment. Both of them are damaging for those involved and for the rest of society.

"What brings about the delinquency is not the academic failure *per se*, but sustained frustration which results from continued failure. . . . When frustration can find no resolution into constructive or productive activity, one response, though not the only one, is aggressive, anti-social behavior."

SOURCE: Michael Brunner, *Reduced Recidivism and Increased Employment Opportunity through Research-based Reading Instruction* (Washington, D.C.: U.S. Department of Justice, 1993), p. 8, https://www.ncjrs.gov/pdffiles1/Digitization/141324NCJRS.pdf

---

If we look at welfare recipients in the United States, an astonishing 90 percent are high school dropouts.[13] But it does not end there. Naturally those who cannot get work tend to be poor. That helps explain why among those who can read only at level 1, 43 percent are relatively poor. Among those who read well—at level 5—only 4 percent are relatively poor.[14]

There is another consequence. Poor education is also strongly correlated with unmarried parenting. Among young women ages 16 to 19 who are at the poverty level and below, those who cannot read well are six times more likely to have a child outside marriage than those who can.[15] Why should this be? There are probably quite a few reasons. I suggest one of them is that illiterate young women have difficulty getting a good job and so are more likely to be tempted to have a baby and to put up with living on welfare benefits in public housing.

Overall, functional illiteracy is strongly connected to crime, unemployment, poverty, and even unmarried parenting. It seems almost trivial to add that being unable to read also means never being able to appreciate history, novels, or biography—in fact, any of the world's literature.

It is not an exaggeration to say that the widespread failure of schooling is a tragedy for the individuals affected and for society (Box 4.4).

Box 4.4
DAMAGE CAUSED WHEN SCHOOLING FAILS

A few statistics highlight the problem in the United States:

- Fifty percent of the chronically unemployed are not functionally literate.[a]
- Two-thirds of students who cannot read proficiently by the end of fourth grade will end up in jail or on welfare.[b]
- Sixty percent of young black men who drop out of school land in prison by their 30s.[c]

---

[a] U.S. Department of Education, in presentation by Susan Sclafani, April 2005, cited by Literacy Texas, Literacy Facts. The statistic is also cited in Hans Meeder, "Preparing America's Future: Enhancing the Quality of Adult Education and Family Literacy," May 2003, www2.ed.gov/about/offices/list/ovae/pi/AdultEd/ncfl.doc.
[b] Cited in "Literary Statistics," Begin to Read website, www.begintoread.com/research/literacystatistics.html.
[c] Geoffrey Canada, "Bringing Change to Scale: The Next Big Reform Challenge," in *Waiting for "Superman": How We Can Save America's Failing Public Schools*, ed. Karl Weber (New York: Public Affairs, 2010), p. 191.

What is going on in the world's schools that brings about such bad outcomes? (Box 4.5 examines how government schooling got started.) What can be done to improve things? We have seen that centrally imposed teaching methods can damage literacy. But there must be more to it than that.

Box 4.5
WHERE DID GOVERNMENT SCHOOLING COME FROM?

We tend to take the dominance of government schooling for granted. But in each country, it is the result of different histories.

In France, the church dominated education until Louis XIV began to challenge it in 1666. The struggle for power between church and state continued right up to the 19th century, when the state finally became dominant. In the middle of that century, the government minister responsible drew out his pocket watch and remarked, "At this moment, all the students of the *lycées* [secondary schools] are explaining the same passage from Virgil."[a]

In Germany, the Catholic Church also initially dominated education, but the challenge of the Protestants in the Reformation temporarily created a vacuum in which private schools thrived. Then the Protestant ascendancy reached the point at which the church used the power and tax-raising capacity of the state to enforce education of the sort it wanted. When the National Socialists came to power in the 1930s, they enforced teaching of Nazi views. Then, after the war, the communists in East Germany enforced teaching of communist views. Three-quarters of the teachers were fired for having signed their previous oath of allegiance to the Nazis.

In the United States, a great diversity of schools operated in the early 19th century, a system that appears to have been quite successful. When Alexis de Tocqueville visited in 1831, he remarked that it was rare to find a New Englander who had not had the advantage of at least an elementary school education.[b] But from the 1830s on, politicians decided that education should be made compulsory, and this mandate led to pressure to make it free—or, rather, paid through taxation. Eventually, all the states introduced compulsory education that they provided free at the schools they controlled. It was a similar story in England.

The sobering thing about the stories of France and Germany is the way education was seen by churches and governments of different sorts as a way of influencing the hearts and minds of children. But even nations that consider themselves liberal democracies are not free of the impulse to control the views and beliefs of the next generation.

---

[a] Andrew J. Coulson, *Market Education: The Unknown History* (New Brunswick, NJ: Transaction, 1999).
[b] Ibid.

I am in San Francisco, where I would like to visit a typical public school. I want to see a school with typical problems—neither a basket case nor a model school. This is more difficult to achieve than it might seem. School boards like to show off their best schools, not their typical ones. In the couple of weeks before I arrived, I wrote emails to the school board asking to visit Balboa High School. It serves a relatively poor part of San Francisco. Its record is better than average, but it is not at the top of the rankings. I did not get a definite "yes" or "no" in reply to my emails, but once I have arrived in San Francisco, I have one more go at it. I call the school directly and ask for the principal. To my surprise, I get straight through, and he says I may visit right away.

The main school building is big, and around the perimeter is a high fence. I enter a hallway with high ceilings and am directed to the reception office, a large, bustling, open-plan room with many people working at desks. The receptionist asks me to wait. While I am sitting there, I hear her take a call on a walkie-talkie. Immediately afterward, she makes a call herself. I hear her say something about "getting an escort." Soon after, she tells me I can go in and see the principal. She shows me into an adjacent office, where Mr. Kerr, relaxed and genial, greets me.

I ask him right away what that conversation concerning an "escort" was all about. He explains that when a student wants to go to the bathroom during a class, he or she has to have an escort to go there and come back. A teacher had phoned reception to request one. The receptionist had telephoned the security personnel to set it up.

Why on earth is such a thing necessary, I ask. He tells me that when he became the principal, the student body told him they did not like this system, which had been created by his predecessor. So Kerr agreed to abolish it and give the children the trust they wanted. But as a result, the toilets were defaced with graffiti and the floors were covered in urine, so he decided to bring the system back.

The story gives some idea of what the school is up against. While we are on the subject of discipline, Kerr also tells me the children are not allowed to wear hats or the colors red or blue on their way to school. Why not? Because red and blue are the colors of two local gangs. If children come to school wearing red or blue, they may be approached by one of the gangs either to be invited to join or else harassed for wearing the "wrong" color.

Safety and discipline are obviously major issues. Another sign of this is that Kerr is proud that the fire alarm is triggered by the children only about once a year. He has been told that in another, even bigger, school in San Francisco, the fire alarm is set off once a week.

Despite this background, the school has improved its academic performance from below average to above average. I ask Kerr what he thinks are the key factors that have helped achieve this. It is no surprise that "making it safe" is the second thing he mentions. And the first?

"Putting in good teachers."

I ask how he did this, but he seems reluctant to say. Eventually, after we talk for a while and tour the school, he lets me have an idea of how it works. Eighty percent of his teachers are exceptional, he says. But 20 percent are not so good, and he would really like to get rid of half of these and replace them with good teachers.

So why not do it?

"It takes years," he replies. It is very difficult and time-consuming to remove a teacher in the public school system. And when finally you manage it, you are obliged to take a replacement from the "consolidated list." This is a list of teachers of the relevant subject who are available to be hired. Doubtless, some good teachers are on the list, but a high proportion are teachers who have been rejected by other schools. That is where fired teachers go: onto the consolidated list. So it is very possible that after finally removing a bad teacher, a principal may be obliged to recruit another one.

Kerr, though, has worked out how to get around this problem—how to game the system. He proudly tells me that he requested an English literature teacher one August, during summer vacation. He was told, "Oh, what a pity you didn't ask in April. We could have offered you plenty of teachers then." None were available in August, which was exactly what Kerr had hoped. Because no one was available, he was allowed to recruit a teacher he knew and thought was good.

"Dance of the lemons"—phrase used to describe the way that bad teachers fired by one school in America are hired by another.

SOURCE: Karl Weber, "Introduction," in *Waiting for "Superman": How We Can Save America's Failing Public Schools*, ed. Karl Weber (New York: Public Affairs, 2010), p. 20.

Kerr's techniques for recruiting better teachers do not always work but they usually do. That is clearly good for Balboa High and its pupils. Its rating has been rising toward a level at which it will be deemed exceptional. But Kerr is a veteran principal. He remarks that novice principals get "hazed." They end up with the teachers that he and other experienced principals have finally managed to fire. The truth is, in this system, bad teachers do not go away. They get recycled. And, of course, the teachers know they are hard to fire—a condition which seems unlikely to prompt a strong work ethic.[16] (See Box. 4.6 for more on the corruption of teaching standards.)

Box 4.6

How to Get On as a Teacher in the United States

> In the early 1990s, Peter Sacks left journalism to teach media studies at a community college—part of the public education system. He demanded effort and good behavior from his students when he began. He gave marks he considered fair, and the average grade he awarded was a C. But he received complaints from the students and demands such as "I need an A in this course to graduate with honors!" As a result, he got poor evaluations from his students. It was highly likely that he would lose his job.
>
> He decided to lower his standards and become wholly indulgent and undemanding. His career as a teacher was at stake. He thought this choice was absurd, but he decided to make a kind of experiment out of changing his approach.
>
> "I did almost anything possible to make them happy, all of the time, no matter how childish or rude their behavior, no matter how poorly they performed in the course, no matter how little effort they gave. . . . If they wanted to read the newspaper while I was addressing the class or if they wanted to get up and leave in the middle of a lecture, go for it."
>
> What was the result? His evaluations by the students became favorable and, in due course, he was granted tenure. In this *Through the Looking Glass* system, he was punished for maintaining high standards and rewarded for letting them go. He concluded, "Nobody in the system had much of a stake in shoring up educational standards . . . just the opposite was the case."
>
> Peter Sacks wrote a book—*Generation X Goes to College*—about his experience. (Peter Sacks is not his real name. He used a nom de plume because he continued to work as a teacher.)

Source: Peter Sacks, *Generation X Goes to College: An Eye-opening Account of Teaching in Postmodern America* (Chicago: Open Court, 1996).

Bearing in mind that the school is rated as above average, I ask: what is the attendance rate? Kerr says it is 94 percent. That does not sound very good to me, and at one point, he says some children there feel that education is something "done to them." I can't help wondering whether the lack of motivation may be partly because there is no clearly identifiable public exam that would have a major effect on the students' careers.

Kerr is clearly appalled at the ignorance of some of the children at his own school. On his desk is a sign reading, "The buck stops here." One of his students asked him what the sign was all about. He told the student that it was the sign that Harry Truman had on his desk.

"Who's Harry Truman?" the student asked.

What about the standard of education generally in the United States? Kerr is gloomy about it. He says that in a survey 30-year-old Americans were asked from which country the United States had achieved independence. Forty percent did not know.

The visit to Balboa and the story of ineffective teaching in France suggest a variety of possible reasons that so many schools around the world are doing badly. But what do the data say? Back at the OECD headquarters in Paris, part of their analysis consists of looking at characteristics of schools and seeing which are linked with good academic achievement. Discipline in the classroom is indeed correlated with better academic outcomes. Or to put in another way, bad discipline is associated with failure.

The best-performing countries tend to have "high-stakes" public exams on which the academic futures of the children depend. To put it the other way, the worst-performing systems tend to avoid high-stakes exams, preferring to announce that everyone is a winner. The best-performing countries also tend to benefit from one thing that is partly cultural: a belief that hard work enables almost any child to achieve success. This idea is particularly common in Asia. In Japan, every child is obliged to learn to play an instrument—and does. There is, of course, a downside to emphasizing hard work and high-stakes exams. In Japan and South Korea, some children work far harder than most Western parents would consider sensible or even humane. The expression "examination hell" is part of normal language in Japan. At the other extreme is a Western view that children either have talent or they don't and that bothering to work hard is less important.

What other factors are there? Andreas Schleicher argues that teacher quality and status make a big difference. Some countries have teachers who are themselves at the bottom end of educational achievement. He also thinks it is useful if children who are doing badly are assigned the best and most effective teachers to bring them up to speed. He emphasizes the importance of motivation for everyone involved: the administrators, the teachers, the children, and their parents. The PISA studies also have found a correlation between the level of autonomy of schools and their achievement.

In brief, the research suggests that the countries with the best outcomes have good classroom discipline, high-stakes exams, a belief that hard work is important and that every child can achieve, able teachers retained in the profession, independence for schools, and a high level of motivation for everyone involved.

But because the systems of the world have generally done so badly, we can infer that something like the opposite commonly occurs: bad classroom discipline, avoidance of high-stakes exams, little belief in hard work or the possibility that every child can achieve, academically low-quality teachers in schools that have little independence, and a lack of motivation among the people concerned. (See Box 4.7.)

Box 4.7
"YOU STAND AT THE FRONT ON THE KNIFE-EDGE OF ANARCHY"

Those words come from an interview by the author with a mature science graduate who went through a teacher training course in England. During his training, he observed many classes in different government schools and did some teaching himself. Here is his account:

All teachers hate poor discipline, but the reality is it's very difficult to keep control in a rough school except by being friendly, getting the kids on your side. Being entertaining is the only way to do it. This is the opposite of what I thought initially (and to what you might think now). As a teacher, you have no natural or assumed authority walking into a classroom. You have to earn it, hence the need for rapid cycling of activities—"fun and games," as the teachers call it. You stand at the front on the knife-edge of anarchy most of the time. When a class "loses it," it's distressing and uncontrollable. I saw it happen often in observation, with many good and experienced teachers. Swearing, constant disruption, laughter, throwing things, chairs pushed over, insulting the teacher, accusing them of racism. In some class groups, this was every single lesson.

(continued on next page)

(continued)

It was frustrating how prescriptive OFSTED [Office for Standards in Education] is about how to teach a subject. It felt like you were running through a formula. At the beginning you had to have a slide with the intended learning outcomes of the class. Lesson plans are required to be in sections of around five minutes. OFSTED likes teachers to change what they are doing often so there is a maximum of five minutes of a teacher talking and asking questions at the front. More than that seemed to be considered bad practice.

There is a trend in schools to de-emphasise knowledge and promote skills. The idea is that knowledge we have now will be out of date so, instead, we should teach skills. This is a disaster for science. A little bit of teamwork, yes. But you need factual stuff!

A big thing these days is AFL—Assessment for Learning. There is continual testing including at primary schools, closely defining what a child can do. Teachers seem to spend as much time on assessment as teaching.

What can be done to make things better? Setting about correcting these faults may well help. But before drawing conclusions, let's look at another possible approach to the question.

Some people in the education business have looked at which countries get the best results with the idea of copying whatever system the country has. So let's try that.

The top six places for functional literacy in the latest PISA study are taken by Shanghai, Hong Kong, Korea, Ireland, Japan, and Singapore (see Table 4.1). Right away, you can't help noticing something about them: five are east Asian.

This observation suggests that there might be something about Asia or Asians that leads to better academic performance. The most obvious thing to anyone who has lived and worked there is the enormous emphasis on hard work and achievement. In Japan, it is seen as one of the prime duties of a mother to ensure that her child does well at school. And when Asians, notably those of Chinese origin, come to the West, they often bring a work ethic with them. They excel in American schools.

If hard work is the cause of the good Asian performance, that is interesting, of course, but it might be difficult to translate into government policy. One cannot just give instructions to "be more motivated and work harder." Something else is special about schooling in the Far East. Yes, there are government schools, to which the vast majority of children go. But it is normal for parents to supplement government teaching with private schooling and tutoring. In the jargon, this is called "shadow education."

In Japan, children often attend government-run schools for the first part of the day and then go on to privately run schools, called *juku*, afterward. This is not just a luxury for super-rich parents. It is widespread. In year three at junior secondary schools, 65 percent of children go to *juku*, 7 percent have tutoring at home, and 15 percent take the cheaper option of correspondence courses.[17] The parents supplement government schooling partly because they want their children to get into the better upper secondary schools, which are most likely to lead to better universities and jobs. But they may also believe that the government schools are not providing a good enough education.

"In a 2008 government survey, two-thirds of parents attributed the growing role of *juku* to shortcomings in public education. Their service is more personalised, and many encourage individual inquisitiveness when the public system treats everyone alike."

Source: "Testing Times: A Controversial Institution Has Some Surprising Merits," *The Economist*, December 31, 2011.

Parents in South Korea, the number two country in the world for functional literacy, spend what has been called a "staggering" amount on shadow education, equivalent to around 80 percent of government expenditures.[18] Supplementary private schools there are called *hagwons*.

According to Andrew Coulson, an education analyst in the United States, "Most students [in Korea] sleep during some or all of their public school classes and then go to private *hagwons* after school until as late as two in the morning."[19] Educator Michael B. Horn has reported from Korea that "parents spend huge sums to send them [their children] to *hagwons* . . . in which students do the 'real' learning."[20]

In Hong Kong, about 85 percent of senior secondary students have some form of private supplementary schooling.[21] The proportion in mainland China does not appear to have been established reliably, but one estimate is that as many as 66 percent of lower secondary school students receive extra private schooling.[22]

Governments and government-funded organizations around the world tend to dislike or resent supplementary schooling and demand that it should be regulated. But as the author of an Asian Development Bank report remarked, "Policy-makers may learn from the shadow. They should ask why it exists in the first place."[23]

The huge amount of supplementary private education in Asia should influence how we regard the PISA results. We cannot reasonably say, "We must learn from the success of Asian government schools," because we know the performance of Asian students has been affected by supplementary schooling.[24] In fact, it would be more logical to say, "The lesson of the relative success of Asian education is that a boost from private education takes these places to the top of the lists."

"Even though it's 'free' at all levels, Greek households spend more for the education of their children (for private tutoring) than any other in the EU."

SOURCE: Aristides Hatzis, "Greece as a Precautionary Tale of the Welfare State," in *After the Welfare State: Politicians Stole Your Future . . . You Can Get It Back*, ed. Tom G. Palmer (Arlington, VA: Students for Liberty, 2012), p. 30.

However, one of the top-performing countries is far away from Asia. It is very different. Finland has a history of being the best-performing country outside Asia in the series of PISA assessments. In the most recent study, it actually comes behind Ireland and Poland for functional literacy, but it is the best outside Asia for science. Finland has no private schools. So what is it doing right?

I asked Andreas Schleicher, the creator of the PISA assessment, what he thought. He said Finland used to have a command-and-control education system that stifled schools. But then, in the 1970s, the economy experienced a major crisis. Gross domestic product fell 18 percent. As a result of this economic and financial crisis, school inspectors were abolished. Schools were consequently given more autonomy, akin to that in charter or "free" schools. Suddenly, Finnish schools came to be judged not by inspectors but by their success in exams.

The story supports the idea that autonomy and that judgment of schools by results might be important. The OECD reports also highlighted the high status and qualifications of the teachers in Finnish schools and their concentration on improving their performance. There is great emphasis on identifying and helping any child that falls behind, too. The schools are also small, which may or may not be significant.

"On average a teacher in the bottom quintile of effectiveness covers only 50 percent of the required curriculum in a school year, while a teacher in the top quintile covers 150 percent."

SOURCE: Karl Weber, "A Nation Still at Risk," cited in Peter Sacks, *Generation X Goes to College: An Eye-opening Account of Teaching in Postmodern America* (Chicago: Open Court, 1996), p. 7.

By chance, while puzzling over these issues, I happened to meet a young Finnish researcher who told me more about Finnish education from the inside. She told me there are elements of competition in the Finnish system. Her own school selected students by ability. When children get to the age of 15 or 16, they face a fork in the road. Either they go to a vocational college or they take a path that leads to a university. It is a high-stakes moment.

I asked the researcher about discipline in the schools. It was as though I had asked about water in the sea. Yes, of course there was discipline. She took it for granted. She said that she herself was the biggest rebel in her class. A keener, more dedicated rebel would be hard to imagine.

She had a less than glowing view of the theme of equality that runs through Finnish education and that many admire so much. For her, it had drawbacks. This is part of an email she sent me:

> There is "equality" even when people clearly have different interests and ambitions. For example until the age of 15–16 all students are divided into different classes based only on their surname or just randomly. Accordingly, students with a passion for a certain subject have to take the very same classes as those people who never do their homework and have zero interest in the subject.
>
> This is especially unfortunate in subjects such as maths and languages which require previous knowledge to learn something new. The brightest students felt discouraged from progressing and the most unmotivated people surely felt that sometimes the classes were too advanced.

The researcher strongly believed that her schools had not stretched her and that she had not had the chance to develop her full potential. She did not think that Finland had preeminently good education; she thought the universities were markedly inferior to British ones.

Several education policy specialists note how homogeneous Finland is. Its population is composed of 3 percent immigrants compared with 9 percent in Britain, 10 percent in France, 12 percent in Germany, and 13 percent in the United States.[25] The academic performance of immigrants is often below average. Japan and Korea also have relatively few immigrants compared with other countries. So perhaps there is nothing wonderful about Finnish education at all. It could be a matter of high-stakes exams, good discipline deriving from the culture, low immigration, or a mixture of these.

It turns out that those are only a few of many reasons that academics doubt whether the Finnish performance is quite as good a guide as the PISA study suggests.[26] This book does not have space to describe them all.

In view of this and the likely reasons for the success of east Asian students, it does not seem sensible simply to copy another country's system. We have, though, found some support for the ideas that discipline, private schooling, and high-stakes exams can help. Is there some other way to find a system of education that could work better?

I am at the Summit Academy in San Lorenzo, California—a low building in a spacious suburban street. It's a calm, pleasant neighborhood, but the children at this school come from the poorer half of society. I meet the genial, bespectacled principal. After a short meeting in his office, I am taken from class to class. As I listen in to the lessons, frankly I am not convinced that the teaching methods are particularly good.

The principal has kindly arranged for me to talk to eight children. He has chosen a mixture of children—"not just the easy ones." Yes, there is Yasmin, bright-eyed and enthusiastic, who sits opposite me and who, I guess, is probably something of an academic star. But there are others at the opposite end of the range.

I ask the principal if he would mind leaving us so the children can speak without worrying about his reaction to what they say. Generously, he agrees.

One of the eight is Michael. He looks Hispanic. He is in eighth grade, which would normally mean that he is about 14, but he was "retained" in fifth grade. In other words, he was held back and obliged to take that year again. So he must be about 15. I ask him what he thinks of Summit Academy. Is it good or bad?

"Not great but good," he replies.

He was previously at a regular public school. I ask him how his life would be different if he was still there. He mutters one word: "Juvie."

I can't hear him very well, but even if I could I wouldn't understand his reply. The others explain. They say he means that if he had stayed at his previous school, he would now be in "juvie"—juvenile hall or juvenile detention.

That's a big difference to make in someone's life. I ask how this school has managed to do that.

"We spend our whole life here!" he says with undisguised regret.

The hours are from 7:30 a.m. until 4:00 p.m. or 5:00 p.m. And then there is homework.

I ask how he came to be at this school. Whose idea was it?

"My mom made me," he complains.

Obviously, he had not wanted to come. Why not? He says he wanted to go to Winton, a public school in the area.[27] Why didn't he want to go to Summit Academy?

"The uniform . . . " he mutters scornfully.

I suggest that he probably also has friends at Winton. He seems to agree.

Why did his mother make him come to this school? He says his sisters came here and his mother saw their grades improve. So she sent him here, too.

What does he expect his future to be? He says he thinks he will go to college, but he does not sound sure about it. He says that when he finishes school, he will become a missionary. After four years of missionary work, he wants to go to Brigham Young University, the Mormon university in Salt Lake City. And after that?

"A lawyer or athlete."

It is hard to know how the rest of Michael's life will develop but, for the time being—in his own opinion—he is not in juvenile detention because of this school. A life that could have gone disastrously wrong from the start has not done so. If his life were the only one to be transformed by this school, its existence would be fully justified. But there are surely others too.

I am still not convinced I have got to the bottom of why Summit Academy has succeeded in changing Michael's life. I ask the others how things are different here. Mohammed, a burly black boy at the end of the row, went to a public school for only one year, but he is eager to tell me the difference. At public school, he says, there were "no lines, no uniforms." Getting around from class to class was "all your responsibility." That sounds as if it could be a good thing, but perhaps he was never told clearly where he was meant to go.

He says he was not supported in his public school as he is here. Here he can go to a teacher at any time. "If you get a bad grade at the public school, you just get a bad grade. But here they follow up," he says.

A much younger, slim black boy adds that in public schools, the teachers "don't care. They don't pay attention so much to how you are doing."

The themes they seem to keep coming back to are greater discipline and teachers who care.

It is tempting simply to conclude, "Oh yes. That makes sense. Let's have more discipline in schools and teachers who care." But it is not that easy. How do you get such things? If you have a command from government that discipline should be better or teachers must care more, it is unlikely to have much impact. There is reason to believe that really good schools do not come through commands from above. So where can they come from?

Perhaps from a structure that improves the incentives and motivation of those involved. The school I am visiting, the Summit Academy in San Lorenzo, is a charter school, a member of the KIPP network of schools that mainly serves lower-income areas.[28] Charter schools are independent schools that receive money from the government according to how many students they have. There is no guarantee that the Summit Academy or any other charter school will attract students. A charter school has to have something that makes parents think it will be good for their child. The school and the teachers will remain in place only if parents think they are doing good work. This may provide a clue to where the motivation comes from.

Would education be better if there were more such schools with the autonomy and incentives of charter schools? Teachers unions in America and Britain (where such schools are called "free schools") campaign passionately against them. But in Sweden, where there is a far greater proportion of such schools, they are widely accepted. Local governments across the political spectrum go so far as to invite free (charter) schools into their area. Swedish socialists and even communists accept free schools. This suggests that they do not have to be a matter of left versus right tribal politics.

One man who is certainly on the left of the political spectrum is filmmaker Davis Guggenheim. In 2008, he directed a biographical film about Barack Obama for the Democratic National Convention. In September the previous year, Guggenheim was driving his children to school for the beginning of the new academic year. His familiar route took him past three Venice, California, public schools. His children weren't going to any of them. They were driving on to a private school. He was embarrassed about this: "Years earlier, my wife and I had researched our neighborhood public school and discovered it wasn't up to snuff. So we did what other parents who can afford it did. We opened up our wallets and paid lots of money so that our kids could get a great education."[29]

He felt guilty that he could pay to get his children into a good school, but poor people could not. So he made a film about it.[30] The film followed five children—all relatively poor—whose parents were trying to get them into charter schools instead of underperforming public schools. One was named Daisy. She was in the fifth grade and so age 10 or 11. Daisy's dream was to be a doctor. But she was due to enter the local public school, from which 6 out of 10 of the children did not even graduate. Her parents feared that she would have little chance of doing well enough to achieve her dream if she went to this school.

There was only one chance for Daisy to fulfill her dream. Down the street was a very successful charter school that had a good record. The difficulty was that it had 135 applicants for only 10 places. The decision about which children would get in was random. It had to be random by law. Entry was decided by a lottery.

Daisy and her father went to the lottery in person. Names were written on pieces of paper and then pulled out of a plastic box. Father and daughter sat there, serious and nervous. One name was read out after another. There were fewer and fewer chances left. Daisy's father felt that her future depended on the result.

He held his daughter's hand and said, "Daisy, cross your fingers!"

More names were read. Only three places were left, then two, then one, then none. She had not got in. The same happened to four of the five children whose fortunes the documentary followed. The film is painful to watch. Hopes are dashed.

It seems awful that the futures of these children should have depended on lotteries. In one case, the issue was decided literally by balls with numbers dancing in the air. The film evokes a sense of outrage. It brings home how desperately keen these parents, at least, were to get their children away from local public schools and into charter schools. The families had so few choices. (See Box 4.8.)

Some may be thinking, "Well, possibly these particular charter schools may have been good, but what about charter schools generally? Are they better overall or were these just exceptions?" The academic papers on the subject get so complex that, after looking at them a while, you can begin to wish you were studying something simpler like nuclear physics. However, one study was particularly well constructed and had a big sample size. It started at the point where the story of Daisy left off. After lotteries such as hers, obviously some children go to the charter schools and the rest go to

Box 4.8
TRAPPED IN A TERRIBLE SYSTEM

"Public education in the United States is a government monopoly. Don't like your public school? Tough. The school is terrible? Tough," journalist John Stossel declared in *Stupid in America*, a television broadcast that appeared on the ABC network in 2006.

As an example of the waste involved in the monopoly, Stossel presented 18-year-old Dorian Cain, of South Carolina.

Cain "was still struggling to read a single sentence in a first-grade-level book when I met him," Stossel reported. "Although his public school had spent nearly $100,000 on him over 12 years, he still could not read."

"Next to the media in general and television in particular, our schools of education are the greatest contribution to the 'dumbing down' of America. No one wants to know the actual results of these policies—whether they really help poor students. The ed school establishment is more concerned with politics—both academic and ideological—than with learning."

SOURCE: Rita Kramer on U.S. teacher training schools in *Ed School Follies: The Miseducation of America's Teachers* (New York: Free Press, 1991), pp. 211, 213.

---

regular public schools. This study followed both kinds of children in New York City.[31] It was a clever study because we know for sure that the children in both cases had motivated parents keen enough to try to get their children into better schools. So, in terms of the parents, we are comparing like with like.

We know quite a lot about the children in this study. They were poorer than average and more likely to be black or Hispanic. These were children who, on average, would do less well than those from richer neighborhoods.

The study followed all the pupils in New York City who had been successful in lotteries and were enrolled in charter schools between 2001–2 and 2007–8. They were compared with others who had been unsuccessful in the lotteries and went on to normal public schools. The students in both groups did better than average for the areas where they lived, probably because they had motivated parents. But how did the ones that got into charter schools fare compared with those who lost out in the lottery—children like Daisy?

Those who went to charter schools gained an average of 3.6 points in math test scores for each year that they attended compared with those who went to public schools. In English, the gain was 2.4 points per year. For a child who attended throughout, from the third to the eighth grade, the total gain in math was 30 points. In English, the gain was 23 points. This is a substantial difference in relation to a minimum score of 650 points to show proficiency and a relatively good score of 685.[32]

These students from Harlem—disproportionately poor and black—had caught up in math with 86 percent of the typical difference between what they would normally achieve in public schools and the results in Scarsdale, an affluent New York suburb. In English, they had made up 66 percent of the gap. To put it another way, charter schools gave the poor in New York City a far better chance of getting on even terms with the rich. It is an important achievement.

This is an impressive study, comparing like with like. But even in this case, academics are ingenious enough to find ways to cast doubt on the results. I would suggest, however, that the sample is so big and the results so dramatic that the quibbling begins to look like an unwillingness to accept what the evidence is telling us.

In the studies I have come across, of varying quality, two kinds of results are predominant both for Sweden and the United States. Some studies show a significant gain achieved by free/charter schools. Some do not. What is rare—in fact, I do not know of any instance—is a study suggesting that free/charter schools damage educational achievement. The overall evidence is that free/charter schools do good. But in any case, they do no harm.

It is very possible, too, that their recorded performance will improve. When they started, both in Sweden and America, they were set up by all sorts of people, some with good ideas and some, no doubt, with bad ones. But a key aspect of free/charter schools is that no one is forced to go to them. So if a school performs badly, it is likely to lose customers and go out of business. Only successful schools are likely to grow (Box 4.9).

It is also worth remembering that the PISA study found that good performance is correlated with autonomy. Free/charter schools are explicitly designed to have more autonomy.

Before concluding that charter schools are the best way to go, is it possible that there is something even better?

Which schools have the very best results according to the PISA study? The analysis in the 2009 edition divided all schools into three categories: public schools, government-dependent private schools,

Box 4.9
HOW DID SWEDEN COME TO HAVE THE HIGHEST PROPORTION OF FREE SCHOOLS IN THE WORLD?

Many people think of Sweden as the ultimate welfare state. They assume that everything is government controlled and government run. But like most countries, it does not fit into the clichés about it when you get a little closer.

I am in a suburb of Stockholm going into a modern school. I walk through a large space like an open-plan office. No children are here because it is after school hours. At the far end is a smaller office where I meet Odd Eiken. Like many Swedes, he is a modest, uncontentious man. But appearances can be misleading. Eiken, when he was a government minister in 1993, introduced reforms that led to the creation of free (charter) schools in Sweden. His reforms have since led to one of the biggest changes in any nation's schooling for 50 years. Sweden now has the highest proportion of free schools in the world.

I ask him how Sweden, of all countries, came to introduce free schools. Several different things happened to make it possible, he says. Small village schools were being closed down by local governments. Parents in those villages wanted to find a way to keep their schools open. That had some influence. Another factor was that some people went to the European Court of Human Rights and argued that it was their human right to have choice in education and that the choice should include private education. The court did not exactly agree, but it was sympathetic. The opinion was influential because Sweden takes the concept of human rights seriously. A third factor was that, after years of left-wing governments, the electorate had a change of view and voted in a more free-market government.

Eiken also recalls an incident that clearly influenced him personally. When he was a child, his mother wanted him to change schools. She was obliged to go to the local government as a supplicant, begging for a favor. She was told, "No. This is the local school to which Odd has been allocated." I guess, though he does not say so, that he felt embarrassed and angry that his mother had felt obliged to humble herself on his behalf. The experience made him see a totalitarian aspect to the education system as it was.

Odd Eiken's bill allowing free schools was passed. What happened then? At first, nothing much. It seemed a nonevent, he says. Yes, some private schools turned themselves into free schools. Then, gradually, a few religious minorities and schools with particular education theories, like Steiner, established free schools. But this was on a modest scale.

Finally, companies began to get going. New schools were created by people who thought they could introduce better management or teaching methods. They began to create strings of schools, which enabled economies of scale. The company for which Eiken now works, Kunskapsskolan, created a pedagogical research and development department. He says his company now has 33 schools in Sweden and

(continued on next page)

(continued)

is still growing.[a] Private companies have turned out to be the driving force behind the burgeoning number of free schools in Sweden. Free schools currently account for 10 percent of schooling in Sweden, Eiken says, and 25 percent in Stockholm. He believes that, in time, a third of schools in Sweden will be free schools.

One welcome result has been open competition between different educational ideas. Previously, government schools had a somewhat uniform theory of teaching. One company, for example, is consciously imitating private schools in Britain with students at desks facing the teacher and lots of team sports. Kunskapsskolan has particular ideas about school design. It believes in having no corridors to discourage bullying and to use space more efficiently. It develops educational resources centrally for use in all schools. Eiken is especially proud of a presentation on the French Revolution.

With this mushrooming of free schools, power lies with the parents to decide which kind of school will prosper. They are doing that simply by choosing which school to send their children to. The competition is intense.

I ask Eiken whether his company ever fires teachers.

"Oh yes!" he says. He says it is vital to be able to fire principals, especially. Even a day with the wrong person in charge can damage a school. It seems it is easier to fire a teacher in Sweden than in America. So much for preconceptions.

What have been key elements in the growth of Swedish free schools?

1. Commercial companies have been allowed to establish them.
2. Local governments are not allowed to refuse planning permission for new schools except on very limited grounds. So former office buildings and warehouses have been converted into schools.
3. Free schools get exactly the same cash per pupil as regular government schools and cannot charge parents at all. Odd Eiken argues that this point has been a key aspect of their growth. There are disadvantages to this policy but, in political terms, the advantage is that opponents cannot argue that free schools are unfair because they have extra funds.[b]

So is it all plain sailing for Swedish free schools? I suggest to Eiken that, over time, governments might impose more regulations and instructions, undermining the very innovation and independence that the schools offer. He replies that this is already happening. A second danger is that, when free schools become a bigger part of the system, the government may reduce the money paid to them, leading to a slippage in standards or facilities.

---

[a] According to the company website, it has 36 schools in Sweden and its educational program operates in five schools in the United Kingdom, one in New York, and one in India, http://www.kunskapsskolan .com/aboutus.4.52570e4b127643a7eac80001100.html.

[b] There are a number of disadvantages. One is that a school may not be able to afford to offer all that the teachers and the parents would like, including, say, classes in another language or a music teacher or the creation of a language laboratory.

and wholly private schools. Government-dependent private schools consistently performed better than public schools. But wholly private schools scored better still. On average, the reading performance of private schools was 34 points higher than that of the public schools, a major difference.

The best-performing schools in the whole world, according to PISA, were the private schools of Shanghai. They had the best scores in all three subjects that PISA looks at. In math, the Shanghai score was in a different league from the rest of the world: 646 points compared with the next highest score of 579 points for private schools in Korea.[33] The average score for OECD public schools was way down at 492 points.

What about those students who are less able? How good are private schools compared with government schools when it comes to teaching children how to read well? Government schools in Australia leave 19.2 percent of their children functionally illiterate. But in the private schools, only 5.4 percent remain so. (See Table 4.2.)

Table 4.2
RATES OF FUNCTIONAL ILLITERACY BY SCHOOL TYPE IN
ADVANCED COUNTRIES WHERE AT LEAST 5 PERCENT OF
CHILDREN GO TO PRIVATE SCHOOLS

	At government schools (%)	At private schools (%)
Spain	3.5	9.3
Portugal	18.9	7.1
Australia	19.2	5.4
Ireland	23.4	5.4
OECD average	**18.6**	**5.1**
United Kingdom	19.2	4.5
United States	19.0	3.1
South Korea	7.1	1.1

SOURCE: Organisation for Economic Co-operation and Development, taken from a table kindly extracted from PISA 2009 by Miyako Ikeda and emailed to the author.

NOTE: I have omitted Japan because the exceptional circumstances there make the data misleading as an indicator of the quality of private education.[34]

Of course, it can be objected that, in many countries, children who go to private schools have wealthier, better-educated, and more strongly motivated parents, and that this is what boosts performance. This is true for many advanced countries. But it is not true for poorer countries like Indonesia and Tanzania, where public education is rationed and the poor buy private education more than the rich do. The effect of a private school education on some American students is reported in Box 4.10.

Box 4.10
BLACK LIVES TRANSFORMED BY PRIVATE SCHOOLS

In 1997, a U.S. charity offered subsidies to low-income children to go to a participating private school of their choice. There was a lottery to decide which children would receive the subsidies and which would not. Academics followed the fortunes of the children. The table shows how they fared.

Proportion going on to full-time colleges

Control group	26.0%
Those offered vouchers to attend private schools	32.5%

Proportion going on to selective four-year colleges, which tend to be more academic

Control group	3.0%
Those offered vouchers to attend private schools	6.9%

It should be noted that the big effect seen among African-Americans was not replicated among the Hispanics who were also part of the study. The paper offers various thoughts on this finding. One idea is that Hispanic parents get their children into college more frequently than do African-American parents, so the Hispanic parents in this study were less powerfully motivated to use the chance to send their children to private schools to possibly increase their children's chances. Separately, private schools made the biggest difference with regard to getting into selective colleges, an indication of reaching a higher academic standard. The proportion of African-Americans going into selective colleges more than doubled when they were offered private schools. Two researchers, Alan B. Krueger and Pei Zhu, argue that the original study of the initial years of the experiment understated the effects. See Krueger and Zhu, "Another Look at the New York City School Voucher Experiment," *American Behavioral Scientist* 47 (2004): 658–98.

Andrew Coulson's review of 150 studies of the performance of public and private schools around the world found that, overwhelmingly, private schools did better.[35] The findings held even after many of the studies adjusted their results to take account of the social and economic position of the parents. Moreover, in cases in which the private schools were at their most independent and the government-run schools were most controlled, the difference was biggest.

The World Bank produced a series of reports comparing private and government education in various developing countries between 1988 and 1994.[36] Often in these cases, the parents of children at the private schools were poorer than the parents of those at government schools. In any case, the researchers controlled for factors including differences in the wealth and educational background of the parents. The study of schools of Colombia and Tanzania, for example, concluded, "Our results are robust. The estimated private advantage is large and empirically important."[37]

These results tie in with some of the main themes of the PISA study. Private schools automatically have more of the autonomy that PISA suggests is important. They are accountable in the sense that, if they perform badly, they lose customers and go out of business. Everyone involved, but particularly the head of the school, is strongly incentivized to succeed. The head is likely to do whatever he or she can think of to ensure that children are learning effectively. That will almost certainly involve maintaining discipline. Of course, the OECD does not endorse private schooling. That would offend the governments of its member countries and would also go against—I would suggest—the organization's unstated political outlook. But almost despite itself, the research points to private education. (See Box 4.11.)

One further advantage of private education is that, if a new teaching method works badly, private schools have a strong incentive to react quickly. This is in contrast to public schools, where a bad idea—such as the "whole-word" method of teaching children to read—can last for decades before being abandoned.

It seems likely that the best results would come if countries moved all the way to private schooling—not just to charter or free schools. The poor could be given subsidized or free education through charitable schooling such as existed in abundance in late 19th century in Britain and elsewhere. Unfortunately, this is not practical politics in most countries.

Box 4.11
VOTING PRIVATE—WHEN THEY KNOW AND WHEN THEY CAN

More than 20 percent of American public school teachers with school-age children enroll them in private schools—almost twice the 11 percent rate for the general public.[a] A British study found that U.K. parents would do the same, if they could afford it.

"If you could afford it, would you send your child to an independent school?"

Yes	57%
No	25%
Don't know/no opinion	18%

SOURCE: Populus opinion poll (U.K., 2012).

While 57 percent of British parents would like to send their children to private schools, only 7 percent do so. In most cases, this seems likely to be because they cannot afford it.

[a] Mark J. Perry, "Why Do Public School Teachers Send Their Own Children to Private Schools at a Rate 2x the National Average?" Carpe Diem blog, October 9, 2013, quoting Professor Walter E. Williams of George Mason University, http://www.aei.org/publication/why-do-public-school -teachers-send-their-own-children-to-private-schools-at-a-rate-2x-the-national-average.

If that is right, what should be done instead? Should we go for free/charter schools as the next-best option?

Perhaps. But the danger is that, over time, governments may impose more and more regulations and controls over charter schools so that they lose the autonomy that made them good.

The Netherlands introduced voucher schooling in 1917.[38] Government money was given to different kinds of independent schools as well as to government schools according to the numbers of students. But in the following decades, rules were made about what schools should teach, how they should teach, how such schools could be created, and so on. A system that once promised independence and competition saw it eaten away over 90 years. How does the Netherlands now score in the PISA tests? Better than average, but it is not outstanding. This performance is consistent with the idea that some

"It would be fortunate if the best method of teaching were to be universally adopted. But who has it and on what authority? Let us therefore demand freedom of teaching."

Source: Frédéric Bastiat, "Freedom," in *The Collected Works of Frédéric Bastiat, vol. 1: The Man and the Statesman—The Correspondence and Articles on Politics*, tr. Jane and Michel Willems (Indianapolis, IN: Liberty Fund, 2011), http://oll.libertyfund.org/titles/2393#Bastiat_1573-01_2277.

residual benefit remains from the reduced level of autonomy that remains.

Another problem with charter schools is that people are bound to object when money from their taxes is spent on schools that teach something they passionately disagree with. In Britain, some individuals argue that no school that teaches creationism should receive public money, for example.

Because of these problems and others, some suggest that private schooling and parental choice can be promoted most successfully through tax credits or tax allowances.[39] In this system, parents pay private schools out of their own pockets and get tax relief for their payments, up to a specified limit.

But what about parents who cannot afford the fees even with tax relief? They can use money paid into scholarship funds by companies and philanthropic individuals who obtain tax relief for their donations. In America, the growth of tax credit programs has been dramatic. The number of children in such programs has risen from 36,000 in 2000 to over 301,000 in 2014.[40] One advantage is that it removes objections such as "I don't want my taxes to be used for teaching creationism." The money used is always the parents' or that of willing donors.

In some countries, critics would be skeptical that such programs would reach the poor. That is why, in Florida for example, politicians have made a point of getting this kind of tax credit funding to the poor and disabled first.

Yet another possible approach is possible, too. In Australia, government subsidies are paid to private schools. Some readers will be astonished by this and wonder how on earth that is politically possible. The answer is simple: the value of the subsidy is inversely related to the wealth of the parents. The poorer the children's parents, the bigger the subsidy. In this indirect way, poorer children are subsidized to get into private schools. The head of one of the leading private schools told me that more than 15 percent of Australian children go to private schools and nearly 24 percent go to private but government-dependent schools, making a total of 39 percent. This helps explain why the system has survived. Private and semi-independent schools and the parents of children attending them are a serious political constituency. You don't easily get elected by attacking the program.

The system also saves the government money. The head told me that each child at a public school costs the government A$13,600, but a child at a private school costs less than half that. Paradoxically, a majority of rich children do not go to private schools. Of the 100 schools with the highest proportion of rich children, 61 were government schools. Perhaps competition from private schools makes the government schools try harder to attract students. Also, some Australian government schools are highly selective and obtain above-average academic results. So rich parents do all they can to get their children into those, obtaining a good education and saving money at the same time. This is a widespread phenomenon around the world: the rich often get the best state education for their children and the poor get the worst. But at least in Australia, the poor have the possibility of going to private or semi-independent schools instead.

How does Australia do on the PISA tests? It comes seventh of the major non-Asian countries in terms of functional literacy. On overall quality of schooling, it came sixth in the earlier 2009 PISA study. So it does pretty well. In fact, when I asked the head of one of the leading private schools in Australia how the subsidy to private schools had survived despite some left-inclined governments in recent decades, he said that one of the reasons is that private schools keep Australia at the upper end of the PISA rankings, and the politicians know that.

It seems that governments can encourage private or independent education in a surprising number of ways:

- Vouchers for free/charter schools
- Tax credits for parents, perhaps with tax credits for companies and philanthropic individuals to help the poor
- Outright subsidies to private schools with higher subsidies being given to schools with poorer parents

Which is best? Each seems to have its advantage and disadvantages:

- *Charter schools/free schools/vouchers.* Sweden shows that these can gradually expand, but the Netherlands demonstrates that their independence can be eroded over the long term.

121

- *Tax credits*. Schools may retain more independence because parents and companies are spending their own money. But this system has not yet achieved a major presence in any country or state.
- *Direct subsidies to private schools*. They sustain a relatively large amount of private schooling in Australia, but such credits may be difficult to introduce where they do not already exist.

In each case, difficulties seem to arise. One of the biggest problems is that bringing about truly widespread private education, and the attendant benefits, seems to take so long. Is there a way in which fast, radical progress could be made? One way might be to introduce free/charter schools using the model of the privatization that took place in many countries in the 1990s. Governments would simply privatize their schools.

In some countries, such as Britain, opinion polls show that most parents would like to send their children to a private school if they could afford it. So it is possible that a political party could attract support by promising that all parents who wanted to send their child to a private school would be able to do so.

Existing government schools could be offered by tender to cooperatives, churches, education companies, charitable trusts, and associations of teachers or parents. Parents would then be able to apply to send their children to any school. The good would prosper and expand and the bad would go out of business. Where schools failed, the buildings could be offered for tender again. Successful companies and other organizations would soon increase the number of schools under their management. Power would be in the hands of parents, not in the hands of governments.

The process could take place over 5 to 10 years. This process might be much quicker than any other method of spreading the benefit of private education. Any program should try to safeguard the system

---

"Much more valuable than copying existing practices is the development of an educational system that can be depended upon to constantly search out and deliver the best methods over the long term."

SOURCE: Andrew Coulson, *Market Education: The Unknown History* (New Brunswick, NJ: Transaction, 1999).

---

from creeping government control, but frankly it would remain a danger.

Why hurry, some might ask. Why not just let slow growth of free/charter schools take place as in Sweden? Slow development would be better than none. But to accept slow development amounts to telling a child at a low-grade government school that will fail to teach him to read, "Bad luck. You were born too early. If you had been born 15 or 30 years later, you might have gone to a good school." It is not something that those who claim to care about children and their futures should be willing to accept.

This idea would represent a revolution in education and would attract opposition. But it is conceivable that a democracy might accept it because it would give choice and power to people.

I don't know whether something on this scale will ever be attempted. In the meantime, the evidence in this chapter suggests that the following policies could improve standards:

- More private schooling should be encouraged through free/charter schools or tax credits or subsidies to poorer students in private schools.
- Schools should have greater autonomy, combined with accountability through public exams.
- School inspection bodies should be abolished and replaced with advisory bodies from which schools can obtain advice for a fee (as in Finland).
- Government legislation should safeguard the autonomy of free/charter and private schools.
- Private companies, as well as teachers or parents, should be allowed to create charter schools. Otherwise, expansion is too slow.
- Local governments must not be allowed to obstruct the creation of charter schools through planning controls and other such techniques.
- Parents should have a choice of schools so that the schools have to compete to attract them.
- Bad schools should not be helped to survive by forcing parents to send their children to them.
- At 15, 16, or 17, most children should get a job combined with vocational training. Only a minority of students should have purely academic higher education.
- Principals and school heads should be able to fire teachers without difficulty and to hire better ones.

5. "Do I Have 'Stupid' Tattooed on My Forehead?"

Social Housing—Apple Pie with Poison in the Filling

I am sitting in a hired car in the accident and emergency parking area of the Hôpital Nord in Marseilles. It is cloudy and drizzling. The small parking lot is crowded, and I am worried I might get in the way of anyone who arrives with an emergency. But this is where I have been told to come.

Soon, a man comes toward me and gets into the passenger seat. He has the air of someone used to dealing with all sorts of people, good and bad, without emotion. His clothes are informal but businesslike. He is a taxi driver, but he is not going to drive me. He told me on the phone that it would be better not to make this journey in a taxi. It might get stoned. The gangs are suspicious of taxis because they might be used by undercover police.

I have asked him to show me a mixture of public housing projects in Marseilles. The local newspapers are packed with reports about five murders that have taken place in the past two weeks, mostly in or near public housing. In one case, a car was torched with a man inside. He had been shot in the head. The killings have generally been part of turf wars between drug-dealing gangs. Extra police have been sent to Marseilles by the tough-talking minister of the interior, Manuel Valls (who later becomes Prime Minister).[1]

My guide, Yves, is a friend of the brother of someone I know. He says we will start with a project where there was an attempted murder last night. He tells me the victim is in the hospital "in a bad way."

The road winds up a hillside in the outer part of Marseilles, where tourists never go. To one side, some blocks of apartments about 12 stories high stand like tombstones, surrounded by rough land. Few people are out. It is bleak. We climb further and turn up a side road into a public housing complex. We have arrived at the edge of a group of three or four wide blocks of apartments grouped together. I pull into a parking space.

"Shall we get out?" I say. "I would like to walk a bit."

Yves looks reluctant, and I am not sure whether he will get out, too. I open my door anyway. He emerges a little later. I lock the door and start walking up the hillside on the left-hand side of the complex. I look at the block of apartments on my right. Yves seems to be following slowly, lagging behind.

"There are plenty of cars parked here," I remark. "It looks like some of the people here are not in poverty."

He mishears me and replies, "Yes, the people are in poverty."

I start trying to explain what I meant, but nervously he interrupts: "Keep your voice down. They will be listening."

I ask him to walk faster so that we look as if we are going somewhere. But still he hangs behind. He is agitated. I climb further up and then turn around to look down on Marseilles beneath us. It is gray and grim. The bustling center seems far away.

Eventually, I give in to Yves's unspoken urging that we should get back to the car. We walk back and get in. He relaxes, and as we start off, he says, "You see the man at the bus stop in the black hoodie? He is the *chouf.*"

I glance out and see a man hunched over with his hands in his pockets, his face barely visible under his hood. "What is a *chouf*?"

"He is the lookout for the gang that controls the housing development. A *chouf* is there all the time. He tells the gang when anyone comes."

"When who comes?"

"The police or someone who wants to buy drugs."

As we drive on down the highway ramp, I exclaim, "But this development … it was designed by an idiot! There is only one entrance! The gang only has to watch this one road and they can protect themselves against the police. It is like a medieval castle. That would have a single entrance, too. The complex is designed to be a castle for a gang!"

I ask Yves the name of the project.

"Solidarité."

Solidarity! How ironic! French politicians and trade unionists frequently appeal to the ideal of "solidarity." It is a central part of French political thought and tradition. The development we have just visited is subsidized housing for the poor, intended to bring this ideal of solidarity into reality. Instead, it is an isolated, threatening place controlled by a criminal gang: the very opposite of solidarity.

Where next?

We drive for quite a while and I have no idea where we are, but Yves tells me the next complex is called Font Vert. Eventually, I see a sign for it as we turn left at a T-junction, and soon after we are right inside. We drive along a narrow road with a big block of apartments immediately on our left. The ground-floor apartments are slightly raised above ground level, but nearly all are tightly shuttered. Even on the first floor, plenty of the apartments have their shutters closed too. Only at the higher levels are they not being used. I remark on this to Yves.

He says matter-of-factly, "They are like prisoners."

We see a woman and child, and I wonder aloud what it is like for them to live in this environment. Are they scared? Do they get abused? Yves says that sometimes a gang stores its drugs in the apartment of a single mother. The woman might get some cash in payment, but in any case she dare not refuse. I guess the gang stores drugs at her place so that, if the dealers' own apartments are raided by the police, no drugs will be found. If the woman's apartment is raided, she won't risk her life by saying who left them with her.

- "A den of thugs."
- "It looked a bit like a concentration camp"—from a veteran of the A.F.N.
- "Very large housing estate with 10 blocks, several drug dealers associated with the Flemish and the Irish, all armed."

SOURCE: Comments about Font Vert on Wikimapia, April 2013. "A.F.N. is probably a reference to an organization involved in the conflict at the end of France's colonial time in north Africa.[2]

Yves says that a gang can suddenly burst into someone's apartment and start using it to deal drugs or guns. I recall a recent newspaper article saying that Kalashnikov rifles change hands in Marseilles for between €1,000 and €1,500 ($1,100 and $1,600).[3]

The block of apartments we are driving alongside is long. Finally, we get to the end of it, and where the narrow road turns left—at the far side of the corner—is a torched car. It is just a charred skeleton. I am startled to see it quietly sitting there as if this were normal. I remark on it. Yves replies that in some places there are dozens like that. Cars are burned for fun.

We leave by the only exit. There is one way in and out. We have not stopped for a second. We certainly have not gotten out of the car.

We drive on to another development, Les Busserines. Yves tells me we must stop on the street outside. He does not want us to go into this one at all. He points to the nearest ground-floor apartment. The windows are shuttered and all possible entrances—all the windows and the front door—are protected with heavy-duty metal bars. It is like a fortress.

We drive on to another development, Marine Bleue. It is, appropriately, painted blue in parts. It sits on a hill and many of its apartments must have fine views. Again, it has one entrance and exit. We drive straight through without stopping.

Finally, we reach La Castellane or, as Yves pronounces it in his Marseilles accent, "La Castellang." It is the most famous estate (public housing development) in Marseilles because Zinédine Zidane was brought up there. Zidane, the son of Algerian immigrants, was arguably the best soccer player of his generation and a French hero. He won the World Cup with France in 1998. He was named World Player of the Year three times. He also famously head-butted another player when playing in the 2006 World Cup final. He was sent out, and the head butt possibly cost France the match. Zidane said his opponent had repeatedly insulted his mother and his sister.

Intriguingly, Zidane feels a strong loyalty to the housing project where he grew up. He once said, "I am still proud to be who I am: first a Kabyle [an ethnic group in Algeria] from La Castellane." La Castellane is mentioned before his identity as a Frenchman.

The development is a huge group of buildings rising up on a hill, a phalanx of tall blocks. The road going up past it is wide and busy. We stop on the far side and look across. Yves tells me that there is, again, one entrance and one exit. He will not go into the complex. He says that if a gang blocked the road, we would be trapped. Once again, he points out the *chouf* standing at the bus stop very close to us. As usual, he is wearing a hoodie.

He tells me a *chouf* is paid €150 ($165) for a shift from 8 a.m. to 1 p.m. "It is much more profitable than going to school and getting a job. They are better off than being a manager. They have Rolex watches, Boss, Prada …"

128

Yves sounds as though he shares their values, which identify these brand names as powerful symbols of success.

I ask if he agrees to pick people up from the projects.

"Rarely," he replies.

Has he had a bad experience?

"Not myself. But I have friends whose cars have been stolen or burned."

I drive us back to our original meeting place at Hôpital Nord. I pay Yves for his time and he gets out. Then I drive to the center of town.

It is drizzling and overcast. I walk to the Old Port, the tourist part of Marseilles with many restaurants surrounding the harbor. They are all full, so I walk away from the port and eventually find an Indian restaurant in which I can have lunch. I write up my notes as I wait for my order to come. Only as I am writing do I realize that during our tour of five housing projects, and after all the talk in the newspapers of a tough security clampdown, I did not see a single police officer.

Of course, not all the public housing in France is as grim as the complexes I saw in Marseilles. Only half an hour away, in Aix-en-Provence, I walked through some reasonably pleasant ones without much trepidation. And some of the public housing in France is positively luxurious, as we will see.

But the variations in quality should not distract us from the fact that in France and around the world, public housing—or, as it is also known, social housing—has been riddled with problems. This is rarely discussed or admitted. The problems include gangs in frightening complexes but go far beyond that, too. Housing is of key importance yet barely noticed or debated. Many people think of social housing as an obviously good thing like apple pie. But it has poison in the filling. And the nine core problems are these:

1. Public housing often contributes to unemployment.

For decades, less well-off people in Britain have received housing benefits, money to help pay their rent. This sounds considerate and reasonable. But if these individuals have been unemployed and then take a job, 65 percent of what they earn disappears in reduced housing benefits. In addition, they lose other benefits, such as tax credits and council (local) tax benefits. As the left-leaning Joseph Rowntree Foundation put it in 2013, "they can face an effective taper rate of 96 percent [in reduced benefits and tax] and be left with four pence from every additional pound of gross earnings" (about 4 cents to the dollar).[4] Someone earning £7 an hour would have to work for 14 hours to be £4 better off. Of course, nobody would work for 14 hours to earn £4. It has been an extraordinary discouragement to extra work.

Then there is the discouragement to working at all. In 2006, the Institute of Fiscal Studies calculated that 3.6 million people who were working would lose less than 30 percent of their net income if they lived on welfare benefits instead. Of those, 1.9 million would be less than 20 percent worse off on benefits.[5] (See Box 5.1.)

Proportion of public housing units in Britain held by someone in full-time work: 23 percent.

Source: "Estate of Mind: Social Housing Is Quietly Making a Comeback," *The Economist*, April 27, 2013.

Under the circumstances, it is remarkable that so many were working at all. What those figures could not show was how many people had decided it was not worth working for such a small financial gain. As the research by Kathryn Edin showed (see Chapter 1), a very large proportion of such people will have other, undeclared income. The problem has gradually gotten worse. The rise in rents between 1979 and 2006, for example, resulted in higher levels of housing benefits and therefore increased the disincentive to work. As a result, housing benefits in Britain have been a major contributor to high unemployment (see Box 5.1).

Something similar, though less extreme, has taken place in the United States. Rent in public housing depends on individual circumstances but usually is 30 percent of income after various adjustments. If someone takes a job, the rent automatically goes up. He or she also has to pay social security payments of 7.5 percent and may lose entitlement to Medicaid and food stamps. There will be income tax, too. Again, public housing has reduced the incentive to work and has added to unemployment.

Some people might be tempted to think, "Well, this one is easy! Just lower the rate at which the rent subsidy is reduced. If someone gets a job, reduce the rent subsidy by only, say, 20 percent. Then people will keep more of their income from working and still have plenty of incentive to work. Problem solved!"

Box 5.1
THE UNEMPLOYMENT TRAP

Rebecca Tunstall, a professor of housing policy at the University of York, wrote in the *New Statesman* magazine about the results of a study she and colleagues completed for the Joseph Rowntree Foundation in Great Britain: "Like many other benefits, and in combination with them, housing benefit creates an unemployment trap."[a] Table B5.1 demonstrates the consequences.

TABLE B5.1
SOCIAL HOUSING AND UNEMPLOYMENT

People with no qualifications *not* in social housing who are unemployed	43 percent
People with no qualifications in social housing who are unemployed	70 percent
Single parents *not* in social housing who are unemployed	35 percent
Single parents in social housing who are unemployed	64 percent

SOURCE: John Hills, "Ends and Means: The Future Roles of Social Housing in England," Economic and Social Research Council Center for Analysis of Social Exclusion, CASE report 34, February 2007, pp. 101 and 102, http://sticerd.lse.ac.uk/dps/case/cr/CASEreport34.pdf.
NOTE: Hills further observed, "The proportion of social tenant householders in paid employment fell from 47 percent to 32 percent between 1981 and 2006" (p. 2).

---

[a] Rebecca Tunstall, "How Housing Traps People in Unemployment," *New Statesman*, March 8, 2013, http://www.newstatesman.com/business/2013/03/how-housing-traps -people-unemployment.

Unfortunately, it is not that easy. If the subsidy reduction were made more gradual, large numbers of extra people would become entitled to it, and so they too would have a reduced incentive to work. The cost of the whole system would jump, too, at least in the short term.[6] This is a difficult knot to unravel. That is why it has been put to one side for so long.

Does this problem apply to all countries with public housing? No. At least, not as severely as in Britain.[7]

How do other countries avoid the problem? In some, housing benefits, or rents, as the case may be, are not adjusted according to income. It's as simple as that. It might sound extremely tough. It means that those who lose their jobs and are hard up must continue to pay full rents and if they can't afford them, they can lose their homes. What countries would be so hard? What countries would treat their people in way that seems so un-welfare-state-like?

One of them is Sweden. If you lose your job in Sweden, you are entitled to generous unemployment benefits as a result of the insurance contributions you have paid while working. You will be able to continue paying your rent. But when the insurance money runs out, you will have to use your savings. If you reach the point at which you can no longer afford the rent, you are likely to lose your home and have to move to something much more modest.

Social housing is different in Sweden. You do not get it on the basis of need. You get it only if you reach the top of a waiting list and can afford the rent.[8] So people in social housing in Sweden are in utterly different circumstances from those in Britain or America. The Swedish model is not unique. According to the Organisation for Economic Co-operation and Development (OECD), the Netherlands, Denmark, and Luxembourg also have "broad-based" allocation of social housing, which means it is aimed at a wide range of people, not just the poor.[9] These countries probably avoid some of the worst unintended consequences of social housing. The crucial point is that, insofar as rents or housing benefits are not adjusted for income, they do not discourage work.

One might ask, "What, then, is the purpose of social housing in these countries? If it provides housing to a broad mix of the population, why should some minority part of the broad mix be in government-subsidized housing while the rest is not? If it confers an advantage on those in social housing, is that not unfair to the others? If it confers no advantage, what is the purpose?"

Frankly it is hard to see one.

There are further problems caused by public housing.

2. Public housing can contribute to the incidence of single parenting.

Why does Sweden have a lower incidence of single parenting than do Britain and the United States? Sweden, after all, is well known for a culture in which the independence of women is celebrated. It is meant to be a land of free living and loving. In Britain, a two-parent family is still held up as the ideal, and America is still quite a Christian country. There is probably no simple answer to this question, but the following story points to one possible factor.

The Pruitt-Igoe Myth was a television documentary that argued that the well-known failure of the Pruitt-Igoe housing project did not mean that all public housing was a bad idea. But in the course of this documentary that favored public housing, former residents of Pruitt-Igoe, in Saint Louis, Missouri, were filmed speaking about fathers who left their families so that the mother and children could qualify for public housing.[10] They also spoke of children denying to officials that their father was living with them. It is a grotesque thought that fathers would leave their families or that children would deny the presence of a father, but the situation can arise because the cost and allocation of public housing in America, as in Britain, is adjusted according to the needs of the tenants.

When housing is allocated on the basis of need, preference tends to be given to single, unemployed parents because they have dependent children. If the rent, or housing benefit, is adjusted according to means and need, then a single unemployed mother will be granted a lower net housing cost than a couple with one working adult is granted. In this way, public housing can make single parenting a more attractive option than it would otherwise be. It can penalize couples.

I have not seen an academic study attempting to measure the impact of public housing allocation on single parenting. But the proportion of single parents in social housing is certainly much higher than in the general population in America and in other countries with similar systems. In Britain, nearly half of all single parents live in social housing whereas only 1/10th of couples do.[11] The logic of the incentives in these countries is that public housing has the potential to increase the incidence of single parenting. But not in Sweden or at least to a far lower extent.[12]

It seems possible, at least, that the difference in the way that public housing is allocated and charged might help explain why Britain and America have more single parenting than Sweden does. Britain and America are, respectively, the European and world capitals of single parenting (see Chapter 6).

3. Public housing creates concentrations of crime and fear.

I saw during my journey around Marseilles how crime can establish itself in public housing. Cabrini Green, in Chicago, is another example of this. It once housed more than 15,000 people. It was described in *USA Today* as "a virtual war zone, the kind of place where little boys were gunned down on their way to school and little girls were sexually assaulted and left for dead in stairwells."[13]

But projects do not have to be gigantic to become crime centers. Dunbar Village in West Palm Beach, Florida, consists of only 226 units. In 2007, a teenager knocked on the door of a young single mother and told her that her car had a flat tire. Nine more teenagers suddenly barged into her apartment, brandishing guns and demanding money. They proceeded to rape and sodomize her multiple times. They beat up her 12-year-old son in the room next door.[14] The details of the story are horrific and do not need to be described here because what really brings home the nature of the complex at that time are the comments made by other residents in the wake of these horrible crimes.

Citoya Greenwood, who lived there with her four-year-old daughter, said, "I try to be in my house no later than seven, and I don't come out. I don't even answer my door anymore." On the Fourth of July, "we didn't know if we was hearing gunshots or fireworks," she told a reporter. Patriciea Matlock said, "So a lady was raped. Big deal. There's too much other crime happening here."[15]

The two teenagers who were charged with committing the crimes were said to be "mostly fatherless, bouncing between homes." The mother of one of them said that she herself was raped twice, at the ages of 7 and 12.

In the year leading up to the multiple rapes of the single mother, police were called 717 times—almost twice a day—to Dunbar Village. Whenever overhead lighting was put in, it was immediately destroyed by gunfire. City officials were considering putting in bulletproof lighting. "Isn't that quite a commentary on what the situation is there?" remarked Molly Douglas, a city commissioner. "I just bow my head sometimes and think we just couldn't possibly have enough officers to take care of all of this."[16]

"Public housing has a long record of looking attractive at the time of the ribbon cutting and then going quickly downhill."

Source: Howard Husock, "Public Housing Developments Bring Hope but History Says Projects Call for Caution," Manhattan Institute for Policy Research website, February 15, 2004, http://www.manhattan-institute.org/html/miarticle.htm?id=4374#.VHRstNKsX9U.

This degree of lawlessness is hard to imagine for those of us living well away from such places. Back in Marseilles, they would understand. A magistrate there remarked, "We have some gang members who refuse to leave prison because they fear being shot as they go out." Interior Minister Manuel Valls referred to "about 40" housing complexes in Marseilles as "sensitive"—a euphemistic expression used in France to mean "dangerous."[17] "It is a war between the law of the state and barbarity," he said. The Marseilles criminal trade in cannabis is concentrated in the public housing projects. A ton of cannabis was seized by police in less than three months at the beginning of 2013, along with 20 rifles, including 10 Kalashnikovs.

Such anecdotal evidence is supported by the statistics. The risk of burglary in public housing in Britain is more than twice as high as in owner-occupied housing: 4.2 percent compared with 1.7 percent, according to official figures.[18] But even this is almost certainly a major understatement. Much of the crime is simply not recorded.

A reporter for the left-leaning *Observer* newspaper went to the Clyde Court complex in Leeds and asked a woman whether she had tried to have an antisocial behavior order (ASBO)—a court injunction against bad behavior—placed on the local gangs who were making her life a nightmare.

"Do I have 'stupid' tattooed on my forehead?" she replied. "The only way to make an ASBO stick is to give evidence in court and if you do that, your life won't be worth living."[19]

"In the areas originally built as flatted council estates [apartment complexes] . . . 18 percent feel unsafe alone even at home or outside in daylight."

SOURCE: John Hills, "Ends and Means: The Future Roles of Social Housing in England," Centre for Analysis of Social Exclusion report 34, Economic and Social Research Council, Swindon, U.K., February 2007, p. 4, http://sticerd.lse.ac.uk/dps/case/cr/CASEreport34.pdf.

Why do so many public housing projects have higher crime levels than elsewhere? It may be partly because of the first two problems of public housing: high levels of unemployment and of single parenting. Both tend to lead to higher levels of crime (see Chapter 7). Then there are the common areas that nobody owns that are typical in such complexes. No one has a strong incentive to protect these areas and keep them in good condition. The burned-out car I saw in Font Vert was just left lying there. If it had been on property that someone owned, it would surely have been removed as quickly as possible. Public housing is, of course, owned by someone, often the local government. But local governments tend not to deal with such problems with the urgency of private owners.

Pretty much everyone now thinks that building massive public housing blocks was a mistake that has contributed to the crime problem. And having only one through road, as in the estates I visited in Marseilles, seems like a terrible blunder. It is hard to know what weight should be given to the different possible causes of crime in public housing. But it is certain that crime is much higher than elsewhere and that many residents live in fear as a result.

4. A huge amount of money spent on public housing is completely wasted.

A significant portion of public housing deteriorates to the point at which it has to be destroyed. In other words, it turns out to be a total waste of time and money.

We have already referred to the failure of the Pruitt-Igoe project in Saint Louis. It was designed by a highly prestigious architect, Minoru Yamaseki, to house 85,000 families. It was built in 1954–56, but it deteriorated until it was 25 percent vacant. It was demolished after just 20 years. The big Cabrini Green project in Chicago, also mentioned earlier, was built in stages between 1942 and 1962. It was closed in 2010.

So many projects have deteriorated badly that it has become U.S. government policy to fund the destruction of some complexes and replace them with new ones. The program is called, without irony, "Hope VI." Before 1995, the units that were demolished had to be replaced one-for-one with new units. But there was not enough money to build the replacements, so the rule "effectively prevented demolition even of very deteriorated developments."[20] Eventually, the rules were relaxed, with the result that 200,000 public housing units were torn down between 1995 and 2008. The number of public housing units dropped from 1.33 million to 1.16 million.

In Britain, a website called Wikia has a list of 64 council housing estates that have been demolished.[21] The source is not official and is probably incomplete, but I cite it because I am unaware of any full, authoritative list. A typical site on the Wikia list is Lee Bank, in Birmingham. This complex was built in the 1960s and was officially opened by Queen Elizabeth. Most of it was demolished in stages between 2000 and 2007. One building on the estate, Charlecote Tower, was destroyed in a controlled explosion in 2000.

In France, construction of the Cité des 4,000 near Paris—so named because the vast project was intended to have 4,000 units—began in 1956.[22] The complex took more than 10 years to build and began to go wrong in the familiar ways that involve crime and physical deterioration. After a child was shot dead there in 1983, President François Mitterrand visited there.[23] Problems continued. After the death by gunfire of an 11-year-old, the complex was also visited by Nicolas Sarkozy, then a tough-talking minister of the interior and later president.

But visits by presidents and ministers did not arrest its decline. The Debussy block was demolished in 1986, the Renoir in 2000, the Ravel and Présov blocks in 2004, the Balzac in 2010, and the "little" Debussy in 2012. There is a poignant contrast between the way these blocks were named after French cultural icons of art, literature, and music and the grim reality of crime and violence that took place in them.

In Béziers, the Capendeguy estate was blown up spectacularly on January 27, 2007. The event has been uploaded a number of times to YouTube, so you can see for yourself the scale of the destruction.[24] It was built 35 years before, in 1972.[25]

The waste that has taken place in public housing has been on a massive scale. I have mentioned only a few examples. As far as I know, nobody has written a full account of all the destruction.

People were taxed to pay for these massive projects. But instead of providing decent accommodation for the poor, as intended, they made life miserable and dangerous for the residents and ultimately had to be destroyed. In some cases, deterioration began within five years of construction.

5. Allocation of public housing can lead to corruption.

In February 2005, it emerged that the French minister of finance, Hervé Gaymard, his wife, and their eight children were living at a prime location not far from the Champs-Elysées at the expense of taxpayers.[26] Gaymard protested that he came from a humble background. He said he was "the son of a shoemaker. . . . I do not have money." He claimed that he needed the apartment. But then it was revealed that he already owned an apartment in Paris, albeit one that was not as big. It was rented out, bringing him money while he had free, luxurious accommodations that he had not declared. He had done nothing illegal, but he had to resign. It then emerged that the budget minister, too, enjoyed an apartment paid for by the government and similarly owned an apartment in Paris that was rented out.

This sort of thing has been a recurring theme in France. Previously, President Jacques Chirac's government was involved in scandals, some involving "the abuse of state-paid apartments."[27] And before that, President Mitterrand's administration was also accused of corruption. As a BBC reporter put it after the Gaymard affair, "the disastrous impression has been reinforced of a self-serving caste of leaders who follow their own moral codes, cut off from the concerns of mere citizens."[28] (See Box 5.2.)

Box 5.2
WHILE RESIDENTS OF FRENCH PUBLIC HOUSING OFTEN LIVE IN HORRIBLE CIRCUMSTANCES, THE ADMINISTRATORS WORK IN LUXURY

In Paris, I meet a specialist in housing, Nicolas Lecaussin, director of development at the Institute of Economic and Fiscal Research. We meet at a café not far from the Arc de Triomphe. He suggests that I might find it interesting to see the office of the national government agency responsible for public and subsidized housing. I don't have to walk far. After our meeting, I walk around the Arc de Triomphe and find Rue Lord Byron, a stone's throw from the Champs-Elysées. It is a narrow street that bends as it goes downhill.

The buildings are elegant—probably constructed in the 19th century. One is particularly wide and reaches up six or seven stories. It has a highly polished brass plaque outside with the words "Union nationale des fédérations d'organismes d'H.L.M." These are the offices of HLM, which stands for *habitations à loyer modéré* ("housing at moderate rent"). Another brass plaque identifies five other organizations, four of which also have HLM in their names.

The role of HLM is to provide housing for the poor. Much of this housing is in the suburbs in drab blocks. But the officials responsible for them are located in one of the fanciest, most expensive parts of Paris and, indeed, the world. The entrance has a decorated metal canopy like a luxury hotel. I step back to look at the building and notice an old sign in the stonework: "Hotel Lord Byron." So the offices were indeed formerly a smart hotel. This does not count as corruption using a narrow definition. But I personally find it sickening.

The corrupt allocation of housing does not happen only at a high level. In November 2012, a regional newspaper reported that "several dozen families have been victims of a huge swindle." They had paid between €1,000 and €1,500 ($1,100 and $1,650) in cash bribes to obtain social housing in Montpellier. The families had then discovered that some of the apartments in question were already occupied. They had been duped. They were victims of a crime but, of course, they were also breaking the law themselves by paying bribes. The total number of people who were tricked will never be known because, as the local newspaper commented, "in admitting it, they confess, de facto, their complicity in corruption." The fact that "dozens" were involved gives us a hint of how commonplace this is.

Also, in the comments made about this story online, no one expressed skepticism about it. On the contrary, everyone concurred that bribery in public housing allocation was widespread. One commented, "I know . . . people who have obtained social housing—a maisonette with a garden—they lived as a couple with nearly €4,000 [per month, presumably, about $4,380] income but with well-placed relations [named individual], the town council and the municipal police, they became entitled to it in less than a month and they are still there. They pay €350 [$380 per month] rent, they have social housing and they go to Cuba each year, never failing to have a week's skiing at Serre Chevalier, and have two Touaregs [a large, luxurious 4x4] parked outside."

The same person claimed to know three other similar cases, all of them among his or her acquaintances and all involving "pulling strings." Another wrote, "There are hundreds and hundreds who have gotten their homes by pulling strings."

I found general acceptance in France that allocation of public housing is often corrupt. No one is surprised if the friends or mistress of a mayor are allocated particularly desirable apartments. The idea that subsidized housing is there to help the less well off certainly exists in France, but it is abused. It has even been claimed that more affluent families rent public housing than rent private housing.[29]

Does this kind of thing happen only in France?

I am now in a taxi in Manhattan being driven to Harlem. The driver is a middle-aged, Hispanic man of ample proportions. He says he has lived in Harlem and the north West Side for 47 years. He remarks that I won't be able to get a taxi from Harlem back to my hotel. Cabs looking for fares don't go there. I ask what the apartments are like in the Ulysses Grant project, which I am intending to visit. He says that they are good. In fact, you could wait a long time to get in there. It would certainly be 3 or 4 years and could even be 9 or 10 . . . unless, that is, you pay someone under the table.

I had not expected to hear of people paying bribes to get into Harlem. He explains that Harlem used to be "bad"—meaning violent and dangerous—in the 1980s, but now it is better. It is far from being fancy, but it is nevertheless in Manhattan and not too far from better areas.

"How much would someone need to pay to jump the waiting list?" I ask.

"Oh . . . $6,000, $7,000," he replies.

Later on during my stay in Manhattan, I ask another taxi driver if he has heard of this sort of thing. He is black and in his 40s, and he says he lives in Newark, New Jersey, 8 miles west of Manhattan.

"Oh yes!" he says. It turns out that he knows plenty about it and can explain the economics of it. An apartment in the Ulysses Grant project might cost $800–$1,000 a month. But it is in a relatively desirable area. An apartment across the road from the project and rented privately would cost $1,600 a month—up to twice as much. So you can save $7,000 or more a year by getting into Ulysses Grant. I ask him what you would have to bribe someone to jump the waiting list. Would it be the $6,000–$7,000 mentioned by the other taxi driver? He thinks that is too much. He suggests a month's pay—perhaps about $3,000.

He adds that one person has been arrested for paying money like this "because it is against the law." You don't say! It is also not exactly what the creators of public housing had in mind.

Of course, the word of two anonymous taxi drivers is not exactly proof perfect. But I have no reason to disbelieve them. It is also worth mentioning that this kind of crime is hard to detect and prove. Both parties to the crime want to keep it secret, as we saw in France. Both have broken the law. But proof does emerge occasionally, as it did in the case mentioned by the taxi driver and again in another country thousands of miles away.

Douglas Norris, a senior client services officer in the housing department of New South Wales, Australia, was a white, middle-aged man, balding from the front of his head. He had a moustache and a tiny beard under his lower lip. The department had 40,000 people on its waiting list.[30] With so many in the queue, priority was given to those in urgent need or over 80 years old. In 2003, Norris was approached by Bruce Murray, a tenant on the property for which he had responsibility. Murray wanted to move from his studio to a one-bedroom apartment.

Norris replied that it could take years to get to the front of the queue. He then allegedly added words to the effect that "you scratch my back and I'll scratch yours." He asked for a payment of A\$500 and promised that, in return, Murray could have a one-bedroom apartment in only two weeks. That is how Norris's little bribery business began.

The Independent Commission Against Corruption subsequently identified seven individuals who had jumped the list by paying Norris.[31] The details of the story show how difficult it is to get hard evidence of corruption of this sort. Obviously, neither the person who gives the bribe nor the one who receives it will report it to the police, and the payment is likely to be in cash. Norris would have gotten away with the scheme indefinitely if not for an informer. Even with an informer, it took an expensive police operation to obtain adequate evidence. So it is impossible to know how widespread this kind of corruption is. We can be fairly confident it happens in France, the United States, and Australia at least.

6. Some social housing subsidizes the rich.

Frank Dobson is a bluff, cheerful member of the British Parliament. He draws a salary of £67,060 (about \$95,000)[32]—more than twice average full-time earnings—plus expenses, and he is automatically a member of the favorable pension program provided to members of parliament.[33] He has had a fairly successful political career, including serving as secretary of state for health from 1997 to 1999. At that time he had a salary of over £72,000 (about \$102,000)—more than three times average earnings at the time—and enjoyed the perks of the office, such as a chauffeur-driven car.

Where would you expect such a well-paid, successful man to live? He actually lives in social housing, in a three-bedroom apartment in a smart mansion block in central London at subsidized rent.[34] We know it is subsidized because he has said that he could not afford to rent privately. "Market rents in our area are phenomenal," he said.

Dobson is getting a subsidy from taxpayers. People who earn less than he is are helping to pay his housing costs. Is this what "social housing" is for?

Bob Crow, leader of a trade union, reportedly had pay and perks worth £140,000 (about \$198,000) in 2011—six times average income.[35] He was living in public housing in London at an estimated rent of

£150 a week ($212)—a small fraction of the open market rent.[36] The subsidy to him from poorer people was even more grotesque.

Are these isolated examples? No. In October 2011, there were 15,000 people in Britain living in social housing despite having earnings of more than £80,000 ($113,000), according to a government report leaked to the *Daily Mail*.[37] Almost a fifth of households in public housing—some 720,000—earn more than the national average wage, according to the report.[38]

Similar stories can be told in France and elsewhere. Where the rent for public housing is not subsidized, it is no scandal that the rich should live there. But where ordinary taxpayers are subsidizing the rich, social housing has become an insult to its original purpose.

7. Social housing can reduce mobility.

Most tenants of social or public housing have obtained their homes only after years of waiting. So they are reluctant to give up the accommodation and the subsidy that is part and parcel of it. They are discouraged from moving to where they might be able to get a job or, perhaps, a better job. They may be discouraged from moving to be near an elderly parent who needs their help.

In New York City, the average tenancy in public housing is 20 years.[39] The turnover of tenancies in London social housing is a mere 3.5 percent a year.[40] These are measures of how public housing can reduce the ability of people to move where it might suit them, damaging their personal freedom, their well-being, and the economy generally.

8. Long waiting lists for public housing cause unfairness: some get it; some don't.

In San Francisco, I did a little tour of some of the housing complexes. Some blocks were boring but otherwise not too bad. One was in a prime area, a development called North Beach Place at the end of the picturesque cable car line that approaches Fisherman's Wharf. These blocks were in good condition, although it may have helped that they were relatively new.

I looked at the San Francisco public housing website to learn more about public housing in the city. The latest developments and refurbishments looked attractive. One could easily get the impression that here, at least, public housing is working.

Still browsing the website, I came to a page with details of the percentage of housing reserved for people in various low-income bands. Below that was a question: "How long is the Public Housing waitlist?"

The answer was this: "The Waiting List is currently CLOSED."

"Waiting lists for social housing are increasing. . . . In England, for instance, housing waiting lists increased . . . to over 1.8 million households in 2011 (an increase of 76 percent since 2000). In France, 1.2 million applicants are registered on waiting lists for social housing and 630,000 in Italy."

SOURCE: Alice Pittini, "Housing Affordability in the EU: Current Situation and Recent Trends," CECODHAS European Social Housing Observatory Research Briefing, year 5, no. 1, Housing Europe Centre, Brussels, Belgium, 2012, p. 8, http://www.iut.nu/Literature/2012/CECODHAS _HousingAffordability2012.pdf.

"Most agencies have long waiting lists for public housing and some no longer accept new applications because of the size of the backlog."

SOURCE: "USA Policy Basics: Introduction to Public Housing," Center on Budget and Policy Priorities website, http://www.cbpp.org/cms/index.cfm?fa=view&id=2528.

Long waiting lists are normal for public housing around the world. Even if public housing were otherwise a successful idea, the problem would remain that many people have to wait many years to get it. And in some cases, such as San Francisco, you cannot even get on the waiting list. It is worth considering why the waiting lists are so long or even closed. Here is one reason:

9. The cost of public housing has risen far beyond what those who created it expected.

When social housing in Britain was given a major push following the Second World War, it was thought that it could be an economical way of building homes. The financial credibility of the government would enable public housing to be built cheaply. The government could borrow at a lower interest rate than individuals could. And after the cost of construction, further costs would be zero because rent would cover the maintenance bills. Indeed, that is more or less how it turned out . . . for a while.[41]

Then three rising costs spoiled the picture. First, many estates (housing projects including amenities such as schools and shops) became riddled with crime and degraded, so the cost of maintaining them rose. Next, people refused to live in these blocks so no rent came in at all. Finally, for several decades inflation was high, and it was politically difficult to raise the rents in line with rising prices. Rents were increased to some extent, but the housing benefit was used to help those who were short of money.

This was a financial time bomb. More and more people were discouraged from working because, if they took a job, they lost their housing benefit. So the number of people receiving housing benefits soared, and the cost rocketed from £400 million ($567 million) in 1980–81 to £12.6 billion ($17.9 billion) in 2003–2004.[42] Social housing that was meant to be self-financing after the initial building cost became a financial disaster. Similar events took place elsewhere in Europe and in Australia, New Zealand, and the United States.

The Public Housing Capital Fund in the United States, which handles money for building and renewing public housing, spent $2.5 billion in 2010, and the operating fund spent nearly twice as much.[43] And these sums were a fraction of the cost of housing vouchers: just under $18 billion. The total federal budget appears to have amounted to $45 billion.[44] But considerable state expenditure must be added to that to arrive at the real annual cost.

An overhang of capital spending also needs to be carried out but has not been yet. The Center on Budget and Policy Priorities, a left-of-center organization in favor of public housing, has calculated that the cost of paying for "unmet needs" in public housing for capital repairs and improvements would be $22 billion.[45] But the center adds that some developments may require more substantial work: "If, for example, 100,000 units were replaced rather than renovated, estimated capital needs would rise from $22 billion to $32 billion." It is a big sum considering that public housing is relatively small in the United States compared with other countries. What is the total cost of public housing in France? I am told that even those who specialize in the subject find the financing impossibly obscure and cannot estimate the total cost. Quite possibly, no one knows. But the sum is likely to be enormous.

***

I have listed a daunting number of problems that tend to arise with social housing. Have any countries managed to avoid them?

It looks as though the best—or perhaps least bad—outcomes have been in countries such as Sweden where public housing has continued to be for everyone and has not been used as a means-tested method of helping the poor. Even so, Sweden has suffered from problems 6, 7, and 8 on the preceding list. And now the European Union appears to be pressing Sweden and others to give up this model and switch toward the means-tested approach that has been such a spectacular failure in Britain and the United States. At a meeting in November 2012, an EU representative faced complaints and criticism from the Netherlands, France, Austria, and Sweden for demanding that public housing should be for only those with low incomes.[46]

In any case, the manifold problems of public housing have led to a significant decline in this aspect of most welfare states. In Britain, the proportion of people living in public housing fell from 31 percent in 1979 to 17 percent in 2012.[47] In the United States, the number of public housing units fell 10 percent in the 12 years from 1995.[48] In Australia, between 2004 and 2010, the proportion of social housing also declined even though the quantity remained more or less constant, because the total amount of housing of all kinds continued its long-term, rapid increase.[49] Germany saw a dramatic fall in social renting as a proportion of all rented property, from 26 percent to 11 percent between 1987 and 2001.[50]

Many tactics have been used to try to save public housing. But there is reason to doubt that any is satisfactory (see Box 5.3).

Whatever ingenious schemes are devised, some problems do not or even cannot go away. In the end, there are only three approaches to public housing, and all of them lead to a dead end:

1. If the *rents* are subsidized, there are sure to be waiting lists, and this will be unfair to those who are excluded. The excluded people will also be paying through their taxes for the subsidies enjoyed by others, adding to the injustice.
2. If the *people* are subsidized by being means tested or needs tested to determine how much help they should receive with the cost of their rent, the financial incentive to work will be reduced, leading to higher unemployment. This will reduce the long-term ability of the poor to get out of poverty.

Box 5.3
POLICIES THAT HAVE BEEN TRIED TO IMPROVE
HOUSING FOR THE POOR

Rent control. This was introduced in Britain as a temporary wartime measure in 1915. It continued until 1980–89, when it was progressively ended.[a] To prevent landlords from evading the controls by evicting tenants, tenants were given long-term security of tenure. The result was that owning property to rent became a terrible investment. Properties ceased to be properly maintained, and the supply of privately rented accommodations available to the poor declined. It was a disastrous policy (Figure B5.3).

FIGURE B5.3
DWELLING STOCK OF PRIVATELY RENTED HOMES IN THE UNITED KINGDOM DURING THE
PERIOD OF RENT CONTROLS (THOUSANDS)

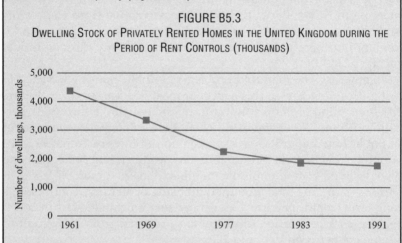

SOURCE: U.K. Office for National Statistics, "Dwelling Stock by Tenure," www.communities
.gov.uk/documents/housing/xls/table-104.xls.
NOTE: Immediately after rent controls were lifted and landlords were permitted to charge market rents and had the secure ability to evict tenants at the end of tenancies, the supply radically increased. The numbers rose to 2,086 in 1999, 3,182 in 2007, and 4,286 in 2012.

Low-rise social housing in mixed areas instead of massive blocks. This kind of housing may well be less prone to crime and degradation. However, pleasant housing in a good area with subsidized rent is bound to create a waiting list. The result will be unfair to most people, who will not be able to get in. If, alternatively, tenants are given money to pay a market rent, they will probably face particularly big unemployment traps because the rent will be high. Or, if neither a rent subsidy nor a tenant subsidy is available, the units might as well be in a private development.

Cheap financing to help poor people buy their own homes. This plan may be of some benefit if the supply of new housing is flexible and can respond to

(continued on next page)

the stimulated demand. Otherwise, the measure just causes higher prices. Policies of this sort also pose a danger: in 1999, U.S. banks were encouraged by the government "to extend home mortgages to individuals whose credit is generally not good enough to qualify for conventional loans."[b] This became known as "sub-prime" lending. Many people who could not afford to buy did so anyway. They subsequently lost their homes. This situation contributed to the financial crisis that began in 2008.

Housing associations. These semi-independent organizations that manage some of the social housing in the United Kingdom are meant to be more flexible and local than city governments, with the result that the management is better. Even if that is true, they do not remove the essential problems with public housing such as unemployment traps and unfairness.

Insistence on providing some "affordable housing" as a condition of allowing private housing development. This practice causes new housing to be less profitable and therefore less attractive to developers. It therefore results in fewer apartments being built than would otherwise be the case. In some cases, entire projects cease to be commercially attractive, and nothing is built at all. As the market in housing is fungible—total supply affects all prices—the net effect is likely to be to make housing on average more expensive than it would otherwise be.

Shared or partial ownership. This enables people to have a stake in ownership. It effectively increases the ability to buy. But if the supply of housing cannot be increased in response to higher demand, it will only result in higher prices.

Compulsory savings accounts that can be used for home purchase. This has been adopted in Singapore. No unemployment trap is created, and there is no unfairness between people in similar positions. As a result of the scheme, there is mass ownership of property in Singapore. Singapore has one of the highest homeownership rates in the world: 90.5 percent.[c] Relatively poor people own their own homes, which provide them with a major asset. But two concerns arise: that it might only work well in a society as well organized as Singapore and that the domination of the system by government reduces personal liberty.

Giving priority in public housing to those who get work combined with personal counseling for those who have problems getting work. These two ideas have been combined in what could be called "the Atlanta experiment." Renee Glover took over the Atlanta Housing Authority in 1994 and created a revolution in U.S. public housing with these policies.[d] The policies reversed the unemployment trap problem because they provided tenants with an incentive to get work instead of the opposite. They also removed bad tenants. The results were remarkable: the employment rate of household heads increased from 18.5 percent in 1994 to 62 percent in 2010. An underclass was turned into a working class.

The idea of giving housing predominantly to those in work rather than to those in need echoes that used in much of Eastern Europe under communist

(continued on next page)

(continued)

rule. In Poland, for example, those who got work often received accommodations that were tied to their jobs.[e] As for giving personal advice to people in their own homes, this is like the approach of Octavia Hill in 19th century Britain. Her estates were financed privately, and the tenants were actively counseled.

The concerns with attempting to replicate the Atlanta experiment are these: that it might take a particular place and special people to get it up and running; that it could create damage to the communities to which troublesome tenants are moved; that it might sustain high costs; and that obtaining democratic support for such "tough love" may be difficult.

Taxing empty property to increase the amount of property available for occupation. This is likely to make property ownership less desirable and thus, in time, reduce the amount of housing created and exacerbate any shortage. It would be better to counteract any reasons that owners might have to leave property empty, contrary to normal commercial incentives. Such reasons are likely to be government regulations or taxes.

Price controls on new property. China has tried to control housing prices by diktat.[f] Predictably, some building projects have been cancelled. These cancellations will certainly lead to less housing than would otherwise have been available. That shortage, in due course, is likely to lead to higher prices—the very opposite of what is wanted. In 2012, *Caixin*, a Chinese newspaper, reported, "Price controls have been blamed for suspensions or cancellations of large numbers of new housing projects, which means new housing supplies are sure to fall over the next few years and push prices higher."[g]

---

[a] Housing Act 1980. For a longer perspective, see Sarah Heath, "The Historical Context of Rent Control in the Private Rented Sector," House of Commons Library Standard Note SN/SP/6747, October 2013, www.parliament.uk/briefing-papers/sn06747.pdf.

[b] Steven A. Holmes, "Fannie Mae Eases Credit to Aid Mortgage Lending," *New York Times*, September 30, 1999, http://www.nytimes.com/1999/09/30/business/fannie-mae-eases-credit-to-aid-mortgage-lending.html.

[c] As of 2013. See "Households and Housing," Department of Statistics Singapore, http://www.singstat.gov.sg/statistics/latest_data.html#20.

[d] Howard Husock, "Reinventing Public Housing," *Washington Times*, November 8, 2010, http://www.washingtontimes.com/news/2010/nov/8/reinventing-public-housing; Howard Husock, "Reinventing Public Housing: Is the Atlanta Model Right for Your City?" Commentary, Manhattan Institute, New York, December 7, 2009. http://www.manhattan-institute.org/html/reinventing-public-housing-atlanta-model-right-your-city-2211.html.

[e] Stanislawa Golinowska, author interview, November 2011.

[f] Liu Shengjun, "Showdown Stage for Housing Controls," *Caixin*, June 13, 2012, p. 3, http://english.caixin.com/2012-06-13/100400466.html. See also Stuart Jackson, "The Door Is Not Shut to Those Looking to Develop in the Middle Kingdom," *The Times* (London), August 25, 2011: "The local government now requires that we and other developers apply for consent to sell completed residential units at a pre-determined price."

[g] Liu, "Showdown Stage for Housing Controls," p. 3.

3. If you do not subsidize either the *rents* or the *people*, then there is no purpose for public housing.

On this analysis, there is no good option. Public housing simply does not make sense. Is there any way out of this three-way trap? Perhaps. It is not public housing, but it addresses the problem that public housing was meant to deal with.

The fundamental thing that most of us want is that the poor should be able to get reasonable housing. People on different political sides can probably agree about that at least.

Let's step back and look at what has actually happened in many advanced countries. The fact is that the opposite has occurred. It has become increasingly difficult for the poor to get housing. Things have gotten worse, not better. They have gotten worse during the past century, during which public housing has been a prominent part of welfare state policy.

On the face of it, this is odd. Advanced countries across the world have seen substantial increases in the incomes of the less well off. The relatively poor can afford many things more easily than before. Food as a proportion of the average budget in the United Kingdom has fallen from over one-third in 1947 to only 11.6 percent in 2013.[51] In America, the cost of food, which took up 42.5 percent of average expenditures in 1901, fell to 13.2 percent just over a century later.[52] For the poor, the drop was even more significant.[53] In Great Britain, annual vacations of only a week were normal in the 1950s. Now the relatively poor are granted, and can afford, vacations of four weeks or more. The proportion of people ages 16–54 who live in households with mobile phones in Britain reached 99 percent in 2012.[54]

The one big, jarring exception to the poor's getting richer is housing. The cost for the average household has jumped from a mere 8.8 percent of expenditure to over one-quarter since 1947.[55] Once again, the impact of this on the poor will have been even greater. That is why the subsidies paid to people for their housing have had to increase, adding to the discouragement to work. The increased cost of housing is at the root of the problem (Figure 5.1).

Why has the cost risen? To look into this, let's compare Germany and Britain. They are surprisingly similar. Since 1970, both have experienced similar population growth.[56] They have had comparable economic growth, albeit at different times. And their population densities are not very different either.[57] (See Table 5.1.)

Figure 5.1

HOUSING HAS LEAPT OVER FOOD AS A MAJOR COST FOR
AVERAGE FAMILIES

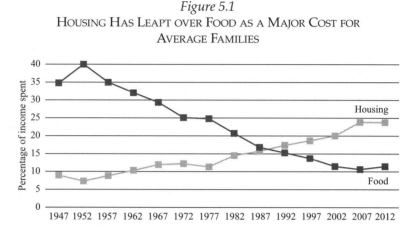

SOURCE: U.K. Office of National Statistics. The raw figures can be found by going to http://www.ons.gov.uk/ons/datasets-and-tables/data-selector.html?table-id=2.5&dataset=mm23 and selecting the categories food and housing.

NOTE: Percentage weightings of food and housing in the British Retail Price Index. The weightings reflect the amount that is estimated to be spent on each category. The weighting of food has fallen partly because people are wealthier and partly because food has become cheaper in real terms.

There is one big difference. In Britain, the cost of housing has soared. In Germany, it has not. In Britain, the average price rose 232 percent in real terms between 1975 and 2014.[58] Over the same period, the cost of German housing actually fell 8 percent (Figure 5.2).

The rise in house prices in Britain has meant that the cost of housing has become a bigger multiple of average salaries. The figure has been volatile but, as the years have gone by, the lowest ratios in the cycle have been higher and so have the highest. In 1981, a Briton on an average salary had to pay 3.5 times his or her salary to buy an average home. That figure rose to a peak of 5.0 times in the late 1990s.[59] At the peak of the following boom in 2007, the ratio reached nearly 6.5.

Among those who rent unfurnished accommodations privately, rent in Britain amounts to just over 30 percent of their income.[60] This is the average. According to the Office of National Statistics, the proportion spent by the poor on housing is more than twice as much as

Table 5.1
HOW MANY PEOPLE PER SQUARE KILOMETER?

Singapore	7,405
Hong Kong	6,787
Malta	1,299
Netherlands	495
Japan	351
United Kingdom	259
Germany	235
Italy	206
Switzerland	198
France	119
Spain	93
Ireland	66
United States	34
New Zealand	17
Canada	4
Australia	3

SOURCE: World Bank online data for 2011, http://data.worldbank.org/indicator
/EN.POP.DNST.
NOTE: 1 square kilometer = 0.3861 square mile.

Figure 5.2
INDEX OF REAL HOUSE PRICES IN GERMANY AND THE UNITED KINGDOM
REBASED TO 100 IN 1975

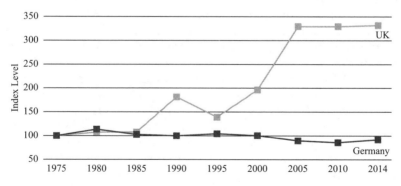

SOURCE: Federal Reserve Bank of Dallas, International House Price Database.
NOTE: In index, first quarter of 1975 = 100.

the proportion spent by the richest.[61] Housing has gone from being a significant cost for the poor to a dominant one. Or, to put it another way, the rising cost of housing has made the poor poorer.

While the ratio of house prices to salaries was rising in Britain, it was falling in Germany.[62] In 2013, the cost of housing, measured per square meter of an apartment, took up a significantly smaller part of a German's net income than in 1991.[63] Another way of measuring this is to look at the cost of 100 square meters (1,080 square feet) of a "typical upscale housing unit" and compare it with average per capita gross domestic product (GDP). In Britain, 100 square meters costs 80 times average per capita GDP in 2014, one of the highest ratios in the world.[64] In Germany, it was only 9.6 times.

"In the 2012 Mercer Cost of Living Survey, no German city ranked among the fifty most expensive expat destinations worldwide."

SOURCE: "Cost of Living in Germany," InterNations website, http://www.internations.org /germany-expats/guide/16008-economy-finance/cost-of-living-in-germany-15974.

Just as the poor have disproportionately suffered from rising prices in Britain, so they have disproportionately benefited from stable prices in Germany. Of all the contrasts in this book, this must count as one of the most important for anyone interested in the living standards of the less well off. What accounts for the contrast in house prices in Britain and Germany? The answer is simple enough to be understood by an 11-year-old. It is a matter of supply and demand. In Britain, the supply of housing has increased very slowly despite substantially increased demand. Therefore, prices have risen. In Germany, supply has increased faster and has met the increased demand.

In 2010, for every 100,000 people in Britain, 15 hectares (37 acres) of land were developed for new housing. In Germany, new development amounted to 50 hectares (123 acres)—more than three times as much.[65] Over the longer term, the rate of building new dwellings per capita in Germany has ranged from 10 to 110 percent a year more than in Britain, according to the European Union.[66] New homes in Britain are also less spacious than in Germany, an average of 76 square meters (820 square feet) compared with 109 square meters (1,170 square feet).[67] Furthermore, the average size of a British family home has been shrinking. It fell by 2 square meters (22 square feet) between 2003 and 2013.[68]

Why is it that supply of new housing in Germany has responded to demand much better than in Britain? Some people like to suggest rapacious builders in Britain hoard land to push up prices to increase their profits. But there is nothing to prevent new entrants in the house-building business from starting up and taking advantage of these supposedly artificial high prices. In any case, it seems unlikely that British builders are any more rapacious than German builders are.

"What's needed is bold action to deliver new homes and lots of them. . . . Millions of young people and families are priced out of a home of their own."

SOURCE: Anne Baxendale, "Fitting the Bill," Shelter policy blog, April 30, 2013, http://blog.shelter .org.uk/2013/04/fitting-the-bill. Shelter is a housing charity in Great Britain.

A more credible explanation is that it is more difficult to obtain permission to build new homes in Britain. Land with permission to build has therefore become extremely valuable. In 2011, in Oxford, for example, it cost £4 million per hectare while agricultural land was worth a mere £16,000 per hectare. Land with permission to build is so rare that it is worth 249 times more than land without permission. Even in far less prosperous areas of Britain, such as Liverpool, land with permission to build is worth over 100 times the value of nearby agricultural land.[69] Barratt, a house-building company, says that, as a rough national guide, land with permission to build is worth 50 times land without permission.[70]

The cost of land with permission to build in England has soared. The average figure tripled in only 16 years, between 1994 and 2010, going from £731,168 to £2,371,549 per hectare.[71] These figures are not just for hotspots like London but the whole of England.[72] The cost has rocketed simply because it is so difficult to obtain the permission.

Housing has been a major part of how welfare states have gone wrong. The poor have been hurt above all. And what has been at the root of this problem? The planning system! It is like a detective story at the end of which you find the villain of the piece is a bureaucrat in a local office who never meant any harm to anyone. The bureaucrat is of course only the instrument of policies that most people, including most politicians, have not thought about very much.

Plenty of countries have their own versions of the British planning problem. The list of countries with price increases of over
90 percent between 1980 and 2008 includes Australia, New Zealand,
Norway, and the Netherlands. Meanwhile, other countries that,
like Germany, have allowed new housing to meet demand include
Switzerland and Japan (see Table 5.2).

The relationship between planning controls and house prices has
been studied by many academics. Over and over again, they have
found the same thing. Even if you look at apparently crowded places
with physical restrictions on development such as Hong Kong and
Manhattan, restrictive planning controls have increased prices.
Kristian Niemietz, after studying a sheaf of studies from around the
world, concluded, "There is overwhelming empirical evidence that
planning restrictions have a substantial impact on housing costs."[73]
The United States provides a useful natural experiment because
planning control there is largely managed by the individual states

Table 5.2
NOT ALL COUNTRIES HAVE PRICED PEOPLE OUT OF HOUSING
CHANGES IN REAL HOUSE PRICES BETWEEN 1980
(OR EARLIEST YEAR AVAILABLE) AND 2008

Countries where prices have gone up less than 20 percent (or fallen), 1980–2008	Countries where prices have gone up by 90 percent or more, 1980–2008
Germany	Australia
Japan	Belgium
Portugal	Finland
South Korea	Ireland
Switzerland	Netherlands
	New Zealand
	Norway
	Spain
	United Kingdom

SOURCE: Organisation for Economic Co-operation and Development, *Economic Policy Reforms 2011: Going for Growth*, Table 4.1.

"The rent is too damn high!"

SOURCE: Name of a minority party in the 2010 election for New York governor, subsequently used as the title of a book by Matthew Yglesias, *The Rent Is Too Damn High: What to Do about It, and Why It Matters More Than You Think* (New York: Simon and Schuster, 2012).

---

and even individual cities. Again, it has been shown that high prices are a response to restrictive planning.

In Houston, Texas, where there are minimal controls, housing is truly affordable and, accordingly, more people have been moving there. Even with a rising population—and therefore increasing demand for housing—Houston has remained affordable. The median home price in recent years has been only 2.3 times median family incomes (2009 figure).[74] This compares with a ratio of 7.1 times in the San Francisco/Oakland area, where there are substantial restrictions on development. In 2006, 11 of 12 states that had price-to-income ratios above 4.0 had some form of restrictive planning.[75] At the other end of the scale, 24 of 25 states where housing was affordable—a ratio below 3.0—did not have restrictive planning.

Further evidence comes from the timing of events. Housing became unaffordable in California 10 years after restrictive planning legislation was passed.[76] In Oregon, it was six years after. In King County, Washington, which includes Seattle, it was four years after a boundary was drawn to prevent urban development. (See Box 5.4 for a French example.)

Some countries have tried to restrain rising house prices in various ways. They have tried taxing houses or restricting the amount of money lent to homebuyers. Such policies do not help in the long term. High prices are telling us that there is unsatisfied demand. The only full answer to unsatisfied demand is increased supply—more housing.

Which leads to a final question: how do countries that allow more building manage it? Germany and Switzerland must have their fair share of people who do not want new buildings to spoil their views or invade their countryside. The answer is that building in these countries is by no means uncontrolled. But two circumstances apply. First, planning control is local; second, taxes are received locally. So local governments have a strong incentive to allow development because taxes imposed on people who are attracted to live

155

Box 5.4
FRENCH WATCH THE PRICE OF PROPERTY "FLY OUT OF REACH"

"Everyone agrees not to give permission for land to be built on," said Nicolas Sarkozy, the former French president.

"But who pays the price? French people who have seen the price of land that that they would like to buy fly out of reach."

Between 1997 and 2010, the price of housing in France jumped 143 percent while wages rose only 33 percent.[a] So property became less affordable.

Why did this happen? Construction costs rose only 44 percent during the time, so that was not the problem. The culprit was the cost of land with planning permission.[b] It rose at least 300 percent.[c]

---

[a] Price of second-hand dwellings from National Institute of Statistics and Economic Studies (INSEE), Paris, using first-quarter figures, http://www.bdm.insee.fr/bdm2/affichageSeries.action?idbank =000817678&bouton=OK&codeGroupe=23. Average annual full-time wages from INSEE, http:// www.bdm.insee.fr/bdm2/affichageSeries.action?idbank=001665118&codeGroupe=1475.

[b] Cost of construction index using first-quarter figures from INSEE, http://www.insee.fr/en/bases -de-donnees/bsweb/serie.asp?idbank=000008630.

[c] I was alerted to the startling contrast between the rise in construction costs and the rise in the cost of land with permission to build by Vincent Bénard, "Libres! Foncier réglementé, familles mal loges," *Contrepoints* (France), October 1, 2012, http://www.contrepoints.org /2012/10/01/98977-libres-foncier-reglemente-familles-mal-logees.[76]

locally form a significant part of their income. At the same time, the new housing is more likely to be in sympathy with what local people will accept because the planning permissions are decided by local governments that want to be re-elected.

The conclusion seems unusually clear. We would all like to see the poor in decent housing. Many attempts to achieve this have focused on public housing, but these efforts have often gone wrong—in some cases, horribly wrong, leading to high rates of unemployment and ghettos of crime. In some countries, housing has become less affordable for the poor, the very opposite of what pretty well everyone wants. The only way to turn this problem around is to make more land available for building by changing the planning system to incentivize local governments to permit it. Such a policy would benefit, above all, the poor.

6. "In Our Liberal Society, There Is a Group of Staunchly Conservative People—Children"

Inconvenient Truths about Parenting

I am in London, going to a talk at the Daiwa Anglo-Japanese Foundation. It has elegant offices in a white stucco terrace facing Regent's Park. On arrival, I am greeted in a polite, deliberate, civilized way. That's how they do things.

The speaker this evening is a young academic from Oxford named Ekaterina Hertog who has done some unusual research. She has made a study of Japanese unmarried parents. Hertog says that it is well known that there is something unusual about Japanese parenting. The number of children born out of wedlock is tiny compared with most of the rest of the world. In most advanced countries, the proportion of births to unmarried women has risen enormously. In Great Britain and the United States, the figure is up to 43 percent. But in Japan, the number has barely passed 2 percent. Hertog set out to discover why.

Some people might respond, "Oh well, Japan is probably socially conservative. That's the reason." But that kind of generalization does not seem to hold water. Hertog says that the divorce rate in Japan has risen substantially, just as it has in other countries. The way Japan has been notably different from other countries has been in its tiny number of unmarried mothers.

For her research, Hertog personally interviewed 68 unmarried mothers in Japan. As if this were not enough, she also interviewed 12 divorced single mothers. One thing soon became very clear. Most of the unmarried mothers felt terrible about having had children out of wedlock. Half of them remained extremely eager to marry the biological fathers of their children. Hertog was astonished by how much they wanted to marry "even the seemingly least attractive ones."

Take Yoshiko. She was clearly a capable woman—a full-time nurse earning more than the man she was living with, who was

157

only working part time. She told this man she was pregnant and, perhaps, she hoped that he would at least offer to get a full-time job to help pay the bills. But no. He said he was willing to get married but only on the following conditions: "I like my life as it is. You work, care for the child and do all the housework. I won't help."

In the West, such an attitude would cause outrage, but Yoshiko was so keen to marry the father of her child that she agreed. In the end, the man did not marry her after all. He decided against it when he discovered that Yoshiko had epilepsy.

You may think that Yoshiko would want nothing further to do with this dreadful character. She was doing well in her job and managing to look after her newborn child. Her boss encouraged her to improve her qualifications by getting a PhD. She was not in desperate need of the man. Yet, even then, Yoshiko told Hertog she would marry him if she could.

Why? And why, as Japanese mothers are so determined to marry the fathers, do they feel it is not so bad to be divorced?

In her talk, Hertog discusses the various possible explanations put forward by senior academics. But I suspect no one has talked to more unwed mothers in Japan than she has. She has reached a clear idea of what is motivating these women. She says that there is a widespread belief in Japan that the best framework for a child to develop successfully is with the two biological parents. The mother is seen as the one with primary responsibility for making sure the child works hard and develops successfully. Meanwhile, the father's job is to provide a role model, especially to boys. He can maintain discipline so that while the children are indulged by the mother, they are kept in order by the father. If the children have problems, such as doing badly at school or being disobedient, it is believed that they can be put right by the concentrated efforts of the mother. Presumably this is made easier if the father is out earning the money.

"To bring a child into existence without a fair prospect of being able, not only to provide food for its body, but instruction and training for its mind is a moral crime, both against the unfortunate offspring and against society."

SOURCE: John Stuart Mill, *On Liberty* (London: Penguin, [1859] 1985), p. 176.

Digging deeper, Hertog quizzed the women about whether they would marry a man who was not the father of the child. She found that they were cautious. They believed another man would not be as good for the child as the biological father would be. One remarked, "These days there is a lot of child abuse, isn't there? Towards others' children. Because this happens often, I am afraid." Hertog reports: "Marrying anyone apart from the child's biological father was often perceived as putting one's own happiness ahead of that of the child."

So it all amounts to a certain understanding of what is best for a child and a certain belief that the mother has to do her best for her children. But why then are Japanese women willing to divorce if they think that married biological parents are so important? Hertog suggests that Japanese women believe that by getting married in the first place, they demonstrate that at least they have tried to give their children the best possible chance in life. There is less blame if they have made the attempt. We should also remember that the Japanese divorce rate, while much higher than it used to be, remains lower than in many Western countries. This is true even though many marriages are between couples who, in Western countries, would not have married in the first place. Overall, the proportion of children brought up by single parents is significantly lower than elsewhere.

"The worst abuse against a child is the absence of a parent."

Sᴏᴜʀᴄᴇ: This is the title that Oxford University sociologist Ekaterina Hertog gave to her study of unmarried Japanese mothers to encapsulate the widespread belief in Japan that parents should be married to each other. The full title is " 'The Worst Abuse against a Child Is the Absence of a Parent': How Japanese Unwed Mothers Evaluate Their Decision to Have a Child outside Wedlock," *Japan Forum* 20 (2008): 193–217.

Japan provides one belief system with regard to parenting. Now let's look at another at the opposite end of the scale. The difference is one of the most dramatic in welfare. In Japan, one in 50 children is born out of wedlock. In Sweden, well over half of children are born that way (Figure 6.1).

I am now in Stockholm, and I have been asking those I interview whether people in Sweden are concerned that unmarried parenting might be bad for the children. The question is usually met with a

Figure 6.1
ONE OF THE BIGGEST CONTRASTS IN THE MODERN WORLD
BIRTHS OUTSIDE MARRIAGE, 2010

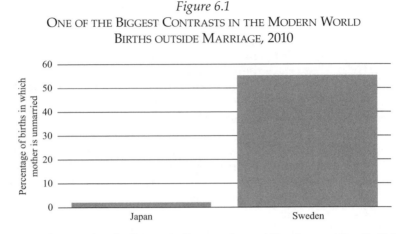

SOURCE: Organisation for Economic Co-operation and Development Family Database, "Share of Births outside Marriage and Teenage Births," http://www.oecd.org/social/family/SF2_4_Births_outside_marriage_and_teenage_births_Jan2013.pdf.

look of puzzlement. It is as though such an idea had never been put to them before. It is outside the normal range of discussion. I also ask whether any research on the subject has been published in Sweden. Again, a look of surprise and uncertainty. It seems the subject is just not on the agenda.

How can that be? The issue is certainly discussed in other Western countries such as Britain and the United States. A possible answer finally emerges in conversation with an academic, Andreas Bergh.[1] He makes a remark that would be astonishing in many countries. He says divorce is "viewed positively" in Sweden. Why is that, I ask. Because it shows women are able to live independently of men, he replies.

"Over time (in marriage), the accumulation of a shared history may become, in itself, a source of meaning, self-definition, and well-being."

SOURCE: Scott M. Stanley, Sarah W. Whitton, and Howard J. Markman, "Maybe I Do: Interpersonal Commitment and Premarital or Nonmarital Cohabitation," *Journal of Family Issues* 25 (2004): 496–519.

I follow up his comment in conversation with other Swedes, trying to establish how they think about the subject. Gradually, I come to believe that the independence and equality of women is viewed as being of such preeminent importance in Swedish society that, if it conflicts with other ideas or goals, it is likely to win. In fact, the point may have been reached at which anything that might interfere with the independence of women is regarded as automatically unconscionable.

That is why, I suspect, there is no appetite in Swedish society to consider the possibility that single parenting might be damaging for the children. It might interfere with the freedom of women. Similarly, it is widely assumed in Sweden that day care from an early age does children no harm. I suggest that the assumption is held because day care enables women to go to work and be independent. In Sweden, parental leave ends when a child is one year old, and people there believe that day care from that age is fine. Many people would applaud this.

Incidentally, some outsiders assume that all the Nordic countries are pretty much the same and that they share similar attitudes. But Finland has a different system and different views, it seems. Financial support for parents there continues until the child is three years old. Many Finns believe that day care before that age can damage a child. It is hard to know whether the rules reflect the different beliefs of people in Sweden and Finland or whether the rules created the beliefs. Perhaps there has been some mixture of rules and beliefs influencing each other. Juho Härkönen, a Finnish sociologist who works in Sweden, suspects that the rules have influenced the beliefs. Human beings have a tendency to believe that behavior that is endorsed by their government and is widespread must be all right. They also, of course, resist any suggestion that they are doing anything wrong themselves.

Now let's go to a place where things are different again: to Rome. I have arrived at a part of the Sapienza University of Rome not far from the city center and the famous tourist sites. I go into an old courtyard and find a throng of students and a lively sense of chaos. Student posters appear all over the place, and there is a slight sense that the students have taken over. I ask directions and walk up a floor or two to where I find a little office. Amid the bustle, Professor Pugliese suddenly comes in. He is an old-fashioned sort of professor, striding around making confident assertions. This turns out to be the shortest interview in all my research because he has to be

161

elsewhere very soon and is going to hand me over to one of his colleagues. In fact, we talk as he is standing in the doorway, obviously in a hurry to go. It is frustrating, but the thing about such professors is that, however assertive and content with themselves they might be, they sometimes make interesting remarks.

I ask him about single parents in Italy and he declares, "In Italy, single mothers are wealthy!" I am puzzled, but he storms on, saying that the upper class in Rome has a lower marriage rate than the rest because being a single mother is a luxury that only the rich can afford. With that, he sweeps out.

After he has gone, I pursue the subject with his colleague and, later, with others. He has pithily highlighted the key point about single parenting in Italy. There is very little support for it from the state. That is why only the rich can afford it.

But why is there so little state help for single parents?

Everyone I speak with takes up the same theme: it is all about the family. The family is the first port of call in the Italian way of thinking about social policy. In principle, it comes before any resort to state welfare. There are important exceptions: pensions, health care, and education. Otherwise, the Italian belief system is focused on the family as the main source of welfare. The family should provide accommodations for those without homes. It should provide care for the elderly. And if a daughter has a baby but no husband, she may well stay with her parents. The family is an attitude of mind, an ideal, and an obligation.

So what happens, I ask, to a young mother who has no man to provide for her and who also, for some reason, cannot get help from her family?

I discover that it depends on where she lives. The issue is handled by each region according to its own ideas. In some regions, women in this situation may be granted accommodations in *case-famiglia* ("family houses"). These are small groups of apartments run by charities or individuals and subsidized by the local government. A parental figure is present. A typical *casa-famiglia* might consist of three apartments joined together with one kitchen and washing machine between them. A single mother would be lucky to get her own private apartment.

Does the mother get a free place at a kindergarten for her child? Perhaps. In some regions, a single mother might get some preference, but it varies and there is no guarantee. Italy has the lowest provision of day care facilities in Europe. It all comes back to the family. The family is expected to look after young children.

The father of the baby, in such cases, is pursued for support and, in theory, must pay substantial amounts. But, of course, the father is not always successfully tracked down and made to pay.

Overall, the picture for a single mother without support from a man or her family is much less attractive than it would be in many other countries. If the mother is entitled to substantive benefits at all, it will be for only up to nine months. Then she must work. It is not an attractive option. That is why only the rich can afford it.

You may not be surprised to hear that the rate of single parenting in Italy is relatively low. Is this due to the culture—the ideal of the family—or is it because the laws make single parenting unattractive? The two things seem to influence each other, and in combination they are powerful.

We have now seen three countries with different ideas and also different kinds of state welfare for single parents. There always seems to be an interplay between the cultures and the welfare systems. This is only a snapshot, of course. All these countries have seen significant changes and they continue to change. Many Italians are concerned that their country is becoming more like Scandinavia. The family is ceasing to be such a cornerstone. A word has been coined to describe what they regard as distressing: defamilization. The rate of unwed parenting has risen from 4.3 percent in 1980 to over one in five in 2007.[2] The proportion of children living in single-parent households has increased to 1 in 10. This is one of the lowest rates of single parenting in the advanced world, but it is still quite a shock for Italy.

In some places, though, there is no concern about the trend. The European Union is positively encouraging things that are part and parcel of it. The EU has a target for increasing the availability of day care outside the home.[3] When people talk of day care, they always mean care that is done by people outside the family. The Organisation for Economic Co-operation and Development (OECD), too, is content that families are losing their grip and that state care is taking their place. These international organizations have taken the view that the Swedish model is best. Their top priority for social policy is similar to Sweden's: enabling independent working women. They are not concerned that there may be consequent damage to children and implicitly they do not believe that people should stay

Figure 6.2
THE WORLDWIDE BOOM IN BIRTHS OUTSIDE MARRIAGE
PERCENTAGE OF CHILDREN BORN OUTSIDE MARRIAGE, 1980 AND 2007

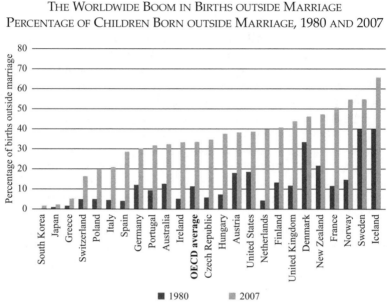

SOURCE: Organisation for Economic Co-operation and Development, *Doing Better for Families* (Paris: OECD Publications, 2011).

married for the sake of the children. The only thing that worries the OECD is that single parents tend to be relatively poor. The OECD's preferred solution to this problem seems to be simply to give them more money.

So the trend around the world is overwhelmingly in favor of "defamilization." The proportion of births outside marriage across the advanced world has jumped to a new level. That has happened in a single generation. In 1980, one in nine children was born outside marriage. By 2007, the proportion had soared to one in three. No doubt since 2007 it has continued its rise. The proportion in England and Wales reached 44.3 percent in 2007 and five years later had moved on to 47.5 percent[4] (see Figure 6.2).

By 2007, 15 percent of children in the advanced world were being brought up by single parents, 11 percent by cohabiting couples, and 72 percent by married couples. Since then the proportion with single parents has increased. In future years, it will inevitably continue to rise as the much higher proportions of children now being born to unmarried parents grow up. True, some of the single parents will marry the fathers or mothers of their children. Some, too, are cohabiting at the time of the birth. But even allowing for this and other such factors, it is sure that the proportion brought up by a single parent will rise. So also will the proportion brought up in households in which one of the adults is not the natural parent.

The trend across the world is emphatic. You might even think it is a force of nature and irresistible, whether for good or ill. But is it?

We should, perhaps, note that the numbers in different countries are still very different from one another (Figure 6.3). In Iceland, two of three births are outside wedlock. In South Korea, only 1 in 66 is.

Figure 6.3
ONE OF THE BIGGEST CONTRASTS IN THE MODERN WORLD
PERCENTAGE OF CHILDREN LIVING WITH ONE PARENT, 2007

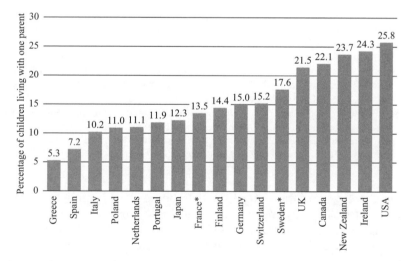

SOURCE: Organisation for Economic Co-operation and Development, *Doing Better for Families* (Paris: OECD Publications, 2011).

NOTE: This is a selection of the countries covered by the OECD statistics. France and Sweden (with asterisks) have the highest rates of children raised by cohabiting couples, 21.0 percent and 30.5 percent, respectively. It is possible that, because cohabiting couples tend to break up more readily than married couples do, the single-parenting figures in these countries will increase.

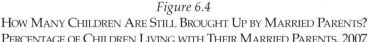

Figure 6.4
HOW MANY CHILDREN ARE STILL BROUGHT UP BY MARRIED PARENTS?
PERCENTAGE OF CHILDREN LIVING WITH THEIR MARRIED PARENTS, 2007

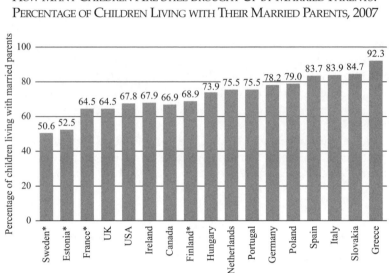

SOURCE: Organisation for Economic Co-operation and Development, *Doing Better for Families* (Paris: OECD Publications, 2011).

NOTE: Selected countries. No figures shown for some countries, such as Japan and Australia. These countries have among the highest proportion of children living with cohabiting parents (marked with asterisks): Sweden, 30.5 percent; Estonia, 23.9 percent; France, 21.0 percent; and Finland, 15.8 percent.

Some of these children are very young, and their parents will divorce. So the percentage of children who spend their whole childhoods with their married parents is sure to be lower. The OECD data fail to distinguish between married couples who are both the natural parents and stepfamilies. So this figure includes stepfamilies.

The extreme variation suggests that being in the modern world does not necessarily mean that mass single parenting is inevitable (Figure 6.4). Perhaps there is not a force of nature and we are at a time in human history in which things could turn out in a variety of ways.

Ironically, Sweden, of all countries, shows that trends in this area can be arrested or even reversed. Births to unmarried women rose quickly between 1980 and 2002.[5] But since then the proportion has plateaued and even fallen back a little. Meanwhile, the marriage rate has rallied—from four per thousand adults at the turn of the century to five in 2011, slightly above the European Union average.[6]

The stories from Japan, Sweden, and Italy show that there are all sorts of different ideas around about parenting. Who is right about the crucial issues of single parenting, divorce, and the care of infants?

For a start, does single parenting tend to damage children, or not?

There are hundreds of studies on this, but let us first pick one that is unusual because it looks at how happy children are. Often, you hear parents say that what they really want for their children, above all else, is for them to be happy.

The research was done by Gundi Knies. Her purpose was to look at whether being poor makes children less happy.[7] She drew on figures from a major long-term study of British families with a sample of 4,900 children. The children, ages 10 and over, were asked to assess their level of happiness.

One can imagine that some researchers associated with the study might have been expecting it to show that being relatively poor makes children unhappy. But that was not the result. Knies found no connection: "Household income is not associated with child life satisfaction in any of the models we estimated." Only when the circumstances were so bad that the child suffered "material deprivation" was happiness affected by income per se.

Knies found a completely different factor had a much bigger impact on the happiness of children. The figures showed that it made a really big difference what kind of family the child came from. Children with two married parents were significantly happier than those from single-parent families. As Knies put it, "The family living context appears to impact hugely on child life satisfaction, living with both biological parents being associated with the greatest happiness."[8]

One of the unusual advantages of this study is that it differentiates between biological parents and stepfamilies. The result is striking. The study indicates that the children living in stepfamilies are significantly less happy than those living with their biological parents. More remarkably still, children living in stepfamilies are also significantly less happy than those living with a single parent.

Incidentally, it is worth mentioning that another finding of this study was that the happiness of the children was quite strongly correlated with whether other children at their school "misbehaved." The more misbehavior, the bigger the damage to their happiness. It seems possible that bad or undisciplined schools may help contribute to making children unhappy as well as causing them to do less well academically.

Because there are so many studies of parenting, it would be easy for an author—including me—to pick studies that suit his purpose. So it is important to go to an overall assessment of what the research about single parenting tells us. A "meta-analysis"—or "study of studies"—pools together, with suitable adjustments, the results of many other studies. Paul Amato, professor of family sociology and demography at Pennsylvania State University, has done several meta-analyses of this subject. What is his assessment?

> Compared with children who grow up in stable, two-parent families, children born outside marriage reach adulthood with less education, earn less income, have lower occupational status, are more likely to be idle (that is, not employed and not in school), are more likely to have a nonmarital birth (among daughters), have more troubled marriages, experience higher rates of divorce, and report more symptoms of depression.[9]

It is a devastating summary. The clear answer is that children are better off with their two married, natural parents.

The next issue on which people have different beliefs is the similar but distinct one of divorce. What about parents who start off married and then get divorced? How do their children fare? Amato says that there are fewer studies of this scenario and that there is "some variation" across the results, although generally the outcomes are comparable. For example, one study with a big sample compared how many children dropped out of high school in the United States. The proportion of children of continuously married parents was 13 percent. The figure jumped to 37 percent for children of unwed parents and fell only slightly to 31 percent for children of divorced parents. The rate for children of divorced parents was better than that for the children of never-married parents but not by very much.

One of the most influential pieces of research into the effect of divorce on children was the California Children of Divorce Project in the 1970s. Academics carefully followed 60 families in which the parents were getting divorced. One of the special things about this study was that the researchers spoke to the children several

Box 6.1
WHAT DO CHILDREN FEEL ABOUT DIVORCE?

"There is one group who are bucking the trend," noted Asta Leppä in the Finnish newspaper, *Helsingin Sanomat.*

"In our liberal society, there is a group of staunchly conservative people who feel that divorces should not be granted except for very weighty reasons. They are children."[a]

Frigide Barjot, French author of *J'éduque mes parents* (which can be loosely translated as "Educating My Parents"), said, "I suffered when my father left my mother. Now the state is trying to organise the separation of mothers and fathers and I don't want children to go through the same thing I went through."[b]

[a] Asta Leppä, "The Mysteries of Divorce, Finnish Style," *Helsingin Sanomat*, February 8, 2013.
[b] Frigide Barjot (a pseudonym for Virginie Tellenne), quoted in Adam Sage, "'God's Nutcase' Frigide Barjot Confronts Hollande on Same-Sex Marriage," *The Times* (London), December 27, 2012.

times over. This sometimes got them closer to what a child was really feeling. Robert, for example, was not visited frequently by his father. At the first interview, he told researchers smilingly, "I have a grand time on his visits" and added, even though he had not been asked, "I see him enough." But, in his third interview, Robert admitted that he missed his father intensely. He longed to see his father every day and was profoundly hurt that his father did not come more often.[10] (See Box 6.1.)

Children have a strong sense of loyalty to their parents. They want to respect and love them. The study found that "children lied bravely to protect them [their parents] and to camouflage their own hurt feelings." This is surely one of the reasons that many parents who divorce often do not understand how painful it is for the children. The children don't tell them. Many divorcing parents believe, or like to believe, that it would be better for the children, as well as themselves, if they divorced. But that is not how most children see it. The study found that fewer than 1 in 10 children was relieved by their parents' decision to divorce even when there was actual physical violence between parents.[11]

The report commented, "Whatever its shortcomings, the family is perceived by the child at this time as having provided the support and protection he needs. The divorce signifies the collapse of that structure, and he feels alone and very frightened."

169

"No matter how well-intentioned parents are, no matter how civilised they feel they are being, their divorce or separation always makes children unhappy. Always. Parents separating is not just a storm but a hurricane that howls through family life . . . wrecking children's security."

SOURCE: Penelope Leach, *Family Breakdown: Helping Children Hang On to Both Their Parents* (London: Unbound, 2014). (Quotation taken from the serialization in the *Daily Mail* (London), June 19, 2014, http://www.dailymail.co.uk/femail/article-2661981/The-toxic-truth-DIVORCE -parents-confront-Dont-kid-Separation-harms-children-And-devastating-new-series-Penelope -Leach-explains-why.html.)

A further issue on which people around the world differ is cohabitation. In some countries, notably Sweden and France, it has become widespread. Supporters of this trend say there is no need for a piece of paper called "marriage." In any case, young children are hardly aware of whether their parents are married or not. They have their parents together and that is the main thing for them. Unfortunately, cohabiting couples are far more likely to break up. One study in the United States found that a quarter of cohabiting parents broke up within just a year of their child's birth. A separate study of first births found that after five years 31 percent of cohabiting couples had split up—almost twice the proportion of married couples (16 percent).[12]

It is actually rare for children to be brought up continuously by co-habiting couples. One study found that less than half of 1 percent of adolescents ages 16 to 18 had spent their entire childhoods with two continuously cohabiting biological parents. Some parents have married, of course. But the majority break up, leaving the child with a single parent. In Britain, Harry Benson of the Marriage Foundation estimates that nearly two-thirds (65 percent) of cohabiting couples who have children are likely to break up by the time a child reaches age 15.[13]

What about single parents who find a new partner? Amato says the studies show that when a single parent remarries, children have problems similar to those of children of single parents. He adds, chillingly, "Stepchildren are overrepresented in official reports of child abuse." Of course, the vast majority of stepparents do not abuse their stepchildren. But a child is at greater risk. The fears of the Japanese single mother quoted by Ekaterina Hertog have some basis in fact.[14]

Children from broken homes are also far more likely to become juvenile delinquents. A review of the evidence in 1998 concluded that the risk of delinquency was double for children from broken homes and that this association was remarkably consistent over time and in different places.[15] A British study of boys in Newcastle found that 53 percent of those who had experienced divorce or separation in the first five years of their lives were convicted of a crime by the age of 30 compared with only 28 percent of the others.[16] In a long-term study of working-class boys in London, 29 percent who came from "disrupted" families were convicted of juvenile crimes compared with 18 percent of children from "intact" but otherwise similar families.[17]

One might hope that this was just a matter of adolescents going through a bad phase after which they would recover. But the same study found that just over a third of boys from the disrupted families had criminal records as adults compared with 22 percent of boys from intact families.

The study also looked into whether the child's prospects are improved if a single mother establishes a relationship with another man. The reverse was the case. The most damaging thing for children appears to be a series of changes in who looks after them. The more changes, the worse the outcome.

"24 percent of prisoners have been in [state] care at some point during their childhood."

Source: U.K. Ministry of Justice, March 2012, quoted in, "Were a Quarter of Prisoners in Care as Children?" Fullfact.org, October 22, 2012, https://fullfact.org/factchecks/were_quarter_prisoners_in_care_as_children-28547.

Much needs to be done to disentangle exactly which circumstances tend to do the most or least damage. But it is overwhelmingly clear that children whose homes break up are dramatically more likely to turn to crime. It follows that in countries where there is a high incidence of broken families, there will be a higher level of crime than there otherwise would have been. The figures suggest that children from broken families are at least 50 percent more likely to commit crimes. So if a country's rate of broken parenting rises from, say 5 percent to 50 percent, it is conceivable that the crime rate will rise by 20 to 25 percent above what it otherwise would have been. And because crime is the ultimate antisocial behavior,

171

it is likely that other kinds of antisocial behavior will also be significantly more common than they would otherwise have been.

Some suggest that the bad effects of single parenting and broken families are not mainly because of single parenting itself but rather because single parents are often poor. But many of the studies already cited separate the impact of being poor from the effect of family breakdown. The study of boys in London, for example, found that broken homes were correlated with a much higher likelihood of crime even after controlling for the parent's being relatively poor and for other possible confounding factors. But to what extent does it make sense to separate the impact of the parent's being poor anyway? Other things being equal, being a single parent brings with it the likelihood of being poorer than someone with a partner or spouse. One income amounts to less than two. Yes, the father may pay money to the mother. But the statistics show that a woman is far more likely to be relatively poor if she is a single parent.

A single mother may also have greater expenses, such as paying for more childcare. Furthermore, it is more expensive for the father and mother to have two separate homes than a single one. Being relatively poor is part and parcel of single parenting, divorce, and separation. As Mayor Bloomberg asserted in an advertisement displayed in New York, "If you finish high school, get a job, and get married before having children, you have a 98 percent chance of not being in poverty."

Our main concern in all of this is the children. The damage to them is of preeminent importance. But bundles of academic studies provide evidence that single parenting and broken homes do not make the adults happy either (see Figure 6.5). An influential review of the parents concluded, "Science tends to confirm Grandma's wisdom. On the whole, man was not meant to live alone and neither was woman. Marriage makes people happier."[18] Or to put it more grimly, single mothers are far more likely to get depressed. One Canadian study with a large sample found that single mothers were about twice as likely to have suffered a period of major depression in the previous year as married mothers. The figures were 15.4 percent for single mothers compared with 6.8 percent for married mothers[19] (see also Figure 6.5).

Single mothers are less healthy too. Another Canadian study found that mothers who had experienced a heart attack or

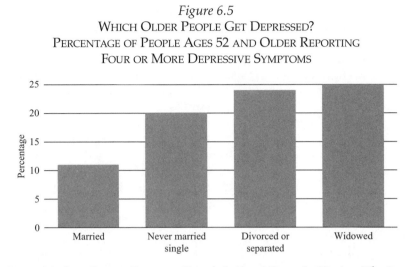

Figure 6.5
WHICH OLDER PEOPLE GET DEPRESSED?
PERCENTAGE OF PEOPLE AGES 52 AND OLDER REPORTING
FOUR OR MORE DEPRESSIVE SYMPTOMS

SOURCE: Andrew Steptoe, Panayotes Demakakos, and Cesar de Oliveira, "The Psychological Well-Being, Health and Functioning of Older People in England" in *The Dynamics of Ageing: Evidence from the English Longitudinal Study of Ageing 2002–10 (Wave 5)*, ed. James Banks, James Nazroo, and Andrew Steptoe (London: Institute of Fiscal Studies, 2012), Chapter 4, http://www.ifs.org.uk/elsa/report12/ch4.pdf.

stroke were 3.3 times more likely to be single mothers than to be "partnered."[20] Married women also live longer: a large-scale long-term study found that among women age 48, 90 percent lived to be at least 65 whereas only 60 percent of the divorced and never-married did.[21]

Fathers, who are usually the ones without custody, are also less happy. The same study found that their longevity was similarly affected. Long-term studies have shown that men's psychological well-being is improved by marriage.[22]

Why does marriage make adults happier? One American sociologist, Linda Waite, found that marriage encourages more healthy behavior.[23] Partners monitor each other's health. Married people are less likely to drink excessively or take illegal drugs. Not surprisingly, men and women who live without adult company are more lonely. Some socialize more to compensate, but they return to a home that contains no other adult who cares about them.

Overall, there seems to be a pretty clear answer on all the related issues of single parenting and divorce. Marriage tends to produce better results for all concerned.

But what is the truth about the other major area in which different countries have contrasting views: day care for infants?

Looking at this subject is a bit like walking onto the battlefield of Waterloo or Gettysburg. The ground is littered with the dead and wounded. Jay Belsky's story reflects just a part of this peril.

Jay Belsky was an able student of child development and worked under Urie Bronfenbrenner, one of the most eminent academics of the time (the late 1970s), on a review of the effects of day care on children.[24] Most people regarded the resulting paper as giving day care the green light. It argued that there was little scientific evidence that day care did harm. The paper was very well received.[25]

Over the next eight years, Belsky was repeatedly asked to write and talk about the subject, and he reported the same message. Then he wrote a review about the effect of the quality of childcare. He found that if caregivers were attentive, stimulating, and affectionate, a child's development could be enhanced. This kind of high-quality care occurred when caregivers were reasonably well trained and the number of children per caregiver was fairly low. This research was applauded and it contributed to his receiving an award for "Distinguished Early Contribution in Developmental Psychology" from the American Psychological Association.[26]

A few years later, in 1986, he was preparing another talk about childcare. He says, "As I worked my way through the newly emerging evidence, I realized I could no longer tell the same story I had been telling."[27] So he reported "a slow steady trickle of disconcerting evidence" linking day care in a child's first year with outcomes such as "insecure infant–parent attachment" and increased levels of aggression and disobedience at three to eight years of age. He concluded that childcare in the first year of life should be regarded as a "risk factor." (A risk factor is not the same as a disaster and may be nullified by other factors.) He delivered his talk to an annual convention of pediatricians and published it in a relatively obscure newsletter.

To his astonishment, his article created a "firestorm." Articles appeared in the *New York Times*, *Washington Post*, *Wall Street Journal*, and *Time* magazine. He was accused of being against day care, of

174

being opposed to women working outside the home, and of being "more or less a misogynist."

"It was rather amazing how quickly supporters and admirers turned me into the devil incarnate almost overnight," he wrote later. He came to realize that he had "run smack into the wall of political correctness before the term was even coined." He had violated "the 11th commandment of the field of child development: 'Thou shalt not speak ill of day care.'"[28]

Belsky later found and reported evidence of actual harm. He was pilloried for doing so. It was as if no one actually cared about what was true. It seemed to him as though to some people the orthodox view was more important than the well being of children.

The extraordinary outcome of the outrage and controversy was that the American government commissioned a major long-term study costing millions of dollars to get to the bottom of the issue. Belsky, as a leader in his field, was commissioned to work on this study, but so were his critics. People with opposing views had to work together.

They fought over the shape of the great study and the interpretation of the findings. Belsky's account of the process sounds like a harrowing marriage counseling session full of angry recriminations. Some called it "the study from Hell." However, at the end of it all, the National Institute of Child Health and Human Development (NICHD) Study of Early Child Care was produced—one of the biggest such studies ever to take place.

What was its conclusion?

There was not just one, unfortunately. There were hundreds, some of which appear, at first sight, to contradict each other. But the green light on day care definitely turned to amber. The research showed that caution was called for. Damage to children was identified. On the other hand, it was not a clear case of "all day care before the age of three is bad." According to the report, many factors influence how a child turns out, and day care is only one of them. It can have a damaging effect, but the effect may be so small as to be insignificant depending on the amount of day care and other circumstances.

Contrary to the earlier emphasis on the quality of day care, the key factor arising from the research seemed to be the quantity of day care.[29] Extensive childcare emerged as a "significant predictor" of "problem behaviors" in kindergarten classes. The greater the quantity of childcare, the more likely the child was to demand lots of attention, get jealous easily, boast, argue a lot, be disruptive, and get into fights. Childcare by a relative came out significantly better than did childcare in a center.

Negative behavior persisted right up to the oldest age assessed by the study: 15 years. The children had "significantly" fewer social skills and weaker work habits. One of the most striking findings was that when children had a lot of day care, the "sensitivity" of the mother to the child was lower. There was more "flatness of emotional engagement with the child," lower sensitivity to the distress of the child, and less stimulation of the child's "cognitive development." The children correspondingly had "less positive engagement" with the mother.[30] In other words, large quantities of day care risked damaging the quality of the interaction between mother and child. Childcare was only one factor, though. The study found that having parents who were relatively poor or unmarried was also a risk factor.[31]

The paper concluded that "the negative effects [of day care] found in these studies are not large," but "even low or moderate risks are significantly multiplied by their widespread prevalence."[32]

Plenty of other research has been undertaken since, of course. A major study by Stanford University and the University of California, Berkeley, in 2005 gathered data from more than 14,000 children in kindergarten, their parents, and their teachers, measuring social behavior and skills, such as aggression and bullying, sharing, cooperation, and engagement in classroom tasks. The study found that "Attendance in preschool centers, even for short periods of time each week, hinders the rate at which young children develop social skills."[33] It also found that the negative impact on social behavior was particularly strong "for black children and children from the poorest families." But the effect was not limited to any one race or class. Middle-class white children who attended preschool suffered lower social skill levels than did similar children who remained at home in the care of a parent. Meanwhile, another study found that children in day care have higher levels of cortisol—a hormone induced by stress—than children being cared for by their mothers.[34]

What about the age from which a child has day care? It is clear from the various studies that the first year is critical, and day care is not appropriate then. Beyond that, the evidence is not so easy or clear. The NICHD study suggests that the total amount of care matters, not so much when it is given. Another study that looked

Box 6.2
WHEN CAN PARENTS PUT THEIR CHILDREN INTO
CHILDCARE WITHOUT HARMING THEM?

Psychologist Penelope Leach argues that it is not possible to give a simple answer, but doing it too early is damaging.

"The most recent studies convincingly suggest that neither a pro-day care nor an anti-day care stance is tenable because the effects of day care on children depend on the caring institution and its personnel and on the age, family experiences and characteristics of individual children being cared for.

"Naturally parents who are seeking more and more day care for younger and younger infants are looking for economic improvement in their own lives, but not many would do so if they believed that they earned money at their children's expense.

"It is clearly and certainly best for babies to have something close to full-time mother care for six months at least—conveniently linked with breast-feeding—and family care for a further year and better two. Using financial or career penalties to blackmail women into leaving infants who are scarcely settled into life outside wombs that are still bleeding is no less than barbarous."[a]

Jill Kirby, who was director of the Centre for Policy Studies in London from 2007 to 2011, argues that the need of children for direct parental care has been pushed to one side:

"The priority for any formulation of childcare policy should be: will this be good for the child's well-being? Sadly this question is very rarely asked. The growing child is simply viewed as an impediment to work."[b]

---

[a] Penelope Leach, *Children First: What Society Must Do—and Is Not Doing—for Our Children Today* (London: Penguin, 1994), pp. 77–79.
[b] Jill Kirby, "Childcare Policy Should Start with Children," *ConservativeHome* blog, October 17, 2012, http://www.conservativehome.com/thecolumnists/2012/10/jill-kirby-childcare-policy-should -start-with-children.html.

specifically at boys in their second year found that boys with moderate or high risk factors were significantly more likely to have problems with "interactions and behaviors" if they had more than 20 hours a week of nonmaternal care.[35] It seems there is no definite age at which an "all clear" sounds. (See Box 6.2.)

The quality of care matters. Unfortunately, there are reasons to be concerned that, in many countries, the quality is deteriorating.

In Sweden, the number of infants cared for per adult has increased dramatically. Jonas Himmelstrand, who studies child-care issues, says that an experienced preschool teacher he talked to re-members that in 1980 the ratio was two and a half young children per adult. But today, the ratio can reach as high as 5.7 children per adult (17 children to 3 adults).[36] In Britain, the government has an-nounced that the number of infants who may be looked after by a child-care provider will be increased from four to six. This obvi-ously reduces the time available for each infant. In several countries, it seems that the initial quality that may have been possible with small numbers of children per adult has become financially more problematic as the numbers have grown.

Himmelstrand has argued that Swedish people, in their exten-sive use of day care, are not genuinely "following their hearts." The same thought has been expressed by Penelope Leach, the British child development specialist, who wrote, "People are expected to feel strongly about their children, but not to act upon those feel-ings."[37] Many mothers feel awful when they first leave their infants at day care. They may quell their emotions because they know that what they are doing is normal. They may assume that, as everyone else is doing it, it must be all right.

It seems possible, to put it no higher, that the feeling that some mothers experience in this situation is an instinct that has evolved because the child truly does want and need her at this time. Hu-mans are, of course, different from monkeys, but it might be worth mentioning one of the most famous experiments in all psychology because it is highly relevant.

Harry Harlow sought to establish what an infant monkey really wants. If previous psychologists like Freud were right, what they wanted from their mothers was milk. To find out, Harlow put baby monkeys into cages with two available surrogate "mothers." One was made of cloth, and the other was made of metal but provided milk. Which would the babies choose? The outcome was clear and poignant. The infant monkeys spent nearly all their time with their cloth mother, "clinging to, climbing on and pushing themselves into the soft folds."[38] But, of course, they need milk. One of the photographs from the experiment shows a little monkey hanging onto the cloth mother with its hind legs and reaching across to take milk from the metal mother. The monkeys were so attached to their cloth surrogate mothers that they did not want to leave them even for milk.

In another experiment, young monkeys were put with their cloth mothers in a room full of toys. After a while, they would eventually climb down from their "mother" to explore, but they would often return to touch her and reconnect. If the cloth mother was removed from the room, all play would stop and "frantic screaming ensued."[39] In essence, this is a sad story of an infant being deprived of its sense of security.

Human infants can also scream when removed from their mothers at an early age. Or else they may go quiet.[40] John Bowlby observed that, when children are separated from their attachment figures for a long time, as in a hospital stay, they quickly descend into passivity and despair. When children know they have a secure attachment figure available, they go out and explore confidently. He argued that when children are denied a stable and enduring attachment relationship—raised, for example, by a succession of foster parents—they are likely to be damaged for life.[41]

Where does all that leave us?

The picture is not clear, and different people will react differently to the evidence. Personally, it leaves me with considerable concern about children being packed off to a large number of childcare sessions before the age of one. I am also somewhat concerned about it for children under two. I feel there is reason to be cautious about it even up to the age of three. Penelope Leach summarized it this way:

> Of course nobody can say, "At such and such an age your child needs you to be around this many hours a day and any fewer will be disastrous for him or her," but it would be fair to say, "The more you are around, the better, and the younger the child, the more it matters."[42]

After reading the research on the subject, I confess that I look back at how my own children were raised and wish we had given them more parental care for longer.

Some may be thinking, "This discussion of day care and parenting is all very well, but what has it got to do with welfare states?"

The relevance is this: welfare states may be influencing the incidence of both single parenting and day care. In this way, they may be affecting the happiness and well being of millions of children and their parents.

Do welfare states affect the rates of single parenting and day care?

Let's take single parenting first. There is plenty of anecdotal evidence of this. But what is needed is a proper academic survey comparing benefits in different countries and analyzing whether these benefits have changed the rate of single parenting.

Fortunately, one researcher has done such a study: Libertad Gonzales at the University of Barcelona. Because her work on this is so significant, I have come to Barcelona mainly for the purpose of talking with her about it.

It is a lovely sunny morning when I reach the part of the university where she works. The buildings are unusual, like military barracks around a rectangular parade ground. I go in and find a series of long corridors with doors into rooms at regular intervals as if they were monks' cells. These are the offices of the academics.

I find Gonzales's door and, after saying hello, she suggests we go outside for a coffee. We find an unpretentious little coffee bar nearby, and I quiz her about her findings. In her studies, she concluded that a difference of €1,000 ($1,100) per year in benefits received by single mothers results in a difference of two percentage points in the rate of single parenting in that country.[43] So, in a given country, an extra €1,000 of benefits would result in the rate of single parenting being, say, 7 percent instead of 5 percent. Her conclusion, despite the caveats that academics tend to add, is pretty clear. Welfare benefit levels do influence the amount of single parenting.

But I want to check out how she arrived at her calculations. I ask her if her figures were based on the people most likely to be affected by benefits—the relatively poor. No, she says. They were based on the overall female population. So her figures, while powerful enough as they stand, understate the effect on the less well off.

Next, I ask her if she included the value of subsidized or free housing given to single parents in certain countries. No, she says, she did not. Again, this means the power of benefits to influence single parenting is likely to be understated because free or subsidized housing can be very valuable. (See Box 6.3.)

As we saw in the previous chapter, the countries with the highest rates of single parenting in the world and in Europe are the United States and Britain. In these countries, the allocation of housing is based primarily on need, so single mothers are favored. There may be no stated priority for single mothers, but there is a de facto priority.[44] Single mothers account for 57 percent of working-age households in public housing in the United States. Only 8 percent of all public housing households are married couples (Box 6.4).[45]

So the evidence from Libertad Gonzales's work is that the benefits offered to single parents increase the rate of single parenting.

Box 6.3
WHO SHOULD PAY WHEN PARENTS FAIL IN THEIR RESPONSIBILITIES?

In his *Re-moralising the Welfare State*, Peter Saunders attacks the assumption that the state should pick up the tab.

"I have discussed the German principle of generational solidarity at a number of seminars and conferences in Britain and Australia, and on every occasion, somebody ventures the opinion that it is 'unfair' to expect grandparents to pick up the tab if the parents fail in their responsibilities to their children," he writes.

"But if it is unreasonable to expect grandparents to contribute to the upkeep of their grandchildren, how much more unreasonable is it to expect complete strangers to do so through their taxes?"[a]

The assumption that the state should pay keeps on appearing in discussion of family issues, he notes:

"Family members helping each other only represents a 'huge saving to the government' if you think the government should be paying and providing for everything."[b]

[a] Peter Saunders, *Re-moralising the Welfare State* (St Leonards, NSW: Centre for Independent Studies, 2013), p. 35.
[b] Saunders, *Re-moralising the Welfare State*, p. 30, citing Adele Horin, "Generation IOU: Parents Fork Out $22 Billion a Year to Help Their Adult Children," *The Age*, July 26, 2012.

Her findings are likely to understate the reality because she did not focus on the poor—those most likely to be affected—and she did not include the impact of subsidized housing, which may well have as much or more impact than cash benefits do. True, some less-focused studies have come to more mixed conclusions. But most, like Gonzales's, do not look particularly at those with low incomes or on the impact of subsidized housing. The country-by-country analysis overwhelmingly suggests that, yes, welfare states can increase the rate of single parenting. Italy, for example, provides barely any benefits for single mothers and has a low incidence of single parenting. Britain has a history of special benefits for single mothers and a much higher rate of single parenting.

As for whether government policies affect the amount of day care, that hardly needs discussion. The incidence of day care for infants is far higher in those countries where the state subsidizes it than in those where it does not. In Sweden, where day care is highly

Box 6.4
"SHOES UNDER THE BED"

Government officials in Britain and the United States from time to time visit the homes of single parents receiving welfare benefits to check that a boyfriend is not living there. They look for such clues as men's shoes under the bed and toilets left with the seat up. If officials find a boyfriend or husband is living with the woman, her benefits will be reduced or withdrawn.

I saw this myself in the United Kingdom when I interviewed and accompanied welfare fraud inspectors in the 1990s. Lisa Conyers shared information about the United States with me in an email. Conyers talked with social workers on Indian reservations (also in the 1990s). These social workers were required to look for items of clothing stored by boyfriends. Hence the phrase they commonly used: "shoes under the bed."

---

subsidized, 92 percent of children ages one to three are in day care—an extraordinary figure and far higher than in most other countries.

To sum up: some welfare states are, by their policies, encouraging single and broken parenting. It is pretty clear that these conditions tend to damage children. Other welfare states are encouraging day care, which is probably of declining quality and may also harm children depending on the quality and circumstances. Overall, to put it bluntly, welfare states are causing unhappiness for millions of children. These children are consequently doing less well at school. A higher proportion of them are becoming criminals, an outcome that ruins their own lives and damages the lives of others. And among adults, too, there is greater unhappiness and loneliness.

Sweden is a wonderful country, but frankly it is in denial about these findings. That is not to argue that the position in Japan is ideal either. There, the position of women is at the opposite extreme, and it surely unduly limits their ability to enjoy and enhance their lives. But the ideas in Japan about the importance of parental care are closer to the mark than are Sweden's. Of the three countries we looked at to begin with, Italy's way of parenting and caring for children seems closest to the best without necessarily being ideal. (See Box 6.5.)

The goal that many of us would probably like to aim for is some way to combine a sense of duty to the children we bring into the world with reasonable respect for the interests of adults. But this isn't easy. On one hand, we want women to be able to pursue careers as

Box 6.5
"CULTURALLY DEAF" TO CHILD ABUSE IN SINGLE MOTHER FAMILIES

Jeremy Sammut, research fellow at the Centre for Independent Studies in Sydney, noted in 2012 that Australia had failed to address the risks that lone, or single, parenting pose to the welfare of children. He wrote[a]:

According to the Australian Institute of Health and Welfare, "a relatively high proportion of substantiations [of reported child abuse and neglect] involved children living in lone mother families." The Australian Institute of Family Studies estimates that child abuse in such households is "about two and half times higher than would be expected given the number of children living in such families."

This problem was created by the Whitlam government when it introduced the single mothers' pension in 1973. This made it possible for women who did not work and did not have bread-winning husbands to raise children at taxpayers' expense. What has ensued is the rise of a dysfunctional underclass of welfare-dependent single mothers with a complex range of personal and social problems, including substance abuse, domestic violence, and an inability to properly parent children. . . .

But we are reluctant to admit this because telling the truth about "diverse" family structures is not politically correct. We are culturally deaf, as it were, to the fact that all "families" are patently not equal when it comes to securing the welfare of children.

---

[a] Jeremy Sammut, "Culturally Deaf to Causes of Child Abuse," *Ideas@TheCentre*, Centre for Independent Studies, April 20, 2012.

they may wish and to be independent. But on the other hand, children appear to benefit from receiving care from their mothers during their early years. Also, we might want to avoid encouraging single parenting by not offering taxpayers' money to subsidize it. In the short term, that means that more single mothers will go out to work and become unable to care for their infants as much as would be ideal.

"We know the statistics: that children who grow up without a father are 5 times more likely to live in poverty and commit crime; 9 times more likely to drop out of school; and 20 times more likely to end up in prison."

SOURCE: Barack Obama in 2008, when he was a candidate for U.S. president, quoted in Heather Mac Donald, "Chicago's Real Crime Story," *City Journal*, Manhattan Institute, Winter 2010, http://www.city-journal.org/2010/20_1_chicago-crime.html. Obama was elected and became president in 2009.

These problems are not easy to resolve. It is certainly desirable that marriage should reestablish itself as the overwhelmingly normal way to bring up children, but even here caution is required. It may not be necessary or respectful of human liberty to create subsidies for marriage. It is probably only necessary to remove as much as possible of the discrimination that exists in some countries against marriage in favor of single parenting. The financial and emotional advantages of marriage and the benefit to the children are clear. They have led people to marriage in the past and should be able to do so again. Marriage should not need government help—only the removal of policies that have undermined it.

This is a difficult area but, bearing in mind the experiences of different countries and the research, here are the policies I would suggest:

- Single mothers should be given no priority over married couples in the allocation of public housing.
- Single and married parents should be given a personal tax allowance for each child. This is better than a cash grant because it automatically encourages at least one parent to work.
- Social insurance (earned through contributions) should provide women—whether with a partner or not—with an income for the first three months after a child's birth.
- If a mother has no partner or husband and has not worked to gain insurance, she should be expected to pay for her own accommodations or else live with her parents. In cases of emergency need, she should be able to seek assistance from charities, subsidized by government, running hostels as in Wisconsin.
- Any state subsidies for day care should be matched by allowances for home care, including by family members. Otherwise, the state is incentivizing parents to have their children looked after by nonfamily members.
- Government subsidies for day care should not be extensive because they might unintentionally encourage single parenting.
- If a single mother works, some of the cost of day care should come from her income so that the natural incentive to prefer childcare provided by family members is not removed. This would also reduce the cost to taxpayers.

184

Some of these policies are normal in various countries. In other countries, they might be highly controversial. But in the end, most people believe the interests of children should have priority. The evidence is that they benefit from having their two natural parents married and with them. They want the loving care of their mother for a large part of their baby and infant years. Children, as Asta Leppä has said, are "staunchly conservative people."

7. "People Used to Be Grateful and Eager. Now the Attitude Is, 'I Want This. You Get It for Me.'"

The Effect of Welfare States on Behavior

It's 1953, and the biggest British sporting event of the year is the Cup Final soccer match between Bolton and Blackpool. Both sides have some of the country's best soccer players playing for them: Nat Lofthouse, for Bolton, is one of the greatest center forwards Britain has ever produced. Stanley Matthews, for Blackpool, is a brilliant right-winger who plays for England, too.

Bolton starts sensationally. Lofthouse scores within 90 seconds and Bolton builds on this beginning. With three-quarters of the match gone, Bolton leads 3–1.[1]

Then Stanley Matthews gets through on the right wing and sends a cross to Stan Mortensen, who scores. The Blackpool team keeps feeding the ball to Matthews because of his ability to dribble past other players. But Bolton is still ahead 3–2 with only two minutes left. Blackpool then gets an equalizer from a free kick. Finally, in injury time (extra time added to make up for time attending to injured players), with only seconds remaining, Matthews again gets through on the right wing and his pass leads to another goal. So Blackpool wins 4–3 at the last moment. It's a sensational game. But for Lofthouse, this must be a moment of great disappointment. How does he react?

If he were a typical modern English player, he would bury his head in his hands, absorbed in his own misery. But this is 1953. Behavior is different. Lofthouse and his fellow Bolton player Malcolm Barrass stand and applaud Matthews, the very man who has robbed them of victory.[2]

Let's go back a little further. It's 1936, and Adolf Hitler is the Führer and Reichskanzler of Germany. The Olympic Games are being held in Berlin, and Hitler wants them to demonstrate the superiority of the Aryan race. But Jesse Owens, a black track and field athlete from the United States, is stealing the show, winning gold in the 100 meters, 200 meters, and the 100-meter relay. He is also entered for the long jump.

In the qualifying heats, Owens commits a foul in his first attempt and comes up short in his second. He is allowed only three goes. If he fails in his last attempt, he will not be in the final. Luz Long, his greatest rival and a German, goes up to him. He suggests that Owens change his marks for the run up. Owens takes his advice and successfully qualifies. He then goes on to win gold, pushing Long into second place. [3]

What does Long do after being defeated, knowing that he himself had helped bring this about? He hurries over to Owens to be the first to congratulate him. Owens and Long run around the stadium together in a joint lap of honor.[4]

Such sporting behavior sometimes still occurs today. But it is surely more unusual. Behind it lies a certain idea of how people should behave. Sir Donald Bradman, considered by many to be the greatest cricket batsman who ever lived, described a part of it:

> When considering the stature of an athlete or for that matter any person, I set great store in certain qualities which I believe to be essential in addition to skill. They are that the person conducts his or her life with dignity, with integrity, courage, and perhaps most of all, with modesty. These virtues are totally compatible with pride, ambition, and competitiveness.[5]

But gradually a change has taken place. In cricket, it was certainly under way by the mid-1960s. That was when sledging made its first appearance in Australia. "Sledging" is the practice of insulting an opposing player to try to put him off his game. A typical tactic is to suggest that the batsman is useless. Another is to make a joke implying that the sledger has had sex with the batsman's wife.[6]

This was a distinct change. Sunil Gavaskar, another of the game's greats, said that in his early years in the game, there was some good-humored banter in key matches.

> But what was banter in days gone by—and which was enjoyed by everyone, including the recipient of it—today has degenerated to downright personal abuse. . . .
>
> I played more than one test match for my country [in fact, he played 125] with and against bowlers who took hundreds of wickets and there was hardly a word uttered in anger on the field. Yes, towards the end of my career I did get referred to a couple of times by a part of the female anatomy and, more than anger, it saddened me to hear that. [7]

188

Some players, such as Shane Warne, one of Australia's most talented spinners, have been proud of their insults. According to Warne, Merv Hughes, another bowler, claimed that a quarter of his wickets were due to sledging.[8] The idea that winning is of prime importance has been taking precedence over the idea that one should behave decently and honorably.

What about honesty in sports? Gary Sobers, another cricketing legend, used to tell the umpire if a ball he caught had bounced on the ground beforehand, with the result that an opponent who might have been declared out was not. He cared more about being honest than about winning. But the idea that one should be honest has faded. Gavaskar commented, "Thanks to the win-at-all-costs theory, appeals are made even though the fielders know that the batsman is not out. There is the other side, of course, where a batsman knows he is out but stays put."[9]

It is striking that those at the forefront of sledging and dishonesty have been from Anglo-Saxon countries: Australia, New Zealand, and Britain. Prominent players best known for opposing that behavior have been from India and the West Indies. Viv Richards from the West Indies, another all-time great, was infuriated by such behavior. When Hughes repeatedly stared him down after bowling in a match in the Caribbean, Richards finally snapped: "This is my island, my culture. Don't you be staring at me. In my culture we just bowl."[10] It is as if the Third World was trying to give the First World a lesson in manners.

Stories of cheating and insulting opponents have spread to many sports. Often the media do not condemn it. That shows how far the change in culture has penetrated. It has even reached the point at which television commentators congratulate players on their cheating. According to one American correspondent, "Complimenting players who trick a referee occurs in every televised NBA [National Basketball Association] game I have ever seen." Naturally, such attitudes are imitated by children. In middle schools, "basketball players train on how to move their body to make it look like they have drawn a foul." Or as one journalist put it, parents "encourage their prepubescent children in Little League to imitate Derek Jeter and Dewayne Wise and fake getting hit by a pitch."[11]

Some people may feel that the sporting gestures of previous generations were silly and misguided. They may think that sledging and cheating are fine and sensible—just part of the modern game. They make excuses such as "everyone does it and you would be a fool not to" or "the reason for the change is just the extra money now."

Stepping back a bit, it is worth recognizing that, at all times and places, people tend to accept what is normal. We are all swept up in the culture of our time. Many people resist the idea that their culture has deteriorated compared with an earlier generation even if the evidence is clear. That is understandable. But I would ask the reader to imagine that we are flying over time and space, trying to observe objectively. As we fly high above, we look down on different countries and cultures in past centuries. Look at how dramatically morals and attitudes have changed.

There are extraordinary contrasts. We see soldiers in the First World War on both sides showing astonishing courage and willingness to face death. We marvel at how they believed they were fighting in a great and glorious cause. The idea of honor keeps cropping up at various times but in different forms. We see aristocrats in the 17th century prepared to fight a duel to the death if their "honor" is impugned. During the reign of Henry IV of France perhaps 10,000 gentlemen died for their honor. The Chevalier d'Andrieux killed 70 men in duels before his 30th birthday.[12] Here the concept of honor seems to have a lot to do with asserting one's status, dignity, and courage.

This idea of honor has something in common with that of Japan in the 19th century and before. Samurai committed suicide—seppuku—if they felt they had been, or would be, dishonored. Again, it seems largely a matter of personal dignity achieved through courage. The Japanese concept of honor persisted into the Second World War. Allied troops in Burma watched in astonishment as a platoon of Japanese soldiers marched in good order into the river to commit suicide to avoid the "dishonor" of capture.[13] The ideas of "giving face" and "loss of face" have been a continuing part of life in East Asia to varying degrees. This concept of personal dignity has included the idea that losing one's temper is undignified.

A somewhat different concept of honor appears in *Othello*, first performed between 1601 and 1604. It includes such themes as doing one's duty, being faithful to one's spouse, courage, and honesty. One of the characters, Cassio, says, "Reputation, reputation, reputation! Oh, I have lost my reputation! I have lost the immortal part of myself, and what remains is bestial."

Two centuries later, 'honor' of another kind appears in *Pride and Prejudice*, published in 1813. One of the characters, Lydia Bennet, has an affair with George Wickham. Jane Austen takes it for granted that Lydia's whole life will be ruined as a result. In fact, the whole family's prospects will be destroyed. Obviously, that is a big contrast with many countries now.

Then there are some completely different systems of belief. If we go across to America in 1917, we find many Quakers refusing to serve in the First World War because they were opposed to all forms of violence. Several other religions have had embedded in them a duty to contribute money or goods to the religious order concerned or to the poor. In Britain, people had to contribute a 10th of their grain to the church. Among modern Mormons, the practice of giving a 10th of one's income remains strong today. In Islam, the prophet Mohammed initiated the *zakat*: money that had to be given by adherents to the poor. In these religions, two ideas seem to be combined: that one should give money as an act of piety—to honor God—and also as an act of kindness. One thing that has influenced believers to be virtuous has been a promise of paradise accompanied by a threat of hell, otherwise.

If we fly back further to the second century AD, we find the Roman aristocracy widely adopting an approach to life that we now call "stoicism." At an outpost of the Roman Empire, we find the emperor himself, Marcus Aurelius, writing down some of this philosophy: "So what is left worth living for? This alone: justice in thought, goodness in action, speech that cannot deceive, and a disposition glad of whatever comes, welcoming it as necessary, as familiar, as flowing from the same source and fountain as yourself."[14] It amounts to an ideal of personal behavior.

Let's swoop forward now to England in 1549. The *Book of Common Prayer* has just been published. The writing of it was guided by Thomas Cranmer, who had been made Archbishop of Canterbury by Henry VIII. It includes a powerful concept of mankind's sinfulness and, implicitly, an insistence that we humans should strive to do better. It includes these words: "We have left undone those things which we ought to have done and we have done those things which we ought not to have done, and there is no health in us."[15] It is hard to imagine a more unequivocal assertion of mankind's sinfulness.

Moving further ahead to 1973, we see the first showing of a L'Oréal advertisement with the tagline "Because I'm worth it."[16] We have gone from a Christian belief in original sin to an assertion of "original virtue" or worth.

The purpose of this journey has been to suggest that cultures, values, and even national characters can and do change. The Italians today bear little relation to Marcus Aurelius. Not many Frenchmen are now keen to fight duels to the death.

I want to suggest that in modern times—and in the course of only one or two generations—attitudes and behavior and so on have also changed or begun to change in some countries. The stories from soccer, athletics, cricket, and basketball at the beginning of the chapter illustrate part of the change that has taken place in some Anglo-Saxon countries from one set of attitudes to another. These are only anecdotes, of course. It is very difficult to prove such changes with objective statistics.

Let's look at another part of modern life. It is not that long ago, in 1946, that the American film *It's a Wonderful Life* had its premiere. The film celebrates a man who behaves kindly and decently. He sacrifices any chance of being famous or rich to do what is decent. Another film, *High Noon*, a classic western starring Gary Cooper, was first shown six years later. It praises a man for his courage in standing alone and facing likely death in a good cause.

Now let's fly forward to 2011. We find another American film in which very different behavior is treated as normal and acceptable. *Bridesmaids* is a comedy in which much of the behavior is mean and selfish. "Gross-outs" proliferate, including vomiting, farting, and defecating.[17] The *Inbetweeners Movie* is another comedy released the same year. A British film this time, it is about a group of teenagers who go on vacation in Greece to get drunk and have sex.[18] The movie shows an almost complete absence of kindness by any of the characters. Instead there are insults and humiliations. Both these films were popular. People who enjoyed them may think that it is ridiculous to take them seriously. They were comedies, not moral lectures. But all films, plays, and novels reflect something of the culture from which they spring, and they probably help spread that culture. The comedies of 60 or 70 years before, such as *Bringing Up Baby* with Cary Grant and Katharine Hepburn, had no such meanness or vulgarity.

I am suggesting that changes in sports and films reflect how to some degree our cultures, attitudes, and beliefs have changed over the past generation or two. If that is right, why has it happened?

There are plenty of possibilities: the development of feminism and women's rights, which, in turn, might perhaps have been encouraged by the reduction in the importance of the physical strength of men as agricultural work and military prowess have become less significant; the vast increase in wealth across the world; the advances of science and the possibly related decline of religion; improved medical techniques and hygiene, which, along with greater wealth, have increased life expectancy; improved contraception, reducing the degree to which women need be concerned about becoming pregnant as a result of sex. There are many candidates.

But one other factor that may have changed behavior in modern societies could be the development of welfare states. How could this work? In a variety of ways.

1. Welfare states → unemployment → crime?

I have argued (Chapter 2) that more people are unemployed because of welfare states. A number of studies indicate that unemployment causes alienation from the rest of society. Younger unemployed males, in particular, can feel resentment and anger. Their resentment may make them feel rebellious and believe that selfishly grabbing what they want is justifiable.

It is true that only a minority of people are unemployed at any one time. But a much bigger—and growing—part of the population has at one time or another been through this depressing and disaffecting experience. Unemployment rates are higher among the young, and young men are known to be more likely to behave antisocially than any other category of men or women.

The ultimate in alienated behavior is crime. Do the unemployed commit more crime? The bare figures are startling. In a study of British prisoners, two-thirds had been unemployed before their imprisonment (see Figure 7.1).[19] This correlation is strong, but it is not immediately clear which thing causes the other. Does being a criminal cause unemployment or the other way around or both? Previously convicted criminals certainly find it harder to get jobs because of their convictions. But does unemployment cause crime?

One indication of what is going on is what criminals themselves say. In one study, over half of prisoners said unemployment was a contributing factor leading to their crimes.

A study in France provides more rigorous evidence. The study looked at changes in unemployment in different areas to see whether rising unemployment led to a consequent increase in crime. It found that "increases in youth unemployment induce increases in crime" and that "this effect is causal for burglaries, thefts, and drug offences."[20] The use of the word "causal" in academic literature is notable because particularly good evidence is needed before the word is used. Normally a study says only that one thing is "correlated" with another. Meanwhile, another study of 402 districts in Germany

Figure 7.1
THE UNEMPLOYED ARE MORE LIKELY TO COMMIT CRIMES
PERCENTAGE UNEMPLOYED IN THE GENERAL POPULATION AND
PERCENTAGE UNEMPLOYED BEFORE IMPRISONMENT IN BRITAIN

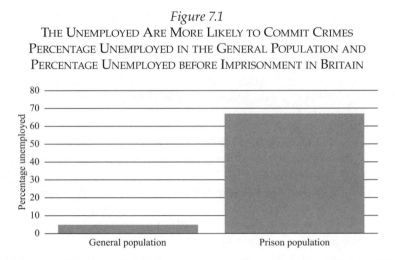

SOURCE: *Reducing Re-offending by Ex-prisoners*, U.K. Social Exclusion Unit, July 2002, http://www.bristol.ac.uk/poverty/downloads/keyofficialdocuments/Reducing%20 Reoffending.pdf..

found that youth unemployment "plays a prominent role in explaining property crime, namely housing burglary."[21] It is true that a causal relationship between unemployment and crime is not supported by all the different kinds of research, but the evidence that does support the idea is extremely strong.[22]

Torching cars has become a New Year's Eve tradition in France. On New Year's Eve 2013, it was considered good news that "only" 1,067 cars had been burned.

SOURCE: David Chazan, "'Only' 1,067 vehicles set ablaze on New Year's Eve in France," *Telegraph* online, January 1, 2014, http://www.telegraph.co.uk/news/worldnews/10546263/Only-1067-vehicles -set-ablaze-on-New-Years-Eve-in-France.html.

One unexpected finding of the research is that the unemployed seem more likely to be the victims of crime too, at least of violent crime. One study—albeit on a small scale and of only male-on-male homicide—found that 70 percent of murder and manslaughter victims were unemployed.[23]

Unemployment does indeed appear to lead to higher levels of crime. So welfare states that cause high unemployment are responsible for a higher level of crime than there would be otherwise. Moreover, crime is the tip of an iceberg of antisocial or uncivil behavior.[24]

2. Single parents and broken families → crime and uncivil behavior

I have also argued that some welfare states have caused more single parenting and broken families (see Chapter 6). I suggested that this has tended to damage the children in many ways and has made them more likely to turn to crime. Some of the statistics on this are dramatic.

A study of U.S. prisoners found that 43 percent had lived in a single-parent household for most of the time they were growing up, and a further 14 percent had lived in households with neither parent.[25] So a majority of prisoners had not spent most of their young years with both their parents. At the time, 1991, this was a big contrast with the average population in the United States. A national long-term study of youths subsequently found "Family background matters. Adolescents raised in families where both parents are present are much less likely to engage in crime."[26]

In Britain, one study found that more than a quarter of prison inmates (27 percent) had been placed in state child protection as a child—a stunningly high statistic considering what a small percentage overall is taken into state care.[27] And, again, family circumstances have been crucial because most times a child is taken into state care, he or she has not been living with both natural parents.[28]

There are some studies in which the significance of single parenting or broken homes appears as a relatively minor factor. However, such studies break down possible factors into multiple categories such as "poor parenting," "lack of parental controls," "lack of parental closeness," and suchlike. This can be misleading by minimizing the fact that these difficulties are more common among single parents.[29]

Some criminologists argue that the key factor explaining different levels of crime around the world and through history is the influence of others who lead people toward crime. That idea is entirely consistent with the theory that an intact family with both natural parents provides a strong influence against crime.[30]

Single parenting is, of course, only one factor. It would be remarkable if its effect could be detected in national crime figures. But just in case, I have looked at whether there is any correlation at all. I have had to use dates that are not ideal. The effect of unwed parenting should probably take at least 12 to 14 years to show through fully in crime levels, and suitable figures with a gap of that length are not at hand. Despite these obstacles, there is indeed a correlation between national rates of single parenting and rates of assault. The R squared figure—indicating the strength of the correlation—is only 0.235, which is relatively low. (See Figure 7.2.) But it is remarkable that there is any correlation at all.

Overall, to the extent that welfare states increase single or broken parenting, they cause crime to be higher than it otherwise would be. Again, it is likely that crime is an indicator of other

Figure 7.2
IS THERE A LINK BETWEEN SINGLE PARENTING AND CRIME?

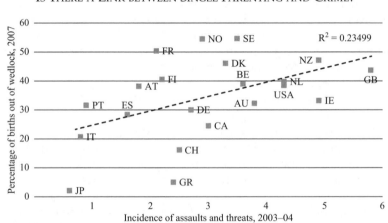

SOURCES: Jan van Dijk, John van Kesteren, and Paul Smit, *Criminal Victimisation in International Perspective* (The Hague: Boom Juridische Uitgevers, 2007), p. 81, http://unicri.it/services/library_documentation/publications/icvs/publications/ICVS2004_05report.pdf. This paper used crime prevalence figures for 2003–2004 and previous surveys. It also used figures from European Survey of Crime and Safety (2005 EU ICS).

For out of wedlock births: Organisation for Economic Co-operation and Development, *Doing Better for Families* (Paris: OECD Publications, 2011). Only advanced countries included. Scotland and Northern Ireland are excluded to avoid overemphasizing the United Kingdom.

NOTE: AT = Austria; AU = Australia; BE = Belgium; CA = Canada; CH = Switzerland; DE = Germany; DK = Denmark; ES = Spain; FI = Finland; FR = France; GB = Great Britain; GR = Greece; IE = Ireland; IT = Italy; JP = Japan; NL = Netherlands; NO = Norway; NZ = New Zealand; PT = Portugal; SE = Sweden; USA = United States.

antisocial behavior. One might add that, to the extent that welfare states encourage and implicitly approve of single parenting, they undermine the sense that parents previously had that they should stay together for the sake of the children. In other words, some welfare states discourage a sense of duty to children.

3. Poor-quality state education → crime and uncivil behavior

An astonishingly high proportion of children—18 percent—have been left functionally illiterate by their schools, as we saw in Chapter 4. I argued there that the remarkably common failure of government schools to teach children to read properly tends to lead to crime. I should add that some criminologists fiercely contest the idea that literacy is linked to crime. They suggest, for example, that criminals tend to be young males of a certain social background and that others from a similar background may be no more literate than the ones who end up in prison.[31] This kind of debate is difficult because so many factors are at work simultaneously.

An Irish study persuasively summed up its conclusions this way: "There is no suggestion that the relationship is a simple causal one. . . . However there is a considerable body of evidence showing that poor literacy skills restrict a range of life choices (particularly employment), and thus become a pre-disposing factor in criminal activities."[32]

If we were in a society in which it was easy to get and keep work despite being illiterate, there would be no reason for poor literacy to cause crime. That was the situation in the early 19th century and before. Now, though, literacy is necessary for most kinds of work. And nowadays, functionally illiterate children are legally required to stay at school even though they cannot follow what is being taught. Is it not inevitable that they become frustrated and irritated?

Tuggy Tug and his gang turned to crime and gang life as a way of getting the self-esteem that all of us seek.[33] Education and employment had been closed off to them mainly because a government school failed them. They had, as the Irish report put it, "a restricted range of 'life choices.'" In fact, Tuggy Tug was affected by all three factors mentioned so far: single parenting, unemployment, and a failed education. If you put these three together, the combination is social dynamite. Welfare states have increased the incidence of all of them.

There is a further way in which government schooling may have affected attitudes and behavior. In many countries it has come to be seen as dogmatic or wrong to teach children values. The idea is that children should discover them on their own. In the United States, this idea gained popularity in the so-called values clarification movement. As Jonathan Haidt has written, "Values clarification . . . urged teachers to refrain from imposing values on anyone. Although the goal of inclusiveness was laudable, it had unintended side effects. It cut children off from the soil of tradition, history, and religion that nourished older conceptions of virtue."[34]

Basic Training for the 20th Century English Gentleman

"If you can keep your head when all about you
Are losing theirs and blaming it on you,
If you can trust yourself when all men doubt you,
But make allowance for their doubting too;
If you can wait and not be tired by waiting,
Or being lied about, don't deal in lies,
Or being hated, don't give way to hating,
And yet don't look too good, nor talk too wise:"

The first verse of "If" by Rudyard Kipling, first published in Rewards and Fairies (London: Macmillan and Co., 1910). After all the "ifs," Kipling concludes, "Yours is the Earth and everything that's in it, And—which is more—you'll be a Man, my son!" The poem is in praise of uncomplaining courage, modesty, decency, self-reliance, and self-control.

The decision not to teach values has not happened everywhere, of course. When I visited the Gan Eng Seng primary school in Singapore, signs were hanging from the dining room ceiling with words in big letters such as "STRIVING," "RESILIENCE," and "AMBITIOUS," along with encouraging sentences such as "Happiness springs from doing good and helping others." Also, some schools still promote religions. In British private schools, some remnant of the values that were traditionally taught there in the past persist, some of which are captured in the Rudyard Kipling poem "If." It is fair to say, too, that some values are taught in schools now in place of the ones that have been dropped. They include racial and religious tolerance.

Some people object to religious schools. Others may not agree with the values promoted by the Singapore school. Yet others may not approve of the values of personal behavior that remain in British private schools. None of us is going to agree with all the values that have ever been taught in either government or independent schools. But it is Orwellian to have the state impose a uniform idea of values or beliefs on all schools. The only way to have variety and freedom in schools is for parents to have the power to choose which schools they want for their children. It seems possible, at least, that, given such a choice, parents would like schools that did esteem personal behavior such as politeness, consideration for others, perseverance, and suchlike.

4. Government interventions in housing → crime and uncivil behavior

Government housing also appears to have had a damaging effect on behavior. This operates in several ways.

First, government-built estates in many countries have become centers of crime and fear (see Chapter 5). In estates such as the ones I saw in Marseilles, one can see in action the theory of some criminologists that a major cause of crime is criminals influencing others to become criminal. In some estates, there is simply no choice but to join a gang.

Second, government housing in some welfare states contributes to unemployment (Chapter 5), which, in turn, encourages crime. Third, government planning controls have made housing far more expensive in some countries than it otherwise would be. Thus poorer people find it more difficult to buy reasonable housing, a situation that may contribute to crime.

The British Ministry of Justice analyzed where prisoners live before going to prison. It found that only 15 percent of the men and 7 percent of the women were owner-occupiers. So only a very small proportion of owner-occupiers commit crimes compared with the rest of the population. This finding does not prove the case, but it does suggest the possibility that home ownership discourages crime.

It is conceivable that the fact of owning a home gives a person a different psychological framework—a sense of having a stake in society and certain self-respect. The country with the highest rate of home ownership, Singapore, is also one with very low levels of crime, although, of course, other factors are also involved.

When young people convicted of crimes were interviewed for one study, more than a third said lack of accommodations was the factor most likely to lead them to reoffend.[35] And people who have served short prison sentences are two to three times more likely to reoffend if they do not have access to suitable housing.[36]

Housing matters. Housing that the poor can afford matters because we want the poor to have good lives, because it can affect unemployment rates, and because it may reduce crime. Unfortunately, government planning controls have made housing unnecessarily expensive in many countries.

5. Means-tested benefits, high taxes, and social security → dishonesty

Some welfare states have encouraged fraud on a massive scale. Kathryn Edin and Laura Lein found that all but one of 379 poor single mothers had a source of income in addition to their welfare benefits (Chapter 1). Most had incomes of a sort that should have been but were not reported to welfare benefit officials. Two of five were working but not reporting their income to the tax authorities. To put it bluntly, they were committing fraud. They knew it, too. That is why Edin found she got to the truth only after welfare recipients were interviewed several times over and convinced that they were not going to be reported.

If such fraud is widespread among recipients of other kinds of means-tested welfare benefits, this amounts to millions of people across the United States and in other countries. These are people who are simply trying to get by, but the circumstances they are in have led them to lie and cheat week by week, month by month, and even year by year.

There is cheating and lying among taxpayers, too. Taxpayers who have salaries from big companies or the government have little opportunity. But the self-employed and small businesses have plenty. They have a strong incentive because the costs of many welfare states have led to high tax and social security rates. I am not aware of research like Edin's on tax evasion, but anyone who has ever paid or received cash for work is aware that it is widespread. Fraud teams report that they detect tax evasion relatively easily. Proving it and mounting a prosecution is the time-consuming part.[37] In the United States, academics have estimated that 18 to 19 percent of income that should be reported isn't.[38] They also found that the rate of evasion has risen dramatically since the end of the Second World

Box 7.1
EXAMPLES FROM THE TOP

The first U.S. president:
"I can't tell a lie, Pa; you know I can't tell a lie. I did cut it with my hatchet."

—Reputed answer of George Washington, age six, when asked if he knew who had chopped down his father's favorite cherry tree. The story may be exaggerated, but for generations it was used to extol the virtue of honesty (see http://en.wikipedia.org/wiki/Parson_Weems).

A recent U.S. president:
"I want to say one thing to the American people. I want you to listen to me. I'm going to say this again. I did not have sexual relations with that woman, Miss Lewinsky. I never told anybody to lie, not a single time—never. These allegations are false. And I need to go back to work for the American people."

—Bill Clinton, January 1998. DNA taken from his semen later proved that President Clinton had misled "the American people." The change in American culture is reflected in the way President Clinton lied and even more in the way he was not wholly disgraced. Efforts were made to impeach him, but he continued in office and was treated with considerable respect in following years.

War. The rate of evasion is linked to the federal income tax rate and the amount of unemployment.

A reflection of this avoidance is the boom in black market economies (see Chapter 8). Many payments for services are being made in cash, evading both sales and value-added taxes and also income taxes. Again, this represents further millions of people who are, to be blunt, lying and cheating.

It seems likely that the more people lie, the less they feel ashamed of it. They come to feel, "Well, everybody else does it. Why should I be the one person who tells the truth?" (See Box 7.1.)

"As many as one-fourth of drivers in the state [California] are using disabled placards fraudulently."

SOURCE: CBS Los Angeles, "CBS2 Investigation Looks into Use of Disabled Parking Placards," CBS Los Angeles website, January 31, 2013, http://losangeles.cbslocal.com/2013/01/31/cbs2 -investigation-reveals-rampant-fraud-in-use-of-disabled-parking-placards. The placards provide for convenient, free parking.

6. State subsidies for single parenting and care for the elderly → the rise of entitlement and the death of duty

I am in Lower Hutt, a sunny little town in New Zealand. I have come to interview Erin McMenamin, the manager of Supergrans, a charity that advises people who are having difficulty coping. Mc-Menamin is a doughty character, the sort who says what she thinks but has a big heart too. I ask: what problems do the people she helps have? She tells me that some have simply never learned how to do things.

She tells me about mothers who can buy flour and vegetables at the store but have no idea what to do with them when they get home. They have never learned to cook. Others have no idea about budgeting or living economically by going to food banks and so on. A large proportion of her clients seem to be single mothers. Some have just escaped from—or need to escape from—a violent partner. She tells me that often "their own mums are young. They have no role models and no support. There is multigenerational ignorance."

I ask about the influence of welfare benefits, and she is typically frank. She says that some people like the lifestyle of not working. When a Supergrans counselor advises single mothers against having another baby, some reply, "If I don't have another baby, I'm going to have to go back to work!"

McMenamin has run Supergrans for a long time, so I ask how things have changed. She says violence and drugs have increased. "The ability to accept where they are has decreased. People used to be grateful and eager. Now the attitude is: 'I want this. You get it for me.'"

So does McMenamin feel less sympathetic than before? She says she is "totally" less sympathetic than when she started, but then the positive side of her nature revives and she adds, "but the better ones outweigh the bad ones—and the bad ones can be turned around."

McMenamin has seen a sense of entitlement develop that was not there before. It is difficult to prove that this has happened or that welfare states have caused it. But it is telling that someone who has been on the front line of welfare for so long has no doubt about it. Many welfare benefits are, indeed, legal entitlements. When people have these entitlements, it is understandable that they should come to think in terms of demanding them.

The psychology of this is different from earlier times when help might be requested from other family members or from a friendly society or charity. Then people probably felt a sense of duty to try to get back to being self-reliant again as soon as possible. But when people receive government money to which they are entitled, no sense of obligation is likely to be felt. There is no awareness that the money comes from other people, some of whom are not rich. The government is perceived as a kind of bottomless pit.

Another testimony comes from Dr. Richard Dumont, 12,000 miles away in Montpelier, France:

> I have seen a decline of politeness and an increase in incivility over the past two decades. When I started, there was what one could call respect for the white gown. Now everything has changed. Doctors, like nurses, too, regularly find themselves being verbally attacked for practically nothing.
>
> A classic scenario: someone describes to us minor symptoms and we ask them to make their own way to the hospital. But they have not got what they wanted, so they explode. The aggression ranges from saying, "I am going to come and smash your face in" to "arseholes," "buggers," or worse. Verbal violence has become routine.
>
> I think these people think of the emergency services as a right and that the moment we do not agree to their demands, they think they can do anything.

Across the channel, in Britain, it is not uncommon to see signs in public buildings such as hospitals and post offices saying that verbal or physical aggression against the staff will result in prosecution.

"Neither we nor our customers are here to be verbally or physically abused.

"Anti-social behaviour will not be tolerated. We will refuse to serve anyone who behaves in an unacceptable way."

Source: Typical sign in public buildings in England. This one was in Hammersmith Town Hall, London.

A sense of entitlement has increased in many countries accompanied by a willingness to complain. Meanwhile, at the other end of the spectrum of attitudes, the sense of duty has declined.

In previous generations, it was common for a couple—even one whose marriage had turned out to be disappointing—to stay together "for the sake of the children." This was thought of as a duty to the children, who should not be expected to pay for the mistakes of their parents. The idea of such a duty has dwindled. The welfare state has played some role in this change.

People used to feel a duty to care for their parents. But welfare states have undermined that sense of duty by assuming responsibility for aged people. As a result, more and more aged people live alone or in institutions in which they tend to be unhappier than they would be with, or close to, their adult children.

The very use of the word "duty" has declined. Patricia Greenfield, a professor at the University of California, Los Angeles, used Google's word count tool, Ngram Viewer, to examine a million books published in the United States between 1800 and 2000 and 350,000 books published in Britain. The use of the word "duty" declined by two-thirds over that time (see Figure 7.3).

It is likely that many reading these words will feel, "Yes, and a good thing too! What a relief to be liberated from the shackles of such an antiquated burden!" But the other side of a duty is a person who benefits. Yes, a duty to visit an aged mother might be a burden for the visitor. But the mother gains the pleasure and comfort of seeing a beloved child.

Figure 7.3

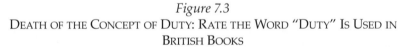

DEATH OF THE CONCEPT OF DUTY: RATE THE WORD "DUTY" IS USED IN BRITISH BOOKS

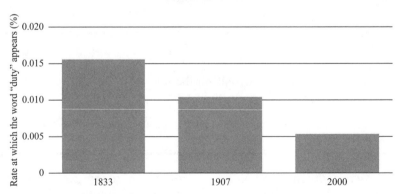

SOURCE: Patricia M. Greenfield, "The Changing Psychology of Culture from 1800 through 2000," *Psychological Science* 24 (2013): 1722–32.

"He every now and then, with evident increase of pain, made a greater effort with his vocal powers, and pronounced distinctly these last words: 'Thank God, I have done my duty'; and this great sentiment he continued to repeat as long as he was able to give it utterance."

SOURCE: From the account by Dr. William Beatty, the ship's surgeon, of the last hours of Admiral Lord Nelson, who was mortally wounded during the Battle of Trafalgar in 1805. Nelson's words reflect the importance he gave to the concept of duty. See http://www.mytimemachine.co.uk /trafalgar.htm.

In France, Pierre Garello, an academic, remarked to me, "France is a very centralized country, but the people are very individualist." By "individualist" the French often mean something akin to self-centered or even selfish. It may be no coincidence that France is both centralized and individualist. It makes perfect sense that, if a centralized government is taking all the decisions about how society is run, the only thing left for the individual to be worried about is his or her own personal interest. Direct, person-to-person kindness is crowded out. The idea of being a civil individual—looking out for others and society generally—is made pointless.

Another possible effect of welfare states may be to lower expectations of one's own behavior and resourcefulness. People may have become so used to the state's providing and deciding things that their confidence in their own ability to fend for themselves or assist others has been reduced.

The idea that one's self-esteem should be based on an idea of oneself as an honorable person who does his or her duty—a concept expressed by people as far apart in cultures as Emperor Marcus Aurelius and Rudyard Kipling—has been under attack. From my own experience in Britain, I know that concepts such as sinfulness, wrong, duty, decency, and honor all existed during my childhood in the 1950s and 1960s. They rarely figure in discussion today. People now expect little of themselves in terms of self-denial and duty. They feel that they have a "right" to do what pleases them. They do not feel shame at their own behavior. "Shame" is another word that has fallen into disuse.

Does this really matter? Perhaps it just seemed a better world to live in when people wanted to do the right thing, to do the best for their country rather than the best for their political career; to do the

right thing by their wives or husbands rather than to leave them because a new lover was more exciting—when there was more reason
to trust one's fellow human beings.

* * *

I have suggested six ways in which welfare states have tended
to change—and usually damage—attitudes and behavior, the real
stuff of a civilization. The routes have been through unemployment,
single parenting, illiteracy, housing, means-tested benefits combined
with high taxes, and the undermining of personal responsibility. In
some cases the evidence is clear. In others, it is hard to prove, but
the logic is there for those willing to follow it. All in all, the effect of
some welfare states, at least, on the spirit, culture, and behavior of
people has been damaging.

Before leaving the subject, let me respond to an objection to this
line of argument that is perfectly reasonable. If welfare states give
so much encouragement to crime and incivility, as I have suggested,
why have the crime figures been falling?

Overall levels of crime have indeed been falling around the
world. Some of the reported drops are astonishing. In New York
City, car thefts have fallen 93 percent.[39] There used to be 500 or
so robberies of banks, building societies (housing loan organizations), and post offices a year in Britain in the 1990s. In 2012, there
were a mere 69.[40] The old-fashioned bank robber is going out of
business. The world appears to be becoming a more law-abiding
place, and governments in several countries have boasted about
how their policing policies have made their countries safer. They
are sometimes irritated when members of the public, in surveys,
say they are still afraid of crime.

Why should crime suddenly be falling? Are people genuinely
more respectful of the law? Are they behaving better? Or is something else going on?

The fall in crime has thrown up a great range of explanations.
Each has its group of intelligent academic supporters (see Box 7.2).

Let's take one of the more common explanations for the fall in
crime: improved defenses against crime through technology and
increased private security. If this is the true cause, it is possible that
the underlying tendency toward crime or willingness to commit it
has not fallen at all. It might even have risen.

Box 7.2
WHY HAS REPORTED CRIME GONE DOWN?
SOME OF THE POSSIBLE EXPLANATIONS

- **The rise of private security**. The number of security guards in Europe increased 90 percent in 10 years. They now outnumber police officers. Cars are fitted with electronic security devices that make them more difficult to steal. The proportion of British households with a burglar alarm rose by half to 29 percent between 1995 and 2011. Bulletproof partitions have been introduced in banks. Video recorders have been installed in shops and in many other places.
- **New technology that has improved policing**. It is now impossible to walk down many city streets without being monitored by a video camera. DNA testing means it is easier to prove someone was at the scene of a major crime. "Predictive" policing has had some success in sending police officers to where trouble is likely.
- **Aging populations**. Young men are the most likely people to commit crimes and as a proportion of the population, their numbers have been decreasing.
- **Reduced lead in gasoline**. The idea might sound absurd but the evidence is surprisingly good.[a]
- **Increased imprisonment**. Increased imprisonment rates per crime committed have been followed by lower crime levels in some countries, and vice versa.[b] However, this idea is fiercely contested.
- **Increased confidence in the rule of law**. A long-term trend over centuries has resulted in people's relying more on the state to enforce justice rather than trying to enforce it themselves.
- **Increased wealth**. Increased wealth is correlated to lower crime levels and may have played a part.
- **Reduction in the number of valuable, easily stolen items**. Thieves used to steal DVD players, but now that they only cost £25 (about $36),[c] they are not worth the trouble and danger. More people have bank accounts and credit cards, so they keep less cash in the home or in their pockets.

---

[a] Kevin Drum, "America's Real Criminal Element: Lead," *Mother Jones*, January/February 2013, http://www.motherjones.com/environment/2013/01/lead-crime-link-gasoline.
[b] David G. Green, "Crime Reduction Factsheet. How Can We Reduce Reoffending by Known Criminals—The Overseas Evidence," http://www.civitas.org.uk/pdf/CrimeReductionFactsheet.pdf.
[c] For the purposes of this book, 1 pound = 1.42 dollars (exchange rate in March 2016.).

The biggest declines have been in property crimes. Those are the sorts of crime most likely to be affected by new technology. Cars are now much more difficult to steal than before. Car thefts have consequently fallen dramatically, but clearly that does not necessarily reflect any improvement in honesty.

The use of video surveillance—closed-circuit television (CCTV) cameras—has soared. It seems that the first town to use a video camera may have been Olean, New York, in 1968.[41] From that small beginning, the use of the cameras has exploded. In the United Kingdom in 2011, it was estimated that there were 1.85 million cameras in use and that the average person on a typical day would be seen by 70 cameras.[42]

Similarly, there has been a rapid growth in the number of private security personnel, mostly security guards. In Canada in 2006, there were more private security personnel than police officers—three for every two, in fact.[43] In the European Union, it has been calculated that the number of security guards jumped by two-thirds in only eight years, between 1999 and 2007. The number rose from 600,000 to "well over" one million.[44]

What about crimes against people?

The most reliable evidence comes from victimization surveys, in which people are asked about crimes they have experienced recently, such as over the past year. The only truly international survey suggests a mixed picture. In some countries, including the United States and Germany, the number of assaults went down between 1989 and 2003–2004. In others, including England and the Netherlands, they went up. (See Figure 7.4.) We should note that any increases are in

Figure 7.4
ASSAULTS APPEAR TO BE INCREASING IN SOME COUNTRIES
PERCENTAGE OF PEOPLE WHO SAID THEY WERE ASSAULTED OR "THREAT-
ENED IN A WAY THAT REALLY FRIGHTENED" THEM IN THE PREVIOUS YEAR

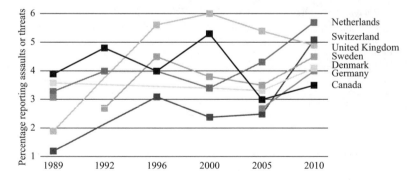

SOURCE: Jan van Dijk, "The International Crime Victims Survey: Latest Results and Prospects," *Criminology in Europe* 11 (2012): 24–33, http://www.esc-eurocrim.org /newsletter/Dec12ESCnewsletter.pdf.

the face of the spread of security cameras and the vast increase in private security guards. More recent international survey figures, for 2010, only allow long-range comparisons for seven advanced countries, but assaults actually increased in six of them: Denmark, Germany, the Netherlands, Sweden, Switzerland, and the United Kingdom. The only exception was Canada.

The United States has a long run of crime statistics that suggests that the incidence of all forms of crime, including violence against other people, has gone down.[45] These figures suggest a peak between 1980 and 1990 and a substantial fall since. However, the latest levels of reported robbery and aggravated assault are still dramatically above the levels in 1960 when the statistics begin. The rate of aggravated assault is more than two and half times higher than it was in 1960 (see Table 7.1).

Table 7.1
VIOLENT CRIME HAS FALLEN BUT IT IS STILL MUCH HIGHER
THAN IN THE EARLY 1960S AND BEFORE
ROBBERIES AND AGGRAVATED ASSAULTS PER
100,000 PEOPLE IN THE UNITED STATES

Year	Robberies	Aggravated assaults
1960	60.1	86.1
1965	71.7	111.3
1970	172.1	164.8
1975	220.8	231.1
1980	251.1	298.5
1985	209.3	304.0
1990	256.3	422.9
1995	220.9	418.3
2000	145.0	324.0
2005	140.8	290.8
2010	119.3	252.8
2011	113.7	241.1

SOURCE: "State-by-State and National Crime Estimates by Year(s)," U.S. Uniform Crime Reporting Statistics, http://www.bjs.gov/ucrdata/Search/Crime/State/Run CrimeStatebyState.cfm. These data are "offenses known to law enforcement" and are not based on victim studies.

Despite substantial falls in overall crime in many countries, the reduction only takes us back to where we were three or four decades ago. Compared with the 1950s or 1930s, most advanced countries remain dramatically more crime ridden.

Looking over the evidence, I would suggest that a rough summary of the history of crime might go like this: Over the centuries, crime appears to have fallen. But the second half of the 20th century saw a remarkable rally. The timing varied somewhat from one place to another. Afterward, property crimes fell, but crime against people did not fall much or even at all in a number of countries.[46]

I would suggest that the role of welfare states in this may have been to contribute to the major rally in the second half of the 20th century. And subsequently, it may cause crime now, especially crimes against the person, to be higher than it otherwise would be. We might also note that among the many ideas that attempt to explain falling overall crime, one is absent. I have seen nowhere the suggestion that the decrease in crime occurred because people have become more decent and honest.

All this is without counting a category of crime that is not recorded even in victim surveys. People do not report crimes they are committing themselves. Surely there has been a vast expansion of fraud in claiming welfare benefits and declaring taxable income.

Have all welfare states had a similar impact on attitudes and behavior? No. Not all welfare states are the same. Not all encourage single parenting to the same extent. Not all have created crime ghettoes in public housing. The incentive to lie about income is much less strong in countries where tax and social insurance payments are lower.

It follows that the impact of welfare states on levels of crime, antisocial behavior, and attitudes has varied considerably. Britain has unfortunately made most of the mistakes that can be made. In the first half of the 20th century, it was a country whose people, rich and poor, were internationally admired for their behavior. Sadly, those days are gone.[47] Other countries have suffered similar effects, but Britain acts as a warning of just how much a nation can be changed by a welfare state.

We should also acknowledge that the people whose behavior and happiness have been most affected by welfare states are the ones who have been most in contact with them and most dependent on them: the less well off. This helps explain an increased division between the poor and the rest— a "coming apart" as Charles Murray has called it.[48] Only less well-off women receive welfare benefits or subsidized housing as a result of divorce or separation. Accordingly, the breakdown of marriage has been most widespread among the less well off. Only those poor enough to claim means-tested benefits have had an incentive to lie or have been discouraged to work. Only those with a low ability to earn have been tempted by benefits to be unemployed instead. To be in a position in which one has an overwhelming temptation to avoid regular work, to lie about income or wealth, and to do informal, unrecognized work instead is a miserable condition for a society to put any of its members in.

The advantage of the continental systems, where most benefit payments are insurance payments, is that there is less incentive to lie about one's means. However, the drawback is that social insurance contributions can be so big that people are again prone to working in the black market to avoid paying them. It is true that the better off also have an incentive to lie, to evade income tax. But most of them are employed by companies or governments and have little scope to do so.

"Watching the ever-increasing costs of the welfare state in Britain and Sweden, we decided to avoid this debilitating system. We noted by the 1970s that when governments undertook primary responsibility for the basic duties of the head of a family, the drive in people weakened. Welfare undermined self-reliance. People did not have to work for their families' well-being. The hand-out became a way of life. The downward spiral was relentless as motivation and productivity went down. People lost the drive to achieve because they paid too much in taxes. They became dependent on the state for their basic needs."

SOURCE: Lee Kuan Yew, *From Third World to First: The Singapore Story, 1965–2000* (New York: HarperCollins, 2000). Lee Kuan Yew was prime minister of Singapore, 1959–90.

All of us, though, are affected by the changes of behavior and attitudes in our society. We are influenced by people we meet. If we come across rudeness and cheating, we are more likely to do the same. Where divorce and single parenting are commonplace, people think it is normal and therefore find nothing wrong or regrettable about it. None of us is immune to the influence. The more cheating there is in sports, the more everyone accepts it. Once a critical mass of people accept the idea that winning is more important than behaving decently, it is difficult for anyone to stand out against that view.

Most of us would agree that these changes in behavior and attitudes are undesirable. We would rather live in a society in which there is less crime and antisocial behavior, in which everyone—not only those in particular parts of town—feels safe walking in the street at night, cars are not torched, and gangs do not terrorize the neighborhood, and in which everyday politeness and consideration are normal. We would prefer a society in which people can trust each other and in which they give and receive help from each other as family or friends. Welfare states have shown a tendency to undermine this kind of society (Figure 7.5). In this way, they have diminished our civilization.

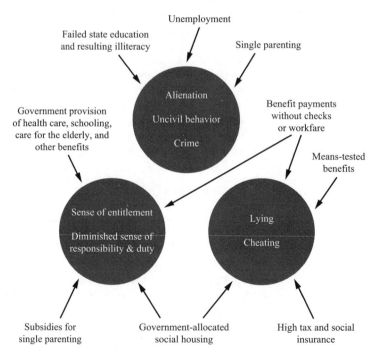

Figure 7.5
HOW WELFARE STATES UNDERMINE SOCIETY

It may seem a Herculean task to try to reverse such tendencies. It may seem pointless even to suggest ways to improve things. Yet there are tasks that can be done. One can at least try simply to remove, as much as possible, the elements of welfare states that have caused the problem. Here are some possibilities:

- Means-tested benefits should have the smallest possible role because they create a temptation to lie.
- Levels of taxation should be as low as possible for the same reason.
- Social insurance should go into personal savings plans rather than to general government income. That way people have less reason to lie about their income.
- Welfare benefits should be kept down to a level at which it is always worthwhile for low-paid employees to work.
- Any special housing or cash benefits for single parents that are not also available to couples should be minimized so that the natural disincentives to single parenting are not reduced too much.
- Single parents should be expected to go to their families for accommodations and support before pursuing government support.
- Diverse, independent schools should be the norm to improve literacy and enable the teaching of a variety of values rather than a uniform dogma or absence of values imposed by government.

It is no good pretending that measures such as these would have an immediate impact. Cultures take years and decades to change. This would only be a start.

8. Not to Be Read by Anyone under the Age of 40

Pensions and Their Unexpected Consequences

I am in Warsaw hurriedly walking along Świętokrzyska Street to get to a meeting. I can see in the middle of the square nearby the extraordinary monster-building given by the Soviet Union to "the people of Poland" but not received with universal pleasure. It is in communist-gothic style with curious details reminiscent of gargoyles.

After a while, I reach some dignified streets from the 19th century and then Krakowskie Przedmieście, a wide main road. On the other side is the presidential palace. I am going to meet a government official but, to be embarrassingly honest about it, as I rush from one appointment to another, I sometimes have not had time to investigate exactly who I am going to see. I know this person is someone working for the government on social security, but I am not entirely sure what she does.

The presidential palace is grand: a wide, elegant, white building of classical design. I tell the guard at the gate who I am going to see and am directed to a particular entrance. I cross a parade ground and go to the door indicated. I am immediately confronted by security procedures like those at an airport but on a smaller scale.

That done, I am told to wait in a small area with a few chairs. Soon, a woman comes down and invites me to follow her back up some stairs. The decor is in a traditional style. She leads me along a corridor and into a large, high-ceilinged room. But this turns out to be just an anteroom. We continue on to the far side, to an impressively solid wooden door. She knocks and we go in. She introduces me to "the minister."

I feel a fool for not having realized I would be meeting someone so senior. The minister is Irena Wóycicka, a woman with severe black hair and bright intelligence.[1] She stands to greet me then goes to sit on an Empire chair behind a massive wooden desk. Friendly and efficient, she quickly assesses my lack of knowledge of the subject and briskly proceeds to tell me a little horror story.

It started long ago, before the Second World War. The Polish copied the kind of social insurance pioneered in Germany by Bismarck. Contributory programs were created covering pensions and other elements of social security for various trades or professions.

During the war, Poland was invaded by both Germany and the Soviet Union. By the end of it all, the Soviets had installed a communist government. This government unified all the different social security programs under its control. The program became, as the minister remarks, "very huge."

An innocent from Britain or America might assume that this very huge system involved large amounts of assistance to the poor and unemployed. But no. Unemployment wasn't the big cost. "Employment was mandatory," the minister crisply explains. So what became very huge?

As the postwar baby boom generation grew up, despite the mandatory employment, there was a lack of jobs for people to do. The government thought that the way to deal with this problem was to get older people to stop working and let younger ones take their jobs. They encouraged older workers to retire early by offering attractive terms. Wóycicka adds, rather defensively, that this sort of tactic was adopted in a number of countries around the world, which is perfectly true. There was a widespread idea that older workers should not keep jobs from young people setting out in life. But Poland seems to have taken the idea further than most. The result was that the cost of pensions was inflated by early retirement on notably generous terms. So pensions became a major component of government spending.

Then things got worse. The communists were ejected from power in 1989. It was an extraordinary time. The new minister of finance, Leszek Balcerowicz, was a radical who loathed communism and appreciated capitalism as only someone who has lived under communism knows how. He masterminded what became known as "shock therapy"—a sudden break with fixed prices and top-down economic control.

Wóycicka remarks that this time of national upheaval would not have been a good moment to change the social security system. In fact, benefits were indexed to maintain their real value. But one result of the big changes in the Polish economy was an increase in unemployment and fear of unemployment. Unemployment benefits were small. So people migrated to where the benefits were bigger: disability pensions and retirement pensions. The cost of both ballooned.

Wóycicka remarks drily, "Poland and the Netherlands were the two champions of disability"—meaning they both had burgeoning numbers of people claiming disability benefits. Naturally, a variety of countermeasures were adopted. The government imposed "bigger control of doctors," benefits ceased to be indefinite, and benefit recipients were checked out every three years. Poland also became a "pensions champion."

The government was determined not to get into unsustainable debt, so the only way to pay for this was dramatically to increase contributions. Total social insurance contributions jumped from 23 percent of wages to 45 percent! The burden on employees was extreme. Naturally, some reforms were made to try to reduce the problem. In 1999, the rules were changed so that, in the future, pensions would be based on contributions instead of salaries. Also, some pension contributions began to be invested in real assets, a "funded" system. But the latter was expensive because, if contributions went into actual investments, then they were not available to pay the pensions of people already retired. More recently, the amount going into funded pensions has been reduced.

It has been proposed that the retirement age should be raised by three months every year. Another proposal is that the women's retirement age should be raised in line with that of men. But raising retirement ages causes a lot of opposition. Eighty percent of the population is against it, Wóycicka says. Nevertheless, as a result of all the measures that have been and are being taken, the cost of Polish pensions is forecast to fall in relation to the size of the economy.

Well, that's good news, certainly. But I leave the minister and the presidential palace with the impression that the government is grappling with a massive problem.

Exactly how big is it? In 2005, the cost of paying government pensions in Poland amounted to 11.4 percent of all economic activity—a staggeringly high proportion.[2] But if that still does not sound like much, let us put it another way. Pensions amounted to more than a quarter of all Polish government spending in 2007—more than twice as much as in Great Britain, the United States, or the Netherlands.

Leaving the presidential palace, I walk along Krakowskie Przedmieście, bustling with cars and trams, and head in the direction of the historic center. I pass Warsaw University, cross a big intersection, and eventually reach a quieter street, Nowy Swiat, lined with traditional shops. At last, I reach my destination: Blikle. This is a charming Polish version of the coffee houses of Vienna but more elegant than most of them with white tablecloths and uniformed staff. This is where two women, Aleksandra Wiktorow and Zofia Czepulis-Rutkowska, have told me to meet them.

They arrive and settle onto a cozy banquette while I sit opposite them. They are friendly and cheerful. Wiktorow is a comfortable, smiling woman who used to have a senior government job. Czepulis-Rutkowska, who speaks better English, clearly has had government experience, too. In the course of our convivial meeting, I ask if they can explain more about the Polish pension horror story.

In the battle to contain the exploding cost, they tell me, pensions stopped being linked to wages. Instead, they were linked to prices, which normally rise more slowly. But at one time, even this was damaging because wages fell. Another ploy was to stop indexing some of the extra money being paid to specially privileged groups such as miners, teachers, construction workers . . . the list seemed long.

Speaking of privileges, they say, do I know about the retirement age for policemen? No. In 1995, they were given the right to retire at the age of 35. Not to be outdone, the military soon obtained the right to retire at 35, too.

"This must have been a great victory for the trade unions," I say.

"Oh no! It was not the trade unions."

Wiktorow and Czepulis-Rutkowska explain that the extraordinarily low retirement ages were negotiated by high-ranking police and military officers. A new government was in power that wanted support from the police and army. It also wanted votes. The support and votes of police officers, soldiers, and generals were effectively bought by committing other people's money for years to come.

"The retirement age for Greek jobs classified as 'arduous' is as early as 55 for men and 50 for women. As this is also the moment when the state begins to shovel out generous pensions, more than 600 Greek professions somehow managed to get themselves classified as 'arduous': hairdressers, radio announcers, waiters, musicians, and on and on and on."

Source: Michael Lewis, "Beware of Greeks Bearing Bonds," *Vanity Fair*, October 1, 2010, http://www.vanityfair.com/business/features/2010/10/greeks-bearing-bonds-201010.

At this point, some readers may be thinking, "This does sound shoddy, but is it really so bad? Does anyone suffer as a result?" Let's look at the consequences of the generous early pensions granted in the past and the exceptionally generous pensions of certain government employees.

Money has to be found to pay for these pensions, and it comes from social insurance. Let's look at someone who pays for them. Take someone employed at a cost to his employer of £11,800 (about $16,760) a year.[3] That figure is after including his employer's social insurance. After the social insurance is removed, the pay of the employee comes down to £10,000 ($14,200) a year, which is a little above the national average.[4] From this amount, the employee's social insurance contributions must be taken, bringing his income down to £8,250 ($11,715). Then there is taxation, which further reduces the take-home pay to £6,750 ($9,585). There is clearly a big drop from the £11,800 cost to the employer down to the £6,750 in the worker's pocket. It is a major wedge (see Chapter 2).

Imagine the frustration in, say, a small town where the boss of a carpentry workshop employs a teenager he has known all his young life. The worker would obviously like more cash in his pocket and the boss is tired of paying a fortune to what probably looks like the bottomless pit of social insurance. Would it not be tempting for him to say, "Well, Dominik, how about I pay you half the money officially and then put the rest directly in your pocket? That way we both gain"? If you think that might be the case, you will not be surprised that the World Bank estimates that the underground economy in Poland amounts to 26 percent of all economic activity.[5]

Of course, not everyone has the opportunity to work for cash on the side. A major company can't do this. But major companies are affected too. A Polish business's rival in Hong Kong, say, can pay lower wages yet still have better-paid employees. Therefore, the company is able to offer products at better prices than the Polish business can, and so it grows, benefiting the Hong Kong economy and all who live there. Such growth passes Poland by.

The Polish situation is unfair too. Money earned by the worker is going to someone else's pension. The current worker will certainly not get anything like a reasonable return on his pension contributions. He could even make a loss. Why? Because the pensionable age is bound to be pushed up. The amounts paid in pensions will have to be subtly reduced compared with national income. Only in such ways will the vast burden of pensions be managed, especially given the fact that people in Poland, as everywhere, are living longer. It all amounts to a kind of theft perpetrated by those who are now retirees against current workers.

To put it bluntly, the postwar generation voted for itself big and early pensions, sometimes with outrageous privileges, and thus it guaranteed that the current generation of workers would be saddled with national debt and pensions with low returns. How should this be seen? Irresponsible? Selfish? As an example of how democracy can be the enemy of justice? Doubtless when the generous pensions were created they were depicted as wonderful, perhaps even rather heroic. They turned out to be plain greedy.

As I leave the charm of the Blikle café and my two genial companions, the burden of Polish pensions seems worse still. I have the impression, though, that the Polish pensions disaster is an extreme case—the unfortunate result of particular circumstances.

Later, I look at the figures for other countries. I discover that Poland is not unique. It is not even the worst case. The cost of pensions amounts to over one-tenth of national output in Poland. In Greece it amounts to 11.9 percent. But Greece is not the worst case either. Pensions amount to an eighth of output in France. But the worst case of all is Italy. The cost is a staggering 14.1 percent of gross domestic product (GDP). In Italy, pensions absorb 29.4 percent of all government spending, crowding out many other spending areas.

Figure 8.1 and Figure 8.2 show plenty of major countries with big pension burdens, but they also show countries with much smaller ones.

I can imagine some people still thinking, "Well, yes, I can see that pension spending has ended up higher than intended in plenty of countries. Clearly some economies are needed. But it is all manageable, isn't it? I'm still not convinced that much harm has been done." What are the real consequences?

1. Current workers are going to get a poor return on their pension contributions.

Poland is an example of a common problem. Europe will simply be unable to pay the pensions it has promised. Pension obligations in 19 of the European Union member countries are about five times

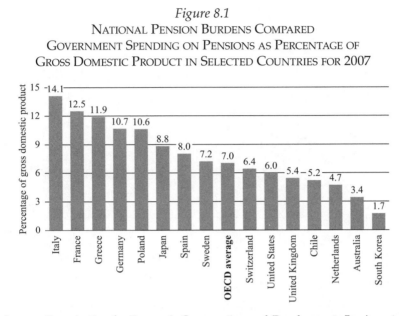

Figure 8.1
NATIONAL PENSION BURDENS COMPARED
GOVERNMENT SPENDING ON PENSIONS AS PERCENTAGE OF
GROSS DOMESTIC PRODUCT IN SELECTED COUNTRIES FOR 2007

SOURCE: Organisation for Economic Co-operation and Development, *Pensions at a Glance 2011: Retirement-Income Systems in OECD and G20 Countries* (Paris: OECD Publishing, 2011), p. 155.

their official gross debt, according to a study commissioned by the European Central Bank.[6]

Europe has the highest proportion of people over age 60 in the world, and the proportion is going to rise dramatically, from 22 percent of the population in 2009 to 35 percent by 2050.[7] The situation is "totally unsustainable," according to Jacob Kirkegaard, a research fellow at the Peterson Institute for International Economics in Washington, D.C.[8] And like any genuinely unsustainable situation, it will not be sustained. The money will not be paid. People currently working will not receive the incomes in retirement that they are theoretically expecting. Younger people will get less or will be paid starting at a later age or both.

The Organisation for Economic Co-operation and Development (OECD), referring to its member countries generally, says, "Many pension reforms will result in large cuts in benefit levels at a given retirement age and might risk a resurgence in old-age poverty."[9]

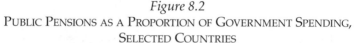

Figure 8.2

PUBLIC PENSIONS AS A PROPORTION OF GOVERNMENT SPENDING,
SELECTED COUNTRIES

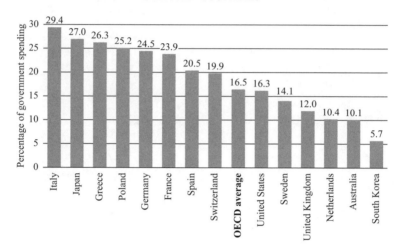

SOURCE: Organisation for Economic Co-operation and Development, *Pensions at a Glance 2011: Retirement-Income Systems in OECD and G20 Countries* (Paris: OECD Publishing, 2011), p. 155.

Furthermore, "Half of OECD countries are already increasing pension ages or will do so." It amounts to a betrayal of promises given to people by governments. But that is not the end of it: "However, most of these hard-won increases [in pension ages] will be outpaced by increases in life-expectancy."[10] In other words, even the cutbacks announced or expected will not be enough (see Box 8.1).

According to Richard Jackson, a specialist in the field, stabilizing government spending on pension payments as a share of GDP would necessitate cutting benefits "in almost every developed country" by between 30 and 60 percent.[11] Yet "workers remain highly dependent on public pensions and entirely unprepared for large benefit reductions." He wrote these words in 2000. Pensions in many countries have been cut back since then, so it is worth looking at his more recent views. According to his most recent estimates, the cost of maintaining the current generosity of pension programs would add an extra 7 percent to government budgets by 2030.[12]

Box 8.1
PENSIONS: FROM CAUTIOUS TO IRRESPONSIBLE

When government pensions were first created in Germany under Bismarck, life expectancy was barely 40 years, and you had to wait until you were 70 to get a small pension. Since then, German life expectancy has almost doubled, but the pensionable age has been reduced to 65 and the value has been increased.[a] A policy that was cautious became irresponsible, presumably because politicians sought votes without caring about the consequences.

Governments are continually "surprised" by the degree to which life expectancy rises. To be surprised once or twice might be forgivable, but the surprise is perennial.

As a result, the reductions in the value of pensions in many countries have been dramatic. For example,

"The pension reforms of 2001 radically changed the German pension system, reducing the generous replacement rate from approximately 70 percent of final salary to a predicted 52 percent by 2030," according to Johan De Deken, assistant professor, Department of Sociology, University of Amsterdam.[b]

---

[a] Dr. Oliver Hartwich, "Fix the Super Roof while the Sun Is Still Shining," *Insights* (New Zealand Initiative), June 15, 2012, http://nzinitiative.org.nz/Media/Insights/June+2012/June+2012.html?uid=49.
[b] Johan de Deken, "Pension Reforms in Germany: Can Occupational and Private Pensions Compensate for the Erosion of Social Insurance?" *Aegon Global Pensions View*, March 2013.

In a desperate attempt to fulfill promises made, younger workers of today and the next generation will be required to pay more money. It does not matter whether the bill is paid through social insurance or tax, it amounts to the same thing: an even bigger subsidy of one generation by the next and with even more damaging results.

In Japan, the government has calculated that the early postwar generation will do perfectly well from the pension system but that those born later will fare worse and those born recently will do worst of all:

> Estimation results show that the net benefit rate is 1.0% for the generation born in 1950, −5.3% for the generation born in 1970 and −13.0% for the generation born in 2010. Thus, the younger generation suffers the larger net burden and intergenerational inequality should not be ignored.[13]

223

"The median ages of Western Europe and Japan, which were 34 and 33 respectively as recently as 1980, will soar to 47 and 52 by 2030, assuming no increase in fertility. In Italy, Spain, and Japan, more than half of all adults will be older than the official retirement age."

SOURCE: Richard Jackson, senior fellow at the Center for Strategic and International Studies. Testimony before the Commission on Security and Cooperation in Europe, June 20, 2011.

It is a kind of rolling rip-off by one generation of the next. In many countries, as in Poland, the postwar baby boom generation voted itself generous pensions. It allowed itself to believe that it was perfectly fine for each generation to fund the pensions of the generation before. Politicians and voters conveniently ignored the obvious fact that life expectancy was rising. They kept the retirement age unchanged. They ignored the fact that the ratio between the numbers of retired people and the numbers of active workers would be utterly transformed.

In France, as recently as 2012, President François Hollande carried through a preelection promise that made the situation even worse: he reduced the age at which people could receive pensions from 62 to 60. He reversed, at least in part, the modest reform of his predecessor, Nicolas Sarkozy. This action demonstrates how difficult it is in a democracy to push through sensible reform. Perhaps the people who happily voted for Hollande and for more money for their own pensions liked to imagine that this was a gain for all French people without consequences. Not so, according to the OECD: "If a pension system is financially unsustainable, the scale of changes needed in the medium or long term will be more sudden and painful."[14]

Despite the Canute-like gesture of President Hollande, the underlying reality is that in France, as elsewhere, future pensions are being cut back. *Marianne*, a French magazine, put it like this:

> Over the years, a succession of reforms of pensions have succeeded each other: the age at which pensions will start has been increased or the conditions have deteriorated and each time it is promised, sworn, that it will be "the last of the last." In particular, the key variable, that of the rate of replacement, that is to say the amount of the pension as a percentage of salary, has not ceased to fall.[15]

And there will be more in that long line of "last" reforms in France. There were 4.2 people of working age for every French pensioner in 2011. This ratio will collapse to 1.9 by 2050, according to *The Economist*.[16] The figures are even worse for Germany.

In France, the pension age will now rise to 67 starting in 2023. Germany is heading toward the same age. It will happen everywhere and to a greater extent than so far announced.

Many advanced countries around the world now have a choice of evils: either break the promises made to those who have made contributions in the past or tax and penalize the next generation to an extraordinary degree. In fact, most countries are doing a mixture.[17] Some must also squeeze spending on every other budget such as education, defense, foreign aid, and so on. It is difficult to cut the health care budget because ageing populations also necessitate more spending there, too.

"Increases in retirement ages are underway or planned in 28 of the 34 OECD countries. These increases, however, are expected to keep pace with improved life expectancy only in 6 countries for men and in 10 countries for women."

SOURCE: Organisation for Economic Co-operation and Development press release, June 11, 2012, citing OECD, *Pensions Outlook 2012* (Paris: OECD Publishing, 2012).

The problem tends to be discussed by the European Union and the OECD as if it were some unfortunate event that has arisen without any human agency. That is not true. The failure to pay pensions as promised and the penalty passed from one generation to the next are the unfortunate creations of the welfare states of the world.

Any young person now entering the workforce has good reason to feel angry with the generation retiring now. The data for the United States in Figure 8.3 give an idea of just how big the intergenerational theft is. The contrast between the gains received by the postwar generation and the losses of the current generation amounts to over $170,000 per person. The contrasts in Poland, France, and Italy are probably even greater.

This new generation will have to pay through the nose to finance the pensions of the old while they themselves get miserable or negative returns on their own contributions. Young people will not

Figure 8.3
EARLY GENERATIONS HAVE RIPPED OFF LATER ONES
DIFFERENCE BETWEEN SOCIAL SECURITY BENEFITS RECEIVED AND
SOCIAL SECURITY TAXES PAID BY A SINGLE MAN, IN 2012 DOLLARS

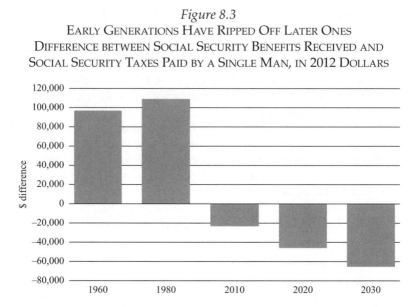

SOURCE: Figures calculated from C. Eugene Steuerle and Caleb Quakenbush, "Social Security and Medicare Taxes and Benefits over a Lifetime: 2012 Update," Urban Institute, Washington, D.C., 2012, http://www.urban.org/UploadedPDF/412660 -Social-Security-and-Medicare-Taxes-and-Benefits-Over-a-Lifetime.pdf.

NOTE: Amounts are based on the average U.S. wage after various adjustments to make the figures comparable. The years shown are when the single man reaches age 65. Negative numbers indicate less money is taken out for the worker than is paid in by him.[18]

demonstrate in the streets or refuse to pay only because of a natural desire to respect their parents coupled with ignorance of what has happened. But the postwar generation—my own generation and before—should be ashamed.

2. Big contributions to fund state pensions have encouraged black markets.

I suggested that the high level of tax and social insurance in Poland is, at least, part of the reason Poland has such a big black market. Could that be true elsewhere too?

The biggest pension burdens are carried by Italy, France, Greece, Germany, Poland, Japan, Spain, and Sweden (see Figure 8.1). So how big are the black markets in these eight countries?

Three of them—Italy, Greece, and Poland—are at the top of the league when it comes to "shadow economies." Two others have above-average underground economies. Two are a little below average. Only Japan is notable in having a relatively big pension burden but a small underground economy. Japan, though, spends less on other welfare state benefits such as disability benefits. So this difference is consistent with the idea that the wedge between the cost to a business of employing someone and the money actually received is a significant influence[19] (see Figure 8.4).

Sweden and Norway are often regarded as civilized, law-abiding countries. But they are also countries with large social contributions and taxation. Sweden has made moves to bring its pension burden under control, but it has still found plenty of other things to spend money on. And yes, Sweden and Norway do indeed have underground economies of above-average size.

Figure 8.4

WHO HAS THE BIGGEST (AND SMALLEST) UNDERGROUND ECONOMY?
SHADOW ECONOMIES AS A PERCENTAGE OF TOTAL ECONOMIC OUTPUT,
SELECTED COUNTRIES

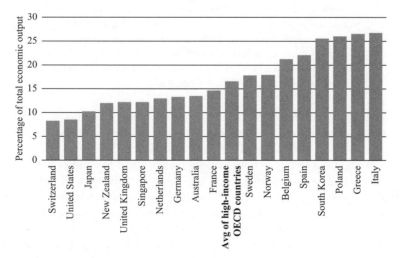

SOURCE: Friedrich Schneider, Andreas Buehn, and Claudio E. Montenegro, "Shadow Economies All over the World: New Estimates for 162 Countries from 1999 to 2007," World Bank Policy Research Working Paper no. 5356, July 2010.

What about the countries that have relatively small pension burdens: South Korea, Australia, the Netherlands, the United Kingdom, the United States, and Switzerland? Strikingly, five of the six also have smaller-than-average underground economies. Korea is the exception. One of the possible explanations for this is that Korea has a dramatically higher proportion of self-employed workers than other countries have. The workers have more opportunity to complete transactions that do not appear on the books.[20]

Does any connection between large pension burdens and large underground economies show up if we look at the national figures? A scattergraph does indeed suggest a modest correlation (see Figure 8.5).

Of course, pension costs by themselves do not wholly account for the size of underground economies. Governments impose heavy taxes and social insurance contributions for other reasons, too. So it is remarkable that pensions are influential enough to show any correlation at all.

Among those who study underground economies, however, the influence of social contributions and taxes will come as no great surprise. According to a World Bank study of black market economies,

> In almost all studies, it has been ascertained that the overall tax and social security contribution burden are among the main causes for the existence of the shadow economy. . . . The bigger the difference between the total cost of labor in the official economy and the after-tax earnings, the greater the incentive to avoid this difference.[21]

And for good measure, the report adds, "Reducing the tax burden is the best policy measure to reduce the shadow economy, followed by a lessening of fiscal and business regulation."[22]

Do we need to ask what is wrong with black market economies? We might as well because there is a Panglossian tendency to think that "whatever exists is fine." But underground economies are inherently unfair. Two people work. One pays a large part of his or her income to the state while the other does not.

Second, black markets encourage dishonesty. Those involved are knowingly and deliberately lying. Once lying becomes normal in one context, the practice is easily transferred to others. Eventually, that leads to a reduction in mutual trust.

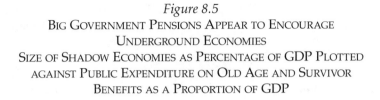

Figure 8.5
Big Government Pensions Appear to Encourage
Underground Economies
Size of Shadow Economies as Percentage of GDP Plotted
against Public Expenditure on Old Age and Survivor
Benefits as a Proportion of GDP

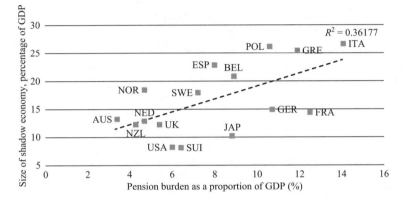

Sources: Organisation for Economic Co-operation and Development, *Pensions at a Glance 2011: Retirement-Income Systems in OECD and G20 Countries* (Paris: OECD Publishing, 2011), p. 155 (figures for 2007), and Friedrich Schneider, Andreas Buehn, and Claudio E. Montenegro, "Shadow Economies All over the World: New Estimates for 162 Countries from 1999 to 2007," World Bank Policy Research Working Paper no. 5356, July 2010 (figures for 2006).

Note: In both cases, these seem to be the latest figures available. I have included all the advanced economies in the OECD list. Big government pension programs create a large tax and social insurance "wedge" that encourages black market economies. Please note that the outlier of South Korea has been omitted. If it were included, the R squared figure would fall from 0.360 to 0.123.

AUS = Australia; BEL = Belgium; ESP = Spain; FRA = France; GER = Germany; GRE = Greece; ITA = Italy; JAP = Japan; NED = Netherlands; NOR = Norway; NZL = New Zealand; POL = Poland; SUI = Switzerland; SWE = Sweden; UK = United Kingdom; USA = United States.

Third, an underground economy makes the problem of funding an overlarge pension system even more difficult!

3. Big state pensions can contribute to unemployment.

The big wedge caused by government pension programs also contributes to unemployment (see Chapter 2).

229

As an experiment, I have tried to see if the boost that big pension burdens give to the wedge—and thus to unemployment—shows through in unemployment levels (see Figure 8.6).

There does indeed appear to be a modest correlation. Again, no one would claim pension burdens are the sole or overwhelming cause of unemployment. But a connection makes sense, and the scattergraph provides evidence to support the idea.

And there is a likely follow-up consequence: when there is unemployment, there is more emigration of working-age people to other countries. Migration from Spain to Germany reached 30,000 in 2012, a 45 percent increase over the previous year. Immigration to Germany from Italy was even higher at 42,000, up 40 percent.[23] These

Figure 8.6
BIG GOVERNMENT PENSION PROGRAMS ARE CORRELATED
WITH UNEMPLOYMENT

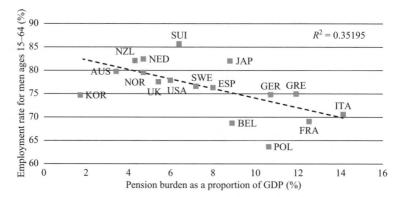

SOURCES: Source for the pension burden: Organisation for Economic Co-operation and Development, *Pensions at a Glance 2011* (Paris: OECD Publishing, 2011), p. 155. Source for the employment rate: "Short-term Labour Market Statistics," OECD.StatExtracts, data for 2007, http://stats.oecd.org/Index.aspx?DatasetCode=STLABOUR.

NOTE: The advantage of using the employment rate of working-age men is that it removes from the equation any cultural variations in the employment rates of women. Note that no country has been excluded from this scattergraph as an outlier.

AUS = Australia; BEL = Belgium; ESP = Spain; FRA = France; GER = Germany; GRE = Greece; ITA = Italy; JAP = Japan; KOR = South Korea; NED = Netherlands; NOR = Norway; NZL = New Zealand; POL = Poland; SUI = Switzerland; SWE = Sweden; UK = United Kingdom; USA = United States.

elevated figures were partly a response to problems that might be temporary. But some migration patterns were established before the 2008 crisis. The number of French people living in other countries has built up over time. It is estimated that 300,000 French people live in London and another 200,000 live in Belgium.[24] This is clearly not because France is a poor country. It is because individuals who cannot get jobs in their own countries or who see their net pay severely reduced by tax and social insurance naturally seek employment elsewhere.

We see a kind of domino effect: dysfunctional, overstretched state pension systems causing high taxes and social contributions, which increase unemployment and then prompt emigration. The emigration is primarily of working men and women. When they move, of course, they no longer pay pension contributions in their own countries. By leaving, they help make the pension crisis back home even worse.

4. In many cases, state pensions have failed to make old people better off.

The ultimate irony is that often the "generous" state pensions have not made people better off in their old age. Millions of people have been given the impression by their governments that a good pension will be paid to them. This has been true in France, Britain, Italy, Germany, and Spain, at least. But the amount that many retirees in these countries are receiving now is less than they were led to expect. Because most people believed their governments, they saved less than they otherwise would have. Thus many people in advanced countries have disturbingly small savings. They are poorer in old age.

More than half of American workers, for example, have less than $25,000 in savings.[25] In Britain, the average savings of people who retired between the ages of 50 and 64 was £91,900 (about $130,500) in 2010, which, if used to buy an annuity, would mean an annual income of £4,000 ($5,680) or less—a pittance.[26] And as this is an average figure, obviously a large proportion of those retirees, probably a majority, had saved less.

What has made this situation even worse in some countries is that some less well-off people of working age have been on welfare benefits that are means tested and paid only to individuals who have little or no savings. This condition has created a perverse incentive

"In countries where people know that the state will not provide for them, saving is a major part of the way of life. In Hong Kong, for example, overall national gross savings were 34 percent of GDP in the 1990s before there were any mandatory or government pension programs. At the same time, the gross savings rates in Germany, France, and Italy were in the region of only 20–22.5 percent."

SOURCE: James Bartholomew, *The Welfare State We're In*, rev. ed. (London: Politicos, 2006), p. 307.

NOTE: I have had to use this old data because, without doing a great deal of digging, I am not aware of a contemporary and reasonably advanced (thus comparable) country without either government pay-as-you-go pensions or compulsory private pension programs. Hong Kong now has a compulsory private program. Countries such as Singapore and Hong Kong with such private programs seem to have higher savings rates than do those with government pay-as-you-go programs. See "Gross Savings (% of GDP)," World Bank website, http://data.worldbank.org /indicator/NY.GNS.ICTR.ZS?page=1.

not to save. Such people have thus become dependent in old age on a state pension that is totally inadequate.

State pensions were created partly to ensure that people would not be poor in old age. But instead, in some cases, they have turned out to be a trick that has led people to save too little and to see out their lives in severely reduced circumstances.

Countries where the old are disproportionately more likely to be poor than the general population include many with large government pension payments. They include Greece, Japan, Spain, and Italy.[27] Poland is the exception. In Poland, the old are less likely to be so poor, but this situation is unlikely to last.

"Even average [German] wage earners with a full career can no longer accumulate sufficient entitlements to be assured of a retirement income above the social assistance level, and hence might still have to depend upon means-tested benefits during their old age. As a consequence, an increasing number of wage earners no longer have an interest in saving to supplement their public pension."

SOURCE: Johan de Deken, "Pension Reforms in Germany: Can Occupational and Private Pensions Compensate for the Erosion of Social Insurance?," *Aegon Global Pensions View*, March 2013. Deken is assistant professor in the Department of Sociology, University of Amsterdam.

5. Public employee pensions are a scandal and a ticking time bomb.

Related to government pension programs for the general population are the programs for government employees. They are related, but different. Bill Lockyer, the state treasurer of California, asserted in 2011 that public employees were not getting particularly generous pensions.[28] Lockyer said the average was $2,500 a month, equivalent to $30,000 a year. It would be a lot of money for many people around the world, but in America that did not seem extravagant.

Daniel Borenstein, a columnist for the *Contra Costa Times*, was surprised by the figure and decided to take a closer look. He found that it was misleading. The "average" cited by the treasurer included public employees who had worked for as few as five years. If, instead, you took only those public service workers getting their full benefits, the average state employee retiring in 2009 was receiving nearly $67,000 a year, a really generous package.

Borenstein then discovered that individuals working for local government in California were receiving even more. In his own county, Contra Costa, the average pension for new retirees was $85,500. Moreover, two-thirds of these retirees were members of the California government pension system and thus were also entitled to social security benefits worth a further $19,000 on average, making a total of over $100,000 a year.

Meanwhile, over on the other side of the country, a local newspaper in Newark, New Jersey, did a similar investigation when a trade union official similarly claimed that government employees had modest pensions. The *Star-Ledger* found that the average for retirees who had served for 25 years was $40,000.[29] Teachers got a better deal, receiving $46,486, and police officers and firefighters did outstandingly well with average pensions of $73,571. These figures can be compared with median pretax earnings in the United States of about $45,500 at that time.[30]

The cost of growing obligations for the pension payments of public sector employees in the United States and elsewhere is a time bomb. It gets little attention partly because public sector employees have every reason not to publicize it. But the damage will become more obvious in due course and, in some cases, it already has.

In Detroit, generous public sector pensions helped provoke a major financial crisis. An emergency manager was appointed and said the cash flow problem made the city insolvent. A lawyer specializing in bankruptcy commented that the lack of funding for the pension fund and health care benefits for the retired "could be the tipping point where the city ends up having to file bankruptcy if there's no concessions made." In New York City, the annual pension contributions jumped from 6 percent of the city's annual spending in 2002 to 18 percent 10 years later. The proportion is still rising. In California, the city of Stockton, with a population of just under 300,000, filed for bankruptcy. What was its biggest debt? An obligation to the California Public Employees Retirement System.[31]

Two economists, Robert Novy-Marx and Josh Rauh, tried to work out the combined effect of all the shortfalls in unfunded state employee pension programs in the United States. They calculated that to fund them properly would require the average U.S. taxpayer to contribute an extra $1,365 a year.

"Potentially huge fiscal liabilities . . . are being passed on to future generations of workers."

SOURCE: Eduard Ponds, Clara Severinson, and Juan Yermo, "Funding in Public Sector Pension Plans: International Evidence," OECD Working Papers on Finance, Insurance and Private Pensions no. 8, May 2011, http://www.oecd.org/finance/private-pensions/47827915.pdf.

In America, we can see that the situation is bad. But America is relatively transparent in its public affairs. We can't be sure just how substantial are the obligations lurking beneath the surface elsewhere around the world. Even the OECD, with all its resources, remarks, "The disclosure of these promises [to public sector workers] is all too often less than transparent, which may be hiding potentially huge fiscal liabilities that are being passed on to future generations of workers."[32] It is rare for the OECD to use such stark language.

Many countries do not publish estimates of these liabilities, but the OECD has tried to work out the figures for a small selection. Looking at this report, you can see that the troubles of the United States are not the worst. There are much bigger unfunded liabilities in France, Finland, Britain, and Germany (see Figure 8.7).

These liabilities are not included in publicly acknowledged national debts. If one adds them to national debts, the figures are truly alarming. In France, the pension debt added to other debts amounted

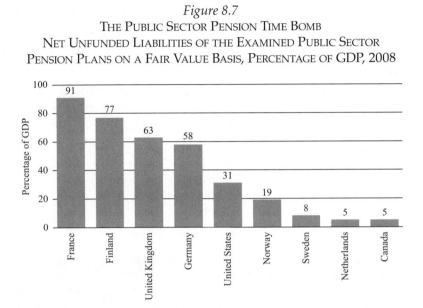

Figure 8.7
THE PUBLIC SECTOR PENSION TIME BOMB
NET UNFUNDED LIABILITIES OF THE EXAMINED PUBLIC SECTOR
PENSION PLANS ON A FAIR VALUE BASIS, PERCENTAGE OF GDP, 2008

SOURCE: Eduard Ponds, Clara Severinson, and Juan Yermo, "Funding in Public Sector Pension Plans: International Evidence," OECD Working Papers on Finance, Insurance and Private Pensions no. 8, May 2011, http://www.oecd.org/finance/private -pensions/47827915.pdf

to 152 percent of GDP in 2008. In Britain, it came to 138 percent. These figures are daunting—the more so because, since 2008, the national debts of most countries have significantly increased. Estimates were not done for Spain, Italy, and Poland, and one might fear that their hidden pension debts are as bad or worse.

6. The cost of big unfunded government pensions can lead to demands to allow more immigration.

A website called Left Foot Forward in Britain carries the headline, "How best to support an ageing population? More immigration."[33] The author cites the well-established concerns that there will be fewer working-age people in the future to support more retired people. Then he quotes a comment from the U.K. Office for Budget Responsibility: "Higher net migration, close to levels that we have seen in recent years, would put downward pressure on borrowing and public sector net debt, as immigrants are more likely to be of working age than the population in general." The conclusion of the article is that "allowing more people of working age into the country would . . . take some of the strain off the welfare state."

It would indeed, at the margin. But the reprieve would be temporary and minor unless the structure of the pension system were changed.[34] It is a strange way to decide on mass immigration, though, isn't it? Create an unsustainable pension system and then try to keep it going a little longer by encouraging mass immigration? Even if it worked, it would be an admission of national incompetence.

* * *

These six problems with government unfunded pension programs are daunting. Those now entering them are sure to get a poor or even a negative return. The burden of government pensions has contributed to the creation of huge underground economies and widespread unemployment. In many cases, they have deceived people, causing them to save too little and to be poor in old age. Public employees have often been granted advantageous terms at the expense of everyone else. The unfunded cost hangs over the finances of many nations—an inheritance of debt for the next generation.

Some of us may be tempted to say, "OK, then. Let's get rid of state pensions altogether. They have obviously failed. Government involvement in saving for old age has done more harm than good."

That may well be true. But it seems unlikely that democracies will be willing to give up all government involvement in pensions. In which case, we need to find a better way of running them. What could that be? Are there any countries that have had more success with pensions? If so, how have they managed it?

One measure of success is whether older people are poor compared with the general population. It is far from being a perfect measure (see the note accompanying Figure 8.8), but it is somewhere to start. On this basis, it appears that the Netherlands has done relatively well. Its older people are less poor compared with the general population than in other countries.[35]

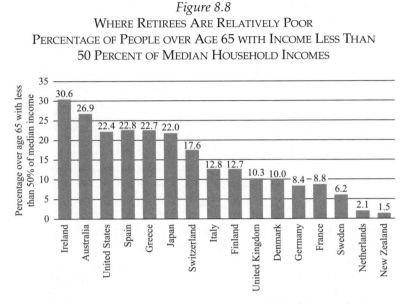

Figure 8.8
WHERE RETIREES ARE RELATIVELY POOR
PERCENTAGE OF PEOPLE OVER AGE 65 WITH INCOME LESS THAN
50 PERCENT OF MEDIAN HOUSEHOLD INCOMES

SOURCE: Organisation for Economic Co-operation and Development, *Pensions at a Glance 2011* (Paris: OECD Publishing, 2011), p. 149.

NOTE: These figures should be treated with caution because accurate income figures are difficult to capture and subject to the honesty or otherwise of tax returns and benefit claims. Also, a country might provide generous pensions that are not sustainable. Meanwhile, someone deemed to be "relatively poor" in Switzerland may well be richer than someone with an average income in Greece.

So what is the Dutch system? First, there is a basic pension paid to everyone who has lived or worked in the country. People become entitled to it at a rate of 2 percent of the full pension for each year they have lived or worked there. The full value amounts to 29 percent of average earnings, so it is basic—not luxurious.

The second element consists of thousands of funded occupational pension programs. They appear to be compulsory for most people. Some programs are run by pension funds and the rest by individual companies.[36] In either case, the value is transferable when someone changes jobs. The pensions are mostly based on the individual's average earnings during his or her working life. The pension funds make real investments, in bonds, stocks, and bank accounts.

It must be admitted that the system has had a few setbacks. Payments were reduced by 1.9 percent on average after the weakness in the financial markets in 2008.[37] Some cutbacks have been as high as 15 percent.[38] Rising life expectancy has also led to increases in the age at which the pensions are payable. But the Dutch system has two big pluses: the government has not built up a huge unfunded liability, and the level of payments is high compared with other systems. Payments from Dutch private pensions amount to 5.2 percent of GDP—one of the highest levels in the world. The Dutch system certainly seems better than average.

The fact that it is "funded"—that is, it has real investments behind it—seems to be a key reason for its success. But if we are going to consider a funded system, there are two other models worth looking at.

I am in Singapore and a think tank there has succeeded in arranging for me to meet Thurman Shanmugaratnam, the deputy prime minister and minister of finance. A taxi deposits me at the side of a busy street in the center of town. I look up and see a modern tower of offices looming over me: the Ministry of Finance. I go in and pass through security before going up in a fast elevator to the floor where Shanmugaratnam works. There I am ushered into a large and, frankly, rather grim internal meeting room. It has chairs but no windows. Suddenly, the minister marches in followed by a small entourage. He is a tall, slim, balding man of Indian heritage with dark areas under his eyes. He radiates active intelligence. He is a prime example of how clever people in Singapore are sometimes fast-tracked to the top. The interview turns into one of the most demanding I have ever done. He deals with issues so quickly and definitively that I have to hurry to think of further questions to ask.

We cover a wide range of subjects, but before long we come to the Singapore pension system. All Singaporeans are obliged to contribute to personal accounts with what is known as the Central Provident Fund. Their money is invested in bonds, stocks, and even gold. They can choose fund managers and individual stocks within certain rules. But it is compulsory for everybody to pay into the program.

Some people in other countries might be unhappy about the compulsory element, I suggest to Shanmugaratnam.

He deals with the objection briskly. The element of compulsion is not what makes the Singapore system different, he declares. Many other countries compulsorily take money from workers to pay for their welfare. What is different about Singapore is that it is transparent, it is funded, and it retains the element of self-reliance. In many Western countries, governments have focused only on the short term. Large and often unquantified liabilities have been built up for the future.

Frankly, all this is hard to deny. I suggest, though, that it is normal for governments to think short term. It is a response to democratic pressure for immediate results. He does not accept that it is inevitable. If a government goes ahead and makes the argument that something makes sense for the long term, the opposition has to deal with that argument, he says. As ever with the Singapore government, the attitude is bold and clear.

"It is fairer and sounder to have each generation pay for itself and each person save for his own pension fund."

SOURCE: Lee Kuan Yew, *From Third World to First: Singapore and the Asian Economic Boom* (New York: HarperBusiness, 2011), p. 105. Lee was the first prime minister of Singapore.

The Central Provident Fund accords with what people believe in, says the minister: doing well through work rather than welfare; the family; building prosperity; and contributing to the community. He points out, perhaps with a little pleasure at the irony, that the fund—the focal point of the Singapore system—developed from arrangements created by Britain when it was the ruling colonial power.[39] He is too polite to add that Singapore has kept and successfully developed this system whereas the "mother country" has taken another direction with inferior results.

How does the Central Provident Fund work? Workers and their employers pay a lot of money into the program to build up a personal fund that the individual can use to pay for housing and health care as well as pensions. Up to the age of 35, the employee must pay in 16 percent of earnings and the employer a further 20 percent. On the face of it, this appears like another damaging wedge—a big gap between the cost of employing someone and the amount the person actually receives. But this case is different because all the money paid in continues to belong to the individual. So he or she need not feel the payments are disappearing. Each individual can see, year by year, how money is building up in the personal account or, to be more precise, accounts.

Part of the contributions goes into the individual's pension fund, known as the Special Account.[40] This part starts at 6 percent of income, rises to a high of 9.5 percent between the ages of 50 and 55, then falls suddenly to 2 percent and declines further thereafter.[41]

Figure 8.9 is a young woman's statement of her account with the Central Provident Fund. You can see she has been employed for less than two years but already she has savings of almost S$15,000 (about US$11,091).[42] The Medisave Account shown on the statement is for health care and the Ordinary Account is normally used to buy housing, although any excess can also be used for other purposes, including investment and education.

Cash in the Special and Medisave accounts attracts an interest rate of at least 5 percent at the time of this writing when total savings

Figure 8.9
ACCOUNT STATEMENT, CENTRAL PROVIDENT FUND

CPF STATEMENT OF ACCOUNT

STATEMENT PERIOD		NAME		ACCOUNT NO.		
JAN TO DEC 2011		HUI				

TRANSACTION DATE	CODE	FOR MTH/ YR OF	REF	ORDINARY ACCOUNT (OA) $	SPECIAL ACCOUNT (SA) $	MEDISAVE ACCOUNT (MA) $
01 JAN	BAL			2,122.54	568.35	707.42
18 JAN	CON	DEC2010	A	598.06	129.94	182.00
17 FEB	CON	JAN2011	A	598.06	129.94	182.00
19 FEB	DPS			−36.00		
15 MAR	CON	FEB2011	A	598.06	129.94	182.00
19 APR	CON	MAR2011	A	598.11	142.97	181.92
18 MAY	CON	APR2011	A	598.11	142.97	181.92
16 JUN	CON	MAY2011	A	598.11	142.97	181.92
15 JUL	CON	JUN2011	A	598.11	142.97	181.92
17 AUG	CON	JUL2011	A	598.11	142.97	181.92
19 SEP	CON	AUG2011	A	598.11	142.97	181.92
17 OCT	CON	SEP2011	A	598.12	155.93	181.95
16 NOV	CON	OCT2011	A	598.12	155.93	181.95
16 DEC	CON	NOV2011	A	598.12	155.93	181.95
31 DEC	INT			134.55	120.07	85.40
31 DEC	BAL			9,398.29	2,403.85	2,976.19

REF A : NATIONAL UNIVERSITY OF SPORE

SOURCE: Author.

NOTE: Hui was 24 at the time of this statement.

in the fund are $60,000 or less.[43] This is a good rate because inflation is very low in Singapore. But savers can choose to make other investments once they have saved a basic minimum in this deposit account.[44] Though the rules are complex, one can gain exposure to stock markets through approved unit trusts run by well-known international companies such as Allianz, Franklin, Fidelity, Templeton, Aberdeen, Schroders, and Legg Mason.[45] In one account, they can also place up to 10 percent of their money in gold funds.

The rules are complex but one can detect a few themes. One is that people should save to provide for themselves. A second is that particularly attractive terms are offered to those who have less money. Third, the government does not want people to blow all the money at retirement and then have nothing to live on.

Unfortunately, we do not have readily at hand comparative statistics to show how well or badly the elderly in Singapore do compared with elsewhere because Singapore is not a member of the OECD. But it appears difficult to reach old age in Singapore without having built up savings. It seems probable, at least, that the elderly are relatively well cared for. It seems even more likely that the current and new generation of workers will do a lot better with their savings than those in the vast majority of Western countries. Exactly as the first Prime Minister of Singapore, Lee Kuan Yew, intended, the old generation is not being unfair to the new.

But there is a third model for funded pensions, too. Back in 1974, Chile had a traditional, unfunded pension program. It suffered from the typical problems of such programs taken to an extreme. Contributions needed to be enormous to pay existing retirees. They amounted to more than half a worker's salary. This gave rise to exactly the sort of problems already described and on a big scale: mass evasion, a large underground economy, and very high unemployment.[46]

Something had to be done. A new system of personal retirement accounts was created. As in Singapore, contributors could choose how to allocate their pension funds. They were similarly able to see the value of their individual plans grow. But there were two key differences: the program was not compulsory, and people did not have to save through a government agency. They could go directly to a fund manager.

It is true that, once this program was in place, a large minority of the population remained outside it and low-paid people became entitled to very modest pensions.[47] However, it is worth remembering that, at the beginning of this process, Chile was an extremely poor country with a pension system already in meltdown, unlike the others we have considered. Moreover, since this system has existed, Chile has grown enormously in prosperity. The pension program is obviously not the only reason, but it may well have contributed.

In 2008, the system was reformed again and the basic state pension element was increased. But the investment part was retained, and in 2012 a study by actuaries Melbourne Mercer with the Australian Centre for Financial Studies ranked the Chilean pension system above those of some advanced countries including the United States, Japan, France, and Germany.

"The major impetus for reform of the Swedish system was the threat of financial disaster."

SOURCE: Edward Palmer, "The Swedish Pension Reform Model: Framework and Issues," World Bank Discussion Paper no. SP 0012, 2000, http://www-wds.worldbank.org/external/default/WDSContentServer/WDSP/IB/2001/12/11/000094946_01110704111524/Rendered/PDF/multi0page.pdf.

Several countries have moved in the same direction. Denmark in the 1980s started increasing the proportion of privately managed, funded pensions. Funded occupational pensions were made all but universal in the 1990s. Since then, personal funded pensions have also been encouraged. In Sweden, reform begun in 1994 also led to the development of pensions backed by investments. It is only a minor part of the system, but at least some pension income is now backed by real investments. Moreover, individuals can choose the fund managers who will look after the money. The Polish also moved toward funded personal pension funds, although this element has subsequently been reduced. (For some dangers, see Box 8.2.)

One of the advantages of personal pensions with actual investments is that people seem happier to declare their incomes and pay their contributions. They understand that the money remains theirs and is not disappearing perhaps never to return.

In Chile, the size of the underground economy admittedly is bigger than that of the average advanced country. It is estimated to be 19.5 percent, compared with a 16.6 percent average for advanced countries. But Chile has a smaller underground economy than Belgium, Spain, and Italy and, compared with the rest of South

Box 8.2
WHAT CAN GO WRONG WITH PERSONAL FUNDED PENSIONS?

The stock market might fall. Over the length of a working life, stock market returns including dividends have been positive in most countries.[a] However, it is worth guarding against the risk that savers of modest means might find they suddenly lose a significant part of their savings just before they retire. One possible answer is to provide better-than-normal cash returns on the first tranche of savings. Only when savings have gone beyond this minimum would people be free to invest in normal investments such as cash deposits, bonds, managed funds, property, gold, or stocks.

Fees and other transaction costs can be high. An important part of the design of the system should be to make sure that contributors can avoid high charges unless they deliberately decide that a high cost fund is what they want.

Individual liberty is constrained by compulsory contributions. True, but this is no worse than existing systems in which money is taken in social insurance and all personal control and ownership is lost.

Governments can raid them. True again, but the risk can be reduced if the whole population has a stake in the system and there are constitutional safeguards.

---

[a] This is the case in Britain and the United States, at least. For the United States, see Michael Tanner, "Still a Better Deal: Private Investment vs. Social Security," *Policy Analysis* 692 (2012): 6–7, http://object.cato.org/sites/cato.org/files/pubs/pdf/PA692.pdf. For the United Kingdom, see the annual report produced by Barclays on equity returns over the long term. Access to the full report is not free, but some relevant data are available at "Your Investment Starts Here," Barclays Stockbrokers website, https://www.barclaysstockbrokers.co.uk/get-started/investment-journey/Pages/your-investment-journey-starts-here.aspx. The data show superior returns for equities over the long term.

America, it is outstanding. It has the smallest underground economy of any country on the continent. The underground economy of Brazil is twice the size. Singapore, meanwhile, has an underground economy of 13.0 percent—below average for advanced countries and probably significantly smaller than that of nearby countries in Southeast Asia.

After all these stories and experiences, what conclusions should we draw?

First and above all, we should conclude that typical state pensions have been among the most disastrous parts of many modern welfare states. One of the key reasons for the multiple problems they have created is that they have been unfunded. Funded pensions have performed better in countries as diverse as the Netherlands, Singapore, and Chile.[48]

What might be the best way to reform?

I would suggest that the majority of pension payments should come from funded pension accounts under the control of each individual. It might work something like this:

- Everyone should have considerable freedom to choose his or her investments.
- The pension funds should be compulsory for everyone in employment. (In some countries, voluntary programs have had poor take-up. If everyone is involved, this provides greater political protection from raids on the investments by governments.)
- Even with universal involvement, the integrity of programs should be heavily protected by law. Experience in Britain, Australia, and Poland has shown that governments find it hard to resist the large pots of money in funded pensions.
- A truly basic pension might also be paid to everyone who has been resident in a country for a long period. This makes means-tested benefits less significant, and means-tested benefits discourage work, honesty, and self-reliance. The Netherlands has this base and New Zealand has started a version of it too.[49]
- The retirement age should rise automatically with life expectancy.
- All public servants should take part in the same pension program as everyone else. Any extra benefits that may be justified for a particular public service job should be transparent and paid outside the pension system. Members of the legislature (Congress) and department heads in the executive branch, above all, should have no special treatment. In addition to the question of fairness, special pensions might cause them to care less about the success of the system used by the general public. Special terms for public servants should be seen for what they are: a form of corruption.

How can a country with an unfunded pension program make the transition?

The method recommended by most specialists is to let the older generation continue with existing pensions while the next generation starts the new system. Those in the middle would have a mixture. It must be admitted that there is a problem of affordability: the new generation must pay, to some extent, both for their own and for their parents' pensions. But this difficulty can be reduced by significantly increasing the retirement age and failing to index pensions to match growth in the economy.

This is not politically easy. But old government pay-as-you-go unfunded pension programs have been a failure. Funded personal pensions would mean elderly people would be better off for generations to come.

9. "While Her Dear Father Lived, Any Change of Condition Must Be Impossible for Her. She Would Never Quit Him."

Who Cares for the Elderly?

Emma Woodhouse lives with her elderly father and cares for him. He is a nervous man, but she comforts and reassures him. They have a family friend, George Knightley, whom Emma has known since she was a child. The two of them enjoy bantering with each other. They have had a few serious disagreements too, but finally they have come to realize that they love each other.

Knightley proposes to Emma. She wants to marry him, but she says no. She cannot go to live with Knightley because she believes she has a duty to her father to stay with him as long as he lives. "While her dear father lived, any change of condition must be impossible for her. She would never quit him."

Knightley does not complain or try to change her mind. He recognizes and accepts her wish to fulfill this duty. Fortunately, they find a way to resolve the problem: Knightley suggests that he could come to live with Emma at her father's home for as long as her father is alive. That way they can marry and Emma can continue caring for her father.

This is the climax of *Emma*, written by Jane Austen and published in 1815. Most people who read it probably do not particularly notice that it is accepted as normal and right that Emma feels she has a duty to her father and that even her suitor accepts that this duty exists.

In another of the most famous 19th-century novels, *Great Expectations* by Charles Dickens, published in 1861, Clara Barley—much further down in the social scale—is pursued by Herbert Pocket. She, too, takes it as normal and right that she should continue to live with and care for her father. He is extremely eccentric and difficult. He "roars" and bangs on the floor. But still she stays with him. She "holds dutifully to her father as long as he lasts," Dickens writes. Only after her father dies does she consent to marry Herbert.

This is not only a matter of women looking after their parents either. In the same novel, John Wemmick, a bill collector, also takes care of his father. Dickens describes the father as "a very old man in a flannel coat; clean, cheerful, comfortable and well cared for, but intensely deaf." Wemmick fires a cannon every day, and the father takes pleasure in being able to hear it.

Children used to live with or near their elderly parents and take care of them around the world. Of course, it did not take place in every case. But it was usual. In Sweden, a detailed study of family life in the 19th century revealed that "at least half of the population [over age 65] had a child living close to them in every age group."[1] At the age of 85, an elderly person had a 50-50 chance of living in close proximity to one or more adult children. Care of elderly parents by their children in Sweden was so orthodox then that it was legally enforceable until 1956.

Until recently, there was also legal and institutional pressure for children in Germany to take responsibility for the care of their parents.[2] In Belgium, there is still a remnant of that requirement—a legal obligation for children to pay for the care of their parents if the parents run out of money. But generally since the 19th century, an extraordinary change has taken place. While in some countries, the idea that children should take responsibility for their parents remains, in others it has almost completely disappeared.

The typical crunch moment is when an elderly woman is widowed. Will she live alone or with one of her children? In Portugal, Spain, and Italy, more than half of women over age 65 who are without a partner live with their children. In Denmark, only 3 percent do. (See Figure 9.1.) The incidence of older women living with their children is 20 times higher in Portugal than in Denmark. The contrast is extreme.

A second set of statistics covers all women over age 65, including those whose partners are still alive (see Figure 9.2). It has the advantage of covering a few extra countries and it shows that, in some countries, adult children are living with both their parents. In these multigenerational households, the elderly are not necessarily frail.

In this chart we see that the Netherlands and Italy are similarly poles apart. Only a fraction of Dutch women over age 65 live with their children—7 percent. In Italy, four times as many do—28 percent.

Why are there such big contrasts in the way people treat the elderly?

It is tempting to say, "Oh well, the Mediterranean countries have a strong tradition of extended families," or "The Catholic countries

248

Figure 9.1
DOES GRANNY LIVE WITH HER CHILDREN WHEN HER HUSBAND DIES?
PERCENTAGE OF WOMEN AGES 65 AND OVER WITHOUT A PARTNER LIVING
WITH THEIR CHILDREN

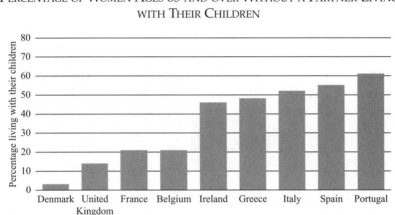

SOURCE: Maria Iacovou, "The Living Arrangements of Elderly Europeans," Institute for Social and Economic Research Working Paper Series 2000–09, February 2000, https://www.iser.essex.ac.uk/research/publications/working-papers/iser/2000 -09.pdf.

are the ones that look after their elderly." But these generalizations are not to be relied on. Most countries—perhaps all—previously had a tradition of children caring for their parents. Japan is a country where it is common for children to live with and care for their elderly parents. More than 61 percent of Japanese women over age 80 live with one of their children.[3] Japan is obviously neither Catholic nor Mediterranean. Moreover, if it were just a matter of Mediterranean culture, why would almost as many women over age 65 live with their children in Austria as in Italy?

Take another measure of family life: in Austria, 7.5 percent of children—not adult children—live in multigenerational households (see Figure 9.3). That is 25 times more than in Sweden. Of course, neither of these countries is Mediterranean.

It could be that a culture, along with political ideas, influences the shape of the welfare state. That, in turn, affects how people treat their elderly, reinforcing or undermining past practice.

If it is not simply a matter of being Catholic or living on the Mediterranean Sea, what other factors could be at work? Let's go back to the contrast between the Netherlands and Italy.

249

Figure 9.2
WHAT PERCENTAGE OF WOMEN OVER AGE 65 LIVE WITH
THEIR CHILDREN?

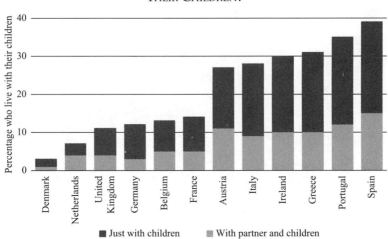

■ Just with children   ▨ With partner and children

SOURCE: Maria Iacovou, "The Living Arrangements of Elderly Europeans," Institute for Social and Economic Research Working Paper Series 2000–09, February 2000, https://www.iser.essex.ac.uk/research/publications/working-papers/iser/2000-09.pdf.

NOTE: The author emphasizes the "inadequacy" of the north–south or Catholic–Protestant differences to explain the contrasts between the countries. Figures from 1994 and 1995.

In the Netherlands, people pay social insurance through their working lifetimes and part of the premium pays for long-term care in a home if it is needed. This is part of the system, and people are consequently encouraged to believe it is normal for the elderly to go into an assisted living home rather than to be cared for by the family. Indeed, it goes against the grain to pay for something and then not use it. That is surely one of the reasons the proportion of people living in assisted living residences in the Netherlands is five times that in Italy, and this reduces the proportion who are cared for by family members. (See Figure 9.4.)

The provision of care for the elderly outside the family has similarly been much greater in Denmark than in Portugal.[4] Denmark was once described as "the envy of the world" for its government-provided care for the elderly.[5] That could help account for why older women are more than 11 times more likely to live with their children in Portugal than in Denmark. In contrast, Japan has kept its provision

Figure 9.3
PERCENTAGE OF CHILDREN LIVING IN MULTIGENERATIONAL HOUSEHOLDS

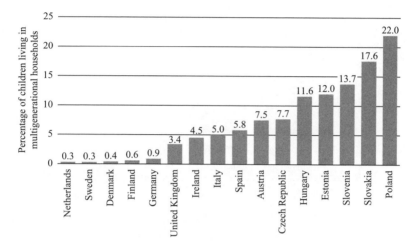

SOURCE: Organisation for Economic Co-operation and Development, *Doing Better for Families* (Paris: OECD Publications, 2011), p. 28.

of institutional care for the elderly comparatively modest. So the continued high level of family care there could well be a response to this history of relatively low government provision.[6]

The idea that the financial arrangements organized by governments affect family care is supported by some academic studies. Gary Engelhardt and Nadia Greenhalgh-Stanley studied the effect of changes in Medicare payments for health care in the home that took place at different times in different places between 1997 and 2000. They concluded that "elderly housing and living arrangements are quite responsive to social insurance benefits."[7]

Ten percent of residents of England and Wales provide unpaid care for someone with an illness or disability.

SOURCE: "Statistical Bulletin: 2011 Census: Key Statistics for England and Wales, March 2011," U.K. Office for National Statistics website, http://www.ons.gov.uk/ons/rel/census/2011-census /key-statistics-for-local-authorities-in-england-and-wales/stb-2011-census-key-statistics-for -england-and-wales.html

Figure 9.4
HOW MANY ARE IN ASSISTED LIVING?
PERCENTAGE OF PEOPLE AGES 65 AND OVER IN ASSISTED
LIVING FACILITIES

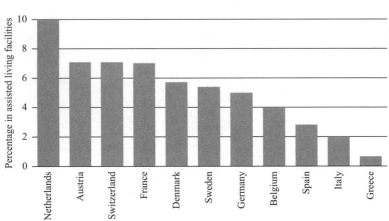

SOURCE: Klaus Haberkern and Marc Szydlik, "State Care Provision, Societal Opinion and Children's Care of Older Parents in 11 European Countries," *Ageing and Society* 30 (2010): 299–323, Table 1.

NOTE: The difference between the Mediterranean countries and the Netherlands is dramatic. But Germany and Belgium also have much lower rates, probably because of current or previous laws requiring adult children to take responsibility.

The overall effect of the changes was to make government provision for the elderly more modest. It seems likely that this is why the proportion of elderly living in multigenerational families in the United States ended a long-running decline and rallied a little, from 17 percent in 1990 to 20 percent in 2008.[8] (See sidebar on page 253.)

If it is true that government policies are framing, however unintentionally, how families live, perhaps governments should be thinking in terms of whether their influence is for good or ill. Do they really wish to diminish the importance of both the immediate and the extended family?

Are government-run care and crowding out the family's role the best thing for the elderly? Governments, especially in Europe, along with the European Union (EU) and the Organisation for Economic Co-operation and Development (OECD), often take it for granted that they are.[9] They support taxing everyone and then giving the money only to those who have government-provided care. But are they right? Is it truly in the interests of the elderly?

The decline in the proportion of elderly living with their children appears to have ended in the United States.

1900: 57 percent
1980: 17 percent
1990: 17 percent
2008: 20 percent

Percentage of Americans ages 65 and over living in a multigenerational family. According to the Pew Research Center, one of the possible explanations is "cuts to Medicare enacted in 1997."

SOURCE: Pew Research Center, "The Return of the Multi-Generational Family Household," Social and Demographic Trends Report, March 18, 2010,

---

How would the elderly *like* to be cared for? The question rarely seems to be asked.

Unusually, it was posed in a Japanese government survey. People were asked where they would like to receive long-term care if they came to need it. One in five wanted to go to a care home, nursing home, or hospital. The vast majority wanted to receive long-term care at home, either independently of their family (46 percent) or with the help of their family (28 percent).[10] It seems that some parents would love to live with or near to their children. But others genuinely do not want to and would rather be independent as long as possible. Some may prefer to put up with a bit of loneliness because they feel they should not be a burden for their children in the prime of their lives.

I wonder what readers of this book would reply if asked where they would like to be living at age, say, 85. Alone? In an institution? With family? Very close to family?[11] Of course, there is a wide spectrum of circumstances. (See Box 9.1.) What is best in one case would not work in another. Some 90-year-old people are still married, hale, and hearty. Others 20 years younger are highly dependent.

Box 9.1
WOULD YOU LIKE TO LIVE HERE?

I am visiting an Anglican retirement village in the suburbs of Sydney. The village is on a big site with its own attractive roads lined with trees. It is like being in a separate world.

There are three kinds of accommodations. Those in relatively good health live independently in well-landscaped, attractively designed apartments. They can buy in services such as laundry and help with cleaning. They can eat in their apartments or go into one of the dining rooms to have meals. They can also take part in organized activities.

For those less able to cope, there are large assisted living facilities. People in these blocks have their own rooms with plenty of their own possessions. They share living rooms and can take part in organized activities. It looks well run. But with plenty of old people gathered together—seeming quiet and perhaps depressed—these homes frankly are not places where I would go, given a choice.

Finally, those residents who are seriously disabled or bedridden go to the on-site nursing home. I was not taken to that building but was told that life expectancy there is significantly shorter than in the assisted living facilities.

There are four basic living arrangements: living with a partner; living with family; being in an institution; and living alone. Let's look at how things go for people in various circumstances.

"Asked where they would like to spend their last days, Americans almost always say at home, surrounded by people they love. . . . In real life, though, . . . more than 30 per cent die in a nursing home . . . and over half end up in a hospital."

SOURCE: "Go Gentle into That Good Night," *The Economist*, March 17, 2012. The article is a review of Ira Byock, *The Best Care Possible: A Physician's Quest to Transform Care through the End of Life* (New York: Avery, 2012).

The Pew Research Center interviewed people ages 65 and older about whether they felt lonely. Among those who lived with others, 8 percent said they were lonely. Among those who lived alone, the proportion was more than three times larger (28 percent). (See Table 9.1.)

It may seem like a statement of the obvious but, just in case there is any doubt, lonely people are not happy.[12] As John Cacioppo and

Table 9.1
ARE OLDER PEOPLE HAPPY LIVING ALONE?

Experience loneliness

Living alone	28%
Living with others	8%

Often feel sad or depressed

Living alone	28%
Living with others	15%

SOURCE: Pew Research Center, "The Return of the Multi-Generational Family Household," Social and Demographic Trends Report, March 18, 2010.

NOTE: Unfortunately, it is not immediately clear in the report whether Pew surveyed people in assisted living facilities and, if so, how they categorized them. Meanwhile in a footnote, the Pew Research Center states that regression analysis models indicate that living arrangements have independent impact on health, depression, and loneliness but not, rather strangely, on reported happiness.

William Patrick put it, "Social isolation is on a par with high blood pressure, obesity, lack of exercise, or smoking as a risk factor for illness and early death."[13] And again, "individuals with the highest baseline scores for loneliness were also the ones most likely to be admitted to a nursing home over a four-year period."[14]

People who live alone are more likely to suffer a decline in both their health and their mental abilities than are those who live with others. So it is no surprise that those living alone are twice as likely to enter a nursing home as others are. This is according to a study of studies—a meta-analysis.[15] It is a massive difference.

Some people may think, "Well, living in a retirement home will mean an elderly person is not lonely. So that would be the best thing." But it is not contact with just anybody that mitigates a feeling of loneliness. It is not even the amount of time spent with other people. It is the nature of relationship: "the individual's ratings of the meaningfulness, or the meaninglessness, of their encounters with other people."[16] When it comes to quality of this sort, the natural intimacy of being with family members and old friends is likely to be best.

The Johanniter aid organization in Germany supplies elderly people with buttons attached to wrist or neck bands. Subscribers, who generally live alone, can press the button in an emergency to summon help. Every day, the organization receives nearly 3,000 emergency calls from their 110,000 customers. In more than half these cases, no one has fallen down or become ill. People have pressed the button just to have someone to talk to.

* * *

"In Hamburg, social workers came across an old woman who hadn't spoken with anyone for two years other than the supermarket checkout woman."

SOURCE: Guido Kleinhubbert and Antje Windmann, "Alone by the Millions: Isolation Crisis Threatens German Seniors," *Spiegel* online international, January 10, 2013, http://www.spiegel.de/international/germany/germany-faces-epidemic-of-lonely-and-isolated-seniors-a-876635.html.

Those who are married are the least lonely and the least likely to go into a nursing home.[17] Living with children is not as good as being married, but the results are much better than living alone. In a study of more than 8,000 people over 10 years, nearly one in five of those living alone went to a nursing home[18] (Figure 9.5). Of those who remained married, fewer than half as many went to a nursing home. Those who lived throughout with one of their children were in between: the chances of going to a nursing home were reduced by a third. These are powerful indicators of the importance of family life to happiness and well being.[19]

What are the results like for those admitted to a nursing home or assisted living? One study in England and Wales compared elderly people in assisted living with those at home—both those living alone and those living with family.[20] The researchers used the Geriatric Mental State exam to gauge levels of depression. They found that 9.3 percent of those living at home were depressed, but the figure soared to 27.1 percent for those living in assisted living facilities—nearly three times as many. The study concluded that "depression was highly prevalent" in assisted living facilities (see Figure 9.6).

The researchers investigated various symptoms of depression. They even asked people if they wished they were dead. A remarkably high proportion of people living at home—12 percent—said

Figure 9.5
HOW MANY WENT TO A NURSING HOME?
PERCENTAGE OF PEOPLE AGES 70 AND OVER ADMITTED INTO A NURSING
HOME DURING A 10-YEAR STUDY

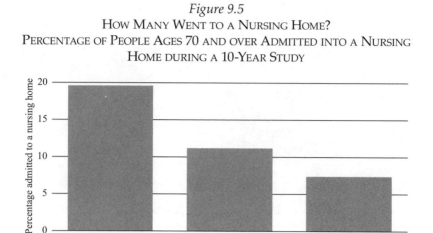

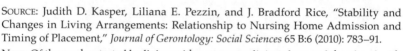

SOURCE: Judith D. Kasper, Liliana E. Pezzin, and J. Bradford Rice, "Stability and Changes in Living Arrangements: Relationship to Nursing Home Admission and Timing of Placement," *Journal of Gerontology: Social Sciences* 65 B:6 (2010): 783–91.

NOTE: Of those who started by living with a spouse or living alone and then lived with an adult child, 12.2 percent eventually went to a nursing home during the 10-year period.

Figure 9.6
WILL GRANNY *REALLY* BE HAPPY IN THE CARE HOME?
RATES OF DEPRESSION AMONG PEOPLE AGES 65 AND OVER LIVING AT
HOME AND LIVING IN ASSISTED LIVING, ENGLAND AND WALES

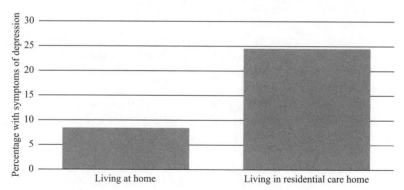

SOURCE: F. A. McDougall et al., "Prevalence and Symptomatology of Depression in Older People Living in Institutions in England and Wales," *Age and Ageing* 36 (2007): 562–68.

257

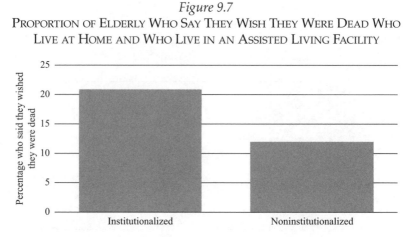

Figure 9.7
PROPORTION OF ELDERLY WHO SAY THEY WISH THEY WERE DEAD WHO
LIVE AT HOME AND WHO LIVE IN AN ASSISTED LIVING FACILITY

SOURCE: F. A. McDougall et al., "Prevalence and Symptomatology of Depression in Older People Living in Institutions in England and Wales," *Age and Ageing* 36 (2007), 562–68.

that they did. We should remember that it is likely that many of them were living alone. Among the elderly who had moved to care homes, however, the proportion wishing they were dead jumped to 21 percent, more than one in five (see Figure 9.7).

That study was of people in assisted living facilities. One would expect depression levels to be worse still in nursing homes. One study was done of residents in a nursing home in Berlin.[21] It found that over a third suffered from minor depression and a further fifth endured major depression so that, in total, 56 percent of residents were depressed.

Academics reading this may well be thinking to themselves, "Hang on! The causation could be the other way around. It could be that depressed people are more likely to go to care homes, not that care homes make them depressed."

This is indeed a theoretical possibility and it would be excellent if someone could pick out the truth with a really long-term study that saw people through a variety of experiences. In the meantime, we must use a little common sense. Yes, it is surely true that people who are depressed are more likely to go to assisted living or a nursing home. Depression and loneliness tend to lead to health problems. But the figures for depression in institutions are on such a major scale that it seems likely that the main thing is that being in assisted living—let alone in a nursing home—causes depression.

We know from many other studies that social interaction is important and contact with loved ones particularly significant. We also know that people like to have some control of their own environments—where they go and when they get up in the morning. Many of us have personal knowledge of people who were cheerful and full of life but who, without any other change in their lives, went to institutions and became depressed. Some of us, sadly, have known people who, soon after admission, died.

On the basis of this and other evidence, it seems that there is a kind of progression from the best circumstance for well-being for the elderly to the worst:

1. Living with a spouse
2. Living with an adult child
3. Living alone—this tends to be lonelier, but the feeling can be mitigated by plenty of social activity
4. Living in a care home—significantly more depressing
5. Living in a nursing home—a majority of people are likely to be depressed

Some people might think, "Well, Granny might not be particularly happy in assisted living or a nursing home, but at least she will be well looked after by professionals." Is that right? Among those who are elderly but not in institutions, between 5 and 10 percent suffer from malnutrition. But, in some studies, up to 60 percent of those in institutions have been found to be malnourished.[22] The study in Berlin previously mentioned found 22.8 percent of nursing home residents malnourished and a further 57.9 percent "at nutritional risk."[23] It is a shock that malnutrition is so common in places that exist for the very purpose of looking after the elderly.

In mitigation, one should mention that depressed elderly people tend to be malnourished and reluctant to eat. However, there is some evidence that, even in hospitals, efforts to help elderly people with their meals may be inadequate. The Care Quality Commission found that 38 percent of inpatients in England said they did not get enough help with eating or only "sometimes" did.[24]

Dame Jo Williams, then the commission's chairman, commented, "Time and again we found cases where . . . people were left without call bells, ignored for hours on end, or not given assistance to do the basics of life, to eat, drink or go to the toilet."[25] In a poll of 1,000 nurses in Britain, almost 30 percent said they would not trust the hospital they worked in to take note of malnutrition if one of their own relatives was a patient.[26] Malnutrition, of course, leads to further problems such as lower resistance to disease and a greater likelihood of injury through falling. (See Box 9.2.)

In one study in America, it was found that 92.5 percent of nursing home residents did not drink enough.[28] Some elderly people need

Box 9.2
CARE FOR THE ELDERLY AT A BRITISH NATIONAL HEALTH
SERVICE HOSPITAL

In late 2012, the Care Quality Commission caused a scandal in Great Britain when its report, *The State of Health Care and Adult Social Care in England*, reported on the poor quality of care that elderly residents received at National Health Service hospitals. Jane Kelly, a reporter for the *Spectator*, put a face on the issue and described one of her experiences as a visitor at an NHS hospital:

"There was a tiny lady of 93, no longer ill but too frail to return home. At first she was very jolly and told me in her fluting, refined voice about her father, who managed a famous biscuit company, and about courting in the Wrens. Over three weeks I saw a change; her voice became faint, she sat with her head hanging down, breakfast untouched. No one helped her to eat. . . . No one thought to investigate how and why she had suddenly become so weak. 'God help me,' she whispered as I held her hand."[a]

And from the commission's report itself:

"Ten percent of NHS hospitals . . . failed to meet standards on treating patients with dignity and respect. Only 2 per cent of private hospitals had the same failings."[b]

The report explained that common themes in the hospitals that did not treat people with respect were "lack of privacy, call bells being out of reach, and staff speaking to patients in a condescending way."

---

[a] Jane Kelly, "It's Time to Admit It: The NHS Is Unable to Look after Our Elderly," *The Spectator*, May 18, 2013, http://www.spectator.co.uk/features/8909201/among-the-bed-blockers.

[b] Jenny Hope and Daniel Martin, "Shameful! Damning Report Reveals the Plight of Neglected, Malnourished Elderly in Hospitals and Care Homes," *Daily Mail* (London), November 23, 2012, http://www.dailymail.co.uk/news/article-2237126/Shameful-Damning-report-reveals-plight -neglected-malnourished-elderly-hospitals-care-homes.html. The figures relate to care of patients generally, but it is widely accepted that those who are elderly, especially those with dementia, tend to be treated with less respect. In any case, the elderly constitute a disproportionately large number of hospital patients. [27]

to be reminded and encouraged to drink many times to get them to take enough.[29] When staff do not have the time, this does not happen.

One indicator of how good nursing homes are at looking after their patients is how frequently they fail to manage medical problems that should be within their capabilities. Congestive heart failure, asthma, and diabetes are examples. An alarmingly high proportion of admissions to hospitals from nursing homes are of this sort, indicating that residents have not been well cared for. In one study in Los Angeles, 45 percent of hospitalizations should not have been necessary.[30] In a study in the state of Georgia, the figure reached 67 percent.

Another indicator of poor-quality care is the incidence of pressure ulcers. The variation is dramatic—anywhere between 2.2 percent and 23.9 percent in American nursing homes, according to an assessment by the Institute for Healthcare Improvement.[31] The vast majority of pressure ulcers can be prevented with the right equipment and care. In one nursing home, the incidence of heel ulcers, one of the most common kinds, was reduced by 95 percent simply by the use of heel protectors.[32] This sort of thing can be prevented relatively easily but, clearly, often isn't.

"Be Nice to Your Kids . . . They'll Choose Your Nursing Home."

Source: Humorous refrigerator magnet.

There is reason to fear that drugs may be used excessively in nursing homes, too. A U.S. government report revealed that 14 percent of residents of nursing homes receive "atypical antipsychotic drugs." An astonishing 88 percent were used for reasons that were "off label"—meaning reasons other than those for which they are intended.[33] Off-label use can be for sound medical reasons, but this should be the exception, not the rule. Such drugs are sometimes used as a "chemical cosh" to make it easier to look after agitated patients. Unfortunately, their use can lead to life-threatening nervous system problems, diabetes, low blood pressure, and dizziness. The government report found that 22 percent of the time these drugs were used they were not administered in accordance with the official standards regarding unnecessary use.[34]

A British study found that more than a quarter of elderly people with dementia were being given antipsychotics (of all types) and that in most cases they were being given them as sedatives.[35] These are drugs that are meant to be given for short periods and as a last resort. Their use is meant to be reviewed regularly, but this was often not done. They can make dementia worse.

"Each day, hundreds of thousands of nursing home residents are given antipsychotic drugs, even though . . . these drugs are inappropriate and life-threatening for the vast majority of residents to whom they are given."

Source: Toby Edelman, senior policy attorney for the Center for Medicare Advocacy, Testimony before the Senate Special Committee on Aging. See "Toby Edelman Statement to Senate Committee Regarding Antipsychotic Drugs in Nursing Facilities," Center for Medicare Advocacy website, April 18, 2012, http://www.medicareadvocacy.org/toby-edelman-testifies-regarding -antipsychotic-drugs-in-nursing-facilities.

I should emphasize that, of course, there are care homes that are run conscientiously and well. But there are also cases in which care is worse than inadequate. It is callous or even cruel. In some cases, people have become suspicious and have set up hidden cameras, discovering some very unpleasant things.[36] A notorious case took place at Winterbourne View, a care home in England. A BBC reporter secretly filmed caregivers pinning patients down, slapping them, dousing them in water, and taunting them. An official report stated that there was "considerable" physical violence against patients and that some required hospital treatment as a result.[37]

The difficulty with this and other such reports is that it is hard to know how common such treatment is. Naturally, while inspectors or relatives are visiting, such behavior stops. It has been found that the elderly are reluctant to report it because they "don't want to make a fuss" or they fear they might be treated even worse in revenge. The same difficulty of measurement goes for bad treatment by caregivers who visit the elderly in their homes to help them get out of bed, to wash them, and to prepare a meal (Box 9.3).

In England, local councils (local governments) are responsible for home visits by caregivers. An inquiry conducted by a trade union, Unison, found that 73 percent of councils authorize visits that last only 15 minutes.[38] The union's spokesman, Heather Wakefield, said,

Imagine trying to provide personal care to an incontinent 94-year-old with dementia, clearing up any mess they have made, feeding them, and giving them medicines, all in just

Box 9.3
A WAY OF MAKING FAMILY CARE EASIER AND BETTER

After the Care Quality Commission found that "A quarter of care provided for the elderly in their own homes is 'unsatisfactory,'" BBC Radio 5 live reporter Rachel Burden interviewed Valerie, an elderly woman who receives care at her home.[a]

Burden first asked Valerie what she thinks of the care she gets.

Valerie says it used to be bad. She remembers a day when the caregiver was late for the first visit, to hoist her out of bed. The caregiver said she was sorry but her car had broken down, and she added that she would not be coming for the second visit at all—to bathe Valerie and give her lunch—because she would have to collect her car.

"Who will come instead?" asked Valerie.

"No one," the caregiver replied.

Burden asks how things have gotten better since that day. Valerie says that about four and half years ago, she was allowed to move to a different system. Instead of the home health care agency being chosen by her local government, she was allowed to use money allocated to her to choose the agency herself. She says she now has much better service from an agency called Nightingale. She has the same caregiver every day except when that person has a day off. When that happens, she is told who will be coming instead.

Valerie says she likes having the same person coming to help her. Some agencies think it is bad for caregivers to become friendly with the elderly people they look after, but elderly people appreciate it, Valerie says. They do not like just anybody coming into their homes.

---

[a] BBC Radio 5, February 13, 2013.

---

15 minutes. There is no time left to have a conversation, let alone provide some compassionate care before rushing out. No wonder home carers tell us they are depressed about the standard of care they are forced to provide.[39]

In theory, those in greatest need, such as the woman described, would be allocated a longer slot of 30 or 45 minutes. But councils are short of money, and the large proportion of them that sometimes provide very short visits suggests that many people may be getting peremptory, inadequate care.

Cost is an important and growing problem, causing a decline in the quality of the care that governments provide. In the United States, the Congressional Budget Office projects that public and private spending on long-term care for the elderly will more than double from 1.3 percent of gross domestic product (GDP) in 2010 to 3.0 percent in 2050.[40] Frankly, they would be lucky to get away with such a modest increase given the aging population. In Japan, the cost of government expenditure alone—following the introduction of a new long-term-care insurance system in 2000—doubled in only six years to reach 1.2 percent of GDP.[41] Denmark starts from a higher base. Its government expenditure already stands at over 2 percent of GDP, so as the population ages, a rise in cost of such proportions or anything like it would be hard to manage.[42]

When governments first started offering care for the elderly, of course, life expectancy was much lower. Moreover, in coming years the number of the most elderly individuals is expected to rise fastest. In Britain, the population over age 80 is set to soar from three million to eight million between 2008 and 2050.[43] The ratio of younger working people to older people is collapsing, with the same implications for elderly care as for pensions. The figures for Japan are forbidding. In 2000, there were 3.9 working-age people for every person over age 65. By 2050, there will only be 1.3.[44] Younger people have got to pay for the pensions of older people and also care for them. There is one bit of good news, however: the elderly are generally healthy for longer than in previous generations.

But the rising cost pressure means that, around the world, savings in the cost of caring for the elderly have been made in every way you can think of. Staffing levels have been reduced, resulting in less personal attention. Waiting lists have been allowed to rise. Priority has been given only to those in the worst condition, so people who, in truth, cannot cope well have been left to fend for themselves. In Australia, the elderly who are deemed to be low priority can wait months before even being assessed.[45]

In a number of countries, homes for the elderly have increasingly been contracted out to private companies to reduce the cost per person. Governments have encouraged the elderly to stay at home with offers of "in-home" support, which is vastly cheaper than institutional care. And when that has not saved enough money, sometimes governments reduce the amount of such support and have provided it only to those in the worst circumstances.

The responses vary from country to country. But everywhere, cost is a major problem and governments accordingly want more elderly people to stay at home. Some politicians claim they have come to realize that people are happier at home. In reality, all have been influenced by the soaring cost.

In the Netherlands, where nursing and assisted living homes dominate, they admit—openly or otherwise—that the cost is getting too high. I talked to Esther Mot, a Dutch economist, who expressed some jealousy that the cost of the German system to the government was not expanding as fast as in the Netherlands.[46] Why is that, I asked. Because in Germany, people are expected to pay more of the cost out of their own pockets, she said.

Vic is a taxi driver in Sydney. He is a Sikh and says that part of his heritage is a belief that children have a duty to look after their parents in old age. The money he earns in Australia will help enable him to fulfill his duty to his parents.

SOURCE: Interview with Vic, who drove the author to an appointment in Sydney.

All of the issues—the cutbacks to government care because of cost and the greater happiness of the elderly in or near their families— seem to lead to one conclusion: that adult children should more frequently take care of their elderly parents. I am not suggesting that this is the best thing in all cases. Far from it. In this particular area of welfare, more than any other, it is dangerous to prescribe any universal rule. But in view of what we know about how sad and lonely elderly people can become in institutions and bearing in mind the worryingly poor care they can receive in assisted living homes, in nursing homes, and when a caregiver visits only once a day, it could, perhaps, be regarded as a moral duty of children to be ready and willing to live with and help care for their parents. This applies above all to the elderly who are widowed or otherwise living alone.

Many people in the West may not like this suggestion. They might regard it as interference in their freedom to live their own lives. They have become accustomed to the idea that social insurance has been paid, so the state should provide. But this approach has simply not proved to be humane, to be kind to the elderly.

Jane Kelly, who has been a hospital visitor and seen old people ignored by their families, wrote this:

> Over the past six decades, we in the developed north took a rather patronising view of people in southern Europe who seemed to cherish family above any civic sense, or those in the developing world relentlessly having babies to care for them in their old age. But our own experiment in cradle to grave care seems to have failed, so maybe they were right all along.[47]

Kelly visited Peter, a 75-year-old disabled man. He had nowhere to go, so the council allocated him a tiny room with a flickering strip light. It didn't even have a kettle. Kelly followed him to this miserable place.[48] To her surprise, Peter mentioned he had a sister in the same city. Kelly phoned her.

"What has it to do with me?" the sister said angrily. "The state should look after him." She added, "You'd better get your finger out!" as if it were Kelly's responsibility to get the state to look after him better.

Kelly asked Peter's sister if she might at least bring her brother a kettle.

She replied, "Will I be recompensed for that?"

We might, each of us, remember that one day we ourselves will probably be old. In the United States, 70 percent of those who reach the age of 65 can expect to need long-term care during their lives.[49] Do we ourselves want to be institutionalized or isolated?

In Sweden, a retiree died in his home in Tumba, a town southwest of Stockholm.[50] His bills continued to be paid by direct debit. His pension was paid by bank transfers directly into his account. The man had relatives, but they were not in regular contact so no one realized that he was dead. Eventually his body was discovered in 2011 because broadband was being installed in the building, so people finally entered his home. The food in the refrigerator was found to date back to the beginning of 2008. His body had been lying there for three years with nobody knowing or caring.

In a similar case in Stockholm, a man was found two years after he had died because some plumbing work needed to be done.[51] One of the people interviewed afterward remarked, "One wonders how many dead, lonely people are lying across the city."

In Japan, the phenomenon of "lonely deaths" has its own special word: *kodokushi*.[52] Inevitably, it is happening increasingly because more people live alone. The number of people over age 65 who live alone in Japan jumped from 880,000 in 1980 to 3.86 million in 2005.[53]

In Germany, Klaus Pawletko, director of Friends of the Elderly in Berlin, has seen a lot of poverty during his career. But he says, "old people actually find being alone much worse than their financial difficulties." He adds, "hardly anyone in Germany talks about that."[54]

266

"The research found that the closer elderly people live to their children, the less lonely they feel. Older people who see their children once a month or less are twice as likely to feel lonely as those who see their children very regularly."

SOURCE: Women's Royal Voluntary Service paper, reported in Rosemary Bennett, "A Friendly Face and a Cup of Tea Takes Edge off Loneliness," the *Times* (London), December 11, 2012, http://www.thetimes.co.uk/tto/public/timesappeal/article3626922.ece. The Women's Royal Voluntary Service has since been renamed the Royal Voluntary Service.

While greater family care for the elderly may be desirable, it must be admitted that there can be problems. An Indian woman tells me that a married woman in her country is expected to look after the elderly parents of her husband. It is one thing to look after one's own elderly parents but to look after someone else's, even a husband's, is bound to be less attractive.

In Japan, where a tradition of women looking after the older generation has continued (albeit less widely than before), there have been surveys indicating a significant proportion of family caregivers admit to feelings of hatred for those they care for.[55]

A wife may be in the prime of her life and wanting to develop a career. She may not want to care for elderly parents, whether they are her husband's or her own. Perhaps this is why the issue is taboo. To advocate caring for elderly parents comes up against some people's idea of feminism—that women should be able to have careers as uninterrupted as those of men. Even in Spain and Italy, women are increasingly taking full-time jobs. Of course, men can be expected to care for their parents, too. But in practice it happens less often.

We should, perhaps, think that it is important for a person—whether a woman or a man—to put a higher priority on caring for an elderly, widowed parent than on a career, at least for a while. In most cases, it should be possible to provide help for an elderly person without sacrificing a whole career. There are all sorts of solutions that can be found. Care can be shared by different family members. Outside help can be brought in. Box 9.4 shows another potential solution.

In Italy, many people try combine family care for their elderly with freedom for the wife by hiring *badanti*—women from poorer countries who are paid to live with elderly people and look after them. They may well live with the extended family, in fact. *Badanti*

Box 9.4
HOME HEALTH CARE: THE IMPORTANCE OF CHOICE

At the United Community Center in Milwaukee, Wisconsin, some of the elderly are residents but others are collected from their homes by bus each day. This helps families stay together because the adult children can go out to work, happy in the knowledge that their mother or father is being looked after during the day. Most of the elderly are Hispanic so, to make them feel at home, the central lounge is designed like a Latin American plaza. There is a balcony and birds in cages. The center offers activities, exercise, and social life.

Ricardo Diaz, the executive director, says his center has good facilities for bathing people, a service that is appreciated because often adult children are embarrassed to help their parents wash. The elderly can also see young children who attend the charter school that is part of the center. They are not in a ghetto entirely reserved for old people.

generally come from nearby countries such as Romania, Moldavia, Ukraine, or Bulgaria, but some come from South America.[56] In Rome, I was told that there are 1.2 million *badanti*, of 1.5 million caregivers in Italy, but some estimates are lower.[57] Something similar happens on a smaller scale in Britain. Many live-in caregivers come from Zimbabwe and other parts of Africa. The difference in Britain is that they usually live with the elderly person and no one else.

The right course of action depends on individual circumstances. Some elderly may genuinely not want—or need—help from their children. Others may be bedbound and affected by dementia or incontinence or both. They may need turning regularly to avoid bedsores. Some may require medication three times a day and may be barely able to speak. Looking after someone in that condition is extremely stressful. To expect a family to do that unaided, at home, would be asking an enormous amount. But the majority of elderly people are in a far better condition, and it is quite possible for them to live with or near their children without being a great burden.

The point that repeatedly emerges when looking at the issue is that there is no universal, best answer. Despite this, it is possible to suggest one clear theme for how governments should approach it: they should do nothing that discourages families from looking after their own. In practical terms, that means equality of treatment between families who look after their elderly and those who do not. At present, many countries effectively favor those who leave strangers to look after their parents. This discourages something that makes elderly people happier and healthier. (For a better option, see Box 9.5.)

There are also positive steps that could be taken. One tactic would be to create compulsory savings accounts that could be used to fund care for the elderly as well as general medical care. A key feature would be that the money could be used to fund care by the family as well as by institutions. If one is to maximize innovation and reduce costs, these savings accounts should be not supplied by governments but by friendly societies, mutual societies, trade unions, professional associations, and for-profit companies. If the funds turned out not to be needed, the money would become part of the person's estate and could be bequeathed like any other asset. Of course, in some cases, the savings would run out. So to cover at least basic care in these circumstances, governments could also require compulsory care insurance. Only when all this provision was exhausted would the state step in. Again, assistance should go to those cared for by their families as much as for those in care homes or alone.

The central idea of removing obstacles to family care should influence other government policies too. If an elderly person wants to live with an adult child, there may not be enough room. Both may

Box 9.5
SPANISH SOLUTIONS

I am in Madrid and Dolores Navarro Ruiz, minister for social and family affairs in the city, is telling me about the help provided for the elderly in Spain. One service is provided specifically in Madrid. Members of her department make regular telephone calls to elderly people on their list who are living at home to check that they are all right. This gives the elderly some reassurance and human contact. It is extremely popular and appreciated.

Another unusual aspect of care there is that Spanish regional governments are required to pay money to families who look after disabled parents. Therefore, there is no discrimination against families looking after their own rather than putting them into institutions. This is in great contrast to most countries, such as France, where money is paid only if the care is provided by someone outside the family. Spain's lack of discrimination may be laudable, but it increases the cost, in the short term at least. The Netherlands tried something similar and was shocked by the rocketing expense. It cut the program back to a fraction of what was originally intended.

need to sell their homes to buy a bigger one together. But this kind of flexibility is discouraged in many countries by high taxes on homes. Accordingly, it is desirable to minimize or abolish taxes on home purchases. It is similarly important that housing should be plentiful and not too expensive because this helps enable family care. In a British survey, half those who said they would not take in an elderly parent needing 24-hour care said lack of space was a reason.[58] Housing is a key issue when it comes to care for the elderly as in other areas of welfare.

"The government and the church both stress the importance of family life but neither dare speak out about the fact that it has completely broken down at both ends of life and is probably no better in the middle. I think that I can stand back to look at this because I am gay and I have always lived alone and look on this as a sort of outsider. Now approaching 70 with both my parents dead, I look back on their life and see one that was supportive of their own parents and of me. I would like to thank God (but as an atheist I cannot) that they did not farm me out to carers [day care] at any age. I did let them down by moving away [for] work, so I did not help them as much as they deserved.

"I have just been talking to a friend who is thinking of moving closer to her two sons but is afraid to be too close. I assured her that this would be impossible. Sometimes it seems we have forgotten what it is to be human."

SOURCE: Online comment signed "Alan Thorpe" in response to an article in the *Times* (London). The comment was made on March 15, 2013, regarding Rosemary Bennett, "Children in Daycare 'Face Mental Health Risk,'" http://www.thetimes.co.uk/tto/health/child-health/article3712099.ece.

One advantage of the scheme described is that it would be less likely to run out of money, as state programs have, causing services to be cut and the elderly to be left in dire circumstances. Furthermore, it would mean that care is not given on the basis of means testing, which can create a perverse incentive not to save. In a means-tested system, people know that, if they spend all their money, the state— or, rather, taxpayers—will pick up the bill. Some means-tested care should be available but only as a last resort and perhaps provided by charities with government support.

The drawback of compulsory savings and insurance accounts, of course, is the element of compulsion. But without compulsion, many would make no provision and then would have to be provided for, through compulsory taxation, by those who have paid in. Effectively in this arrangement, one form of compulsion—saving—would replace another—tax. And the requirement to save, unlike being taxed, would provide some freedom, dignity, and choice if we need help. The saved money could also be used flexibly to provide what is really needed in individual circumstances.

Such a system would not be perfect. No system of care for the elderly will ever be so. But it would result in millions of elderly people enjoying a happier old age.

10. "All Animals Are Equal, But Some Animals Are More Equal Than Others."[1]

The Public Sector

The public sector provides large portions of the services provided by welfare states around the world. It supplies education nearly everywhere, health care in varying degrees, and pensions usually.

The public sector is often depicted as worthy and admirable. Here is David Cameron, speaking in 2006, before he became British prime minister:

> Public service—the concept of working for the good of the community—is a high ideal. We see it in our doctors and nurses, our police officers and our soldiers. But we also see it in many, many areas of our civil service and local government.[2]

Journalists, too, tend to treat the public sector with respect. In this case, Eduardo Porter in the *New York Times* argues that it is better than the private sector:

> Our track record suggests that handing over responsibility for social goals to private enterprise is providing us with social goods of lower quality, distributed more inequitably and at a higher cost than if government delivered or paid for them directly.[3]

Some people praise the public sector and add in condemnation of private enterprise as an alternative provider. They say that it is wrong for companies to make profits from educating children or caring for the sick. Often public servants are thought of as decent people doing their best for others while receiving low incomes. Is that fair? (See Figure 10.1.)

We're in a room full of teachers in New York City.[4] Some are reading books. Others are doing crossword puzzles. A few are playing

Figure 10.1
"TRUST ME. I'M A CIVIL SERVANT."
PROPORTION OF PEOPLE WHO SAY THAT THEIR PUBLIC ADMINISTRATION
FUNCTIONS WELL

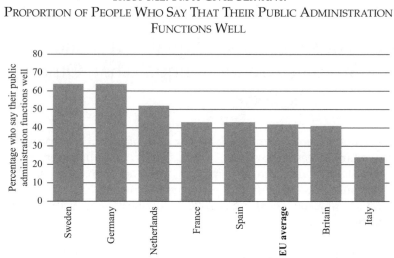

SOURCE: *Italy Today: Social Picture and Trends 2010* (Milan: Censis, 2011), p. 55, using Eurobarometer data.

chess. Yet others are debating with each other. One is painting a watercolor. Another is planning a vacation. They are spending the whole day in this room. They are not teaching any classes at all.

Every day they come to this room at the same time that other teachers go to schools. They leave at the same time too. They are paid the same. They have the same vacation entitlements too. The only difference is that they are not teaching.

There are plenty of rooms like this in New York City—enough to contain more than 700 teachers. The cost to taxpayers of paying for these nonteaching teachers is between $35 million and $65 million a year.[5] But why aren't they teaching?

Some of them are considered by their former schools to be incompetent or lazy. Some have been accused of improper conduct such as sexual harassment of students. Others have been accused of crimes. For these or other reasons, they are not allowed to teach.

The rooms in which the teachers sit all day are officially described as "temporary reassignment centers." Colloquially, they are called "rubber rooms" because staying in them can make you go crazy and a "rubber room" is slang for a padded cell.

Of course, it is understandable that some teachers should be sus-pended while accusations are resolved. But why are there so many? Because these teachers are in limbo for a long time. Typically their cases take two to five years to be resolved. Why does it take so long? The explanation is that there are many layers of state laws and agree-ments with unions that severely restrict the ability of schools to fire teachers.

This is how the rubber rooms were in 2009. Since then, the ones in New York City have been closed. After their existence became a public scandal, the mayor and the union made a deal: cases would be dealt with more quickly, but the teachers could stay at home. Yet even after this deal, the cases were still not dealt with very much faster. The problem did not go away. It was only made less visible—swept under the carpet.

Is the New York City experience a one-off?

No. Firing teachers is difficult in many American states.[6] In Illinois, one in 2,500 is removed (see Figure 10.2). For comparison, the figure for doctors is one in 57 and for attorneys one in 97. Teach-ers are close to being impossible to fire. In New York State, disciplin-ary hearings for teachers last eight times longer than the average

Figure 10.2
LOST CREDENTIALS BY PROFESSION
PERCENTAGE IN EACH PROFESSION WHO LOST THEIR CREDENTIALS IN
ILLINOIS

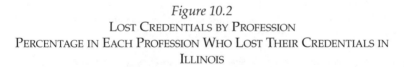
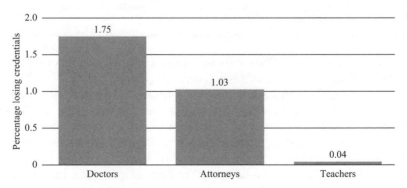

SOURCE: Karl Weber, "A Nation Still at Risk," in *Waiting for "Superman": How We Can Save America's Failing Public Schools*, ed. Karl Weber (New York: Public Affairs, 2010), p. 7.

NOTE: The figures in the source data have been changed into percentages.

U.S. criminal case. The total cost to taxpayers of the teachers who are waiting for these hearings is $65 million a year.[7]

Because it is so difficult and expensive to fire teachers, schools are reluctant even to try. If a school finally manages to get rid of a bad teacher, he or she joins a pile of teachers who must be hired when other schools need new teachers. Bad teachers don't get fired. They get recycled. And if a school has to lay off a teacher, it has to fire the most recent recruit regardless of merit.

Michelle Epperson won the title of Teacher of the Year in the Sacramento City Unified School District. Soon after, she was laid off along with 400 others when the number of teachers was cut due to shortage of money.[8] Why did they pick the Teacher of the Year? Because she had less seniority than other teachers did.

Stephen Wright, a tenured teacher at Downers Grove School District in Illinois, was warned by the district against "improper touching" of female students. He had also asked his classes for synonyms for oral sex and asked students why semen tastes salty. For these and "other confirmed improprieties" the district eventually fired him. The cost to the school district was $134,799 in legal fees. Within a year, Wright was back teaching in another school.

According to a local newspaper, "none of the tenured teachers fired in the last decade have had subsequent action taken to revoke or suspend their teaching certificate [in Illinois]."

SOURCE: Scott Reeder, "Teachers Get Fired, but Don't Leave Classroom," Hidden Violations website, http://hiddenviolations.com/stories/?prcss=display&id=358596; see also http://hidden violations.com/pdf/7.pdf. The case was heard in 2002.

Some may think, "Does it matter much if some good teachers are fired and some not-so-good ones have jobs for life?"

Eric Hanushek and Steve Rivkin examined the difference made by teacher quality. He concluded that if students had good teachers instead of average ones for three or four years in a row, the effect was as big as the difference in attainment between students who were entitled to free or reduced-price lunches and those who were not. That, of course, is the holy grail of education: to give decent opportunities to the poor. Hanushek and Rivkin also found that, if the bottom 5–10 percent of teachers were replaced with average ones, the United States would move from being below average in international comparisons to being one of the best.[9]

276

Let's put it more bluntly and emotionally: the difficulty in firing low-quality teachers damages the education of American children. Above all, it affects the children of the poor—those who cannot afford to move to a prosperous neighborhood to get their children into a better school with better teachers.

How has it happened that teachers are so difficult to fire, damaging the futures of millions of children? Because teacher trade unions have used their power to make it this way. The rules are designed for the benefit of union members, not children. This is not public service as praised by David Cameron—a form of philanthropy. It is selfishness.

"Getting bad teachers out of the classroom is essential if kids are to be educated effectively. Yet the formal rules prevent it."

Source: Terry M. Moe, *Special Interest: Teachers Unions and America's Public Schools* (Washington, D.C.: Brookings Institution, 2011).

Some may think, "But this is not a public sector problem. This is a union problem." Yet the two things are connected.

How have unions achieved so much power in education? By taking advantage of the fact that education is virtually a government monopoly in the United States. The American teachers unions provide a case study of how the public sector can combine with unionization to cause harm to the public.[10] In America, first, the public sector established monopoly of supply in education. Second, because of this monopoly, teachers unions were, in due course, able to become powerful. This took place through the 1960s and 1970s.[11] Third, they used their numbers and money from dues to obtain political power. Between 1989 and 2010, the two big teachers unions—the National Education Association and the American Federation of Teachers—together made bigger political contributions than unions representing any other trade or profession. They gave twice as much as the Teamsters Union, for example. A full 95 percent of these donations went to the Democratic Party.[12] Fourth, they used their power to promote their interests, getting for themselves better pay and conditions and making it difficult for teachers to be fired. This raised the cost of education and damaged the interests of children. (See Box 10.1.)

The contrast with the private sector is this: in private enterprise, companies that produce services at a higher price and lower quality do not survive. If unions force a company to pay higher wages and

Box 10.1
POWER IN THE WRONG HANDS

A. J. Duffy, president of the most powerful union in California—the United Teachers of Los Angeles—reveled in adopting a gangster style of dress. He wore two-tone shoes and suits with wide lapels. Behind his desk was a picture of Marlon Brando playing a Mafia boss in *The Godfather*.[a] Duffy led a boycott of the *Los Angeles Times*, which dared publish a series of articles in which test scores were used to assess the effectiveness of teachers.[b]

In 2011, Neil O'Brien, then director of Policy Exchange, a London-based think tank, had these thoughts on his country's National Union of Teachers when it was objecting to reform of teachers' pensions:

"Unfortunately, considerable power—the National Union of Teachers especially—seems to have ended up in the hands of Leninists. . . . The ultra left has survived in the trade union movement despite its disappearance from mainstream politics. . . . Some unions have become a sort of Jurassic Park, in which otherwise extinct ideologies can live again."[c]

---

[a] Author interview with Lance Izumi, who works for the Pacific Research Institute in San Francisco.
[b] Jason Song and Jason Felch, "Union Leader Calls on LA Teachers to Boycott *Times*," *Los Angeles Times*, August 15, 2010, http://articles.latimes.com/2010/aug/15/local/la-me-teachers-react-20100816.
[c] Neil O'Brien, "Reform of Teachers' Pensions Is Fair. Unsurprisingly, the Ultra-Left Don't See It That Way," *Telegraph* blog (London), June 28, 2011, http://blogs.telegraph.co.uk/news/neilobrien1/100094388/reform-of-teachers-pensions-is-fair-unsurprisingly-the-ultra-left-dont-see-it-that-way.

---

reduce the quality of what is offered, the company goes bust. Consequently, the union loses the power it established. But in the public sector, no matter how badly a government monopoly fails, it continues in place. Therefore, unions can be as demanding as they like. This is how unions have come to be much more powerful in the public sector than in the private sector. It is why the issues of union power and the public sector are connected.

Some people will be thinking that the case of American teachers is an extreme one. That may be true. Children's lives are damaged. That causes anger. But the story demonstrates that it is wrong to assume that the public sector is always and inherently philanthropic. Many individual American teachers are philanthropic. But collectively they are not.[13]

I would ask those who have a gut reaction in favor of the public sector to bear with me. Of course, there are decent, hard-working people within it. But it is only right, if we truly want the best results for the public—such as the best education for children—to look at ways in which the public sector has let the philanthropic ideal down. It is quite a list.

1. The public sector has a tendency to give itself special privileges.

Let us take public sector pensions. All across the United States, police officers receive special pensions. In most states, firefighters do, too. There is a considerable range of occupations in the public sector that get such special pensions. In about half the states, wildlife conservation officers receive special consideration. Park or forest rangers get special pension terms in a similar proportion of states. In seven states, a "motor vehicle inspector" gets favored treatment and, in three states, so does a "dispatcher."[14]

The proportion of public employees who receive special treatment is rising. The idea of what is "arduous" in public service keeps on expanding. In Florida, the number of categories of workers entitled to special pension terms was increased on five occasions between 1993 and 2011. The numbers of workers entitled to them rose 53 percent.[15] In California, in 2000, the number of employees eligible for enhanced or early retirement jumped 30 percent and the number eligible only for regular retirement plans fell.[16]

See Figure 10.3 and Box 10.2 for some other public privileges.

Figure 10.3
FRENCH PUBLIC SECTOR WORKERS RETIRE YOUNGER

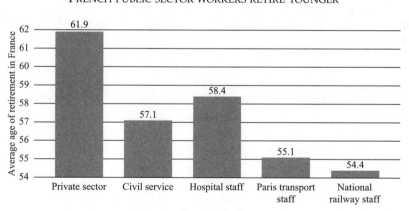

Source: "Le public part toujours à la retraite beaucoup plus tôt que le privé," *Le Figaro*, March 24, 2013, http://www.lefigaro.fr/retrait/2013/03/23/05004 -20130323ARTFIG00413-le-public-part-toujours-plus-tot-a-la-retrait-que-le-privé .php. The article cites *Le Monde* as the original source.

Box 10.2
THE PRIVILEGED WORLD OF SENIOR PUBLIC SERVANTS

Jacques Attali was an adviser to François Mitterrand, the French president, from 1981 to 1991. After the communist regimes of Eastern Europe began to fall in 1989, Attali was made head of a new bank set up by Western governments even though his background was not in banking. The European Bank for Reconstruction and Development was meant to offer financing to help Eastern European countries rebuild themselves. Before long, it became a scandal. The *Financial Times* reported that the bank had spent £55 million ($78 million)[a] on the refurbishment of its offices—the second set of offices it had occupied.[b] Of that money, £750,000 (about $1.07 million) had been spent on replacing one kind of marble with another. The bank's expenditure on itself was more than its entire lending during 1991 and 1992, its first two years of operation. As a result of this and other revelations of extraordinary self-indulgence, Attali eventually resigned. But there was no punishment or fine. He was allowed to keep the salary he had been paid of £250,000 ($355,000) a year, tax free. He also had traveled by private jet at the expense of the bank.

Attali was later involved in another scandal known as Angolagate. Yet, despite these two scandals in his curriculum vitae, in 2007 President Sarkozy made him president of a commission to study obstacles to economic growth. Senior public servants sometimes seem to keep getting public sector appointments almost regardless of their behavior.

Aurélie Boullet, wrote under the pen name Zoé Shepard about her experience as a high-flying young civil servant. She had passed tough exams to get her job, but once she was in the post, she was scandalized by how little she and her colleagues were expected to work.

She wrote, "I asked myself exactly where I had landed . . . an absurd universe in which the people who do the least declare that they are overwhelmed and where one works for 35 hours not in a week but in a month."[c]

Boullet was also angered by the substantial salaries and benefits given to the bureaucrats while front-line public servants, such as nurses, teachers, social workers, and the police, were starved of cash.[d]

---

[a] For the purposes of this book, 1 pound = 1.42 U.S. dollars (exchange rate during March 2016).
[b] See Richard Thomson, "Attali Runs out of Credit: The EBRD President Was Finally Forced to Yield to Calls for His Head," *Independent* (London), June 27, 2006, http://www.independent.co.uk/news/business/attali-runs-out-of-credit-the-ebrd-president-was-finally-forced-to-yield-to-calls-for-his-head-writes-richard-thomson-1494218.html.
[c] Zoé Shepard, *Absolument dé-bor-dée! Ou le paradox du fonctionnaire* (Paris: Albin Michel, 2010), pp. 23–4. Translated, the first part of the title is "Absolutely Snowed Under."
[d] Andrew Malone, "Will the Emperor of Excess Bankrupt France?," *Daily Mail* (London), October 27, 2011, http://www.dailymail.co.uk/news/article-2053994/Nicolas-Sarkozy-Will-Emperor-Excess-bankrupt-France.html.

There are many jobs in the private sector that could be considered equally arduous. Builders have demanding physical jobs but get no special pensions. Private investigators experience stress, like police investigators, but get no privileged pensions. Those working with the mentally ill on behalf of charities receive no privileges and often very low pay. The public sector seems quick to regard its employees as "special"—more special and deserving than other people.

In many cases, the public sector regards all its employees as special. All civil servants in Britain—teachers, local council administrators, cleaners, and so on—are entitled to pensions of a defined value related to salary, which is inflation indexed. Such favorable terms are practically unknown to the rest of the workforce. In Ontario, Canada, nearly all public sector workers have pensions based on their salaries, but only just over half of employees in the private sector do.[17] In many other countries, public sector workers again have better pension plans than everyone else. Who funds these better plans? The rest of the public, of course. It all amounts to a transfer of wealth from the general public to public sector.

In addition to this, workers in the public sector are less likely to face compulsory layoffs. We saw that U.S. teachers are almost impossible to fire. A study in Ontario found that public sector workers are less than a fifth as likely as workers in the private sector to be fired.[18]

Some will be thinking, "Yes, but the security of public sector jobs and the generosity of their pensions merely compensate them for being less well paid." It is true that average pay in the public sector in many countries is below that in the private sector. But the public sector often includes a higher proportion of low-paid jobs such as cleaning and clerical work. The Fraser Institute did a study comparing pay for people of similar qualifications and ages doing similar work in Ontario. The conclusion was that those in the public sector are paid 14 percent more.[19] In the United States, another study found that public sector workers in similar jobs were paid between 3 and 19 percent more than those in the private sector.[20]

Policy Exchange, a British think tank, looked at public sector pay and concluded, "When controlling for the differences like age, experience and qualifications, the hourly pay premium for a public sector worker was 8.8 per cent as of December 2010."[21] In Greece, the wages of workers in the government-run railways averaged €65,000 ($71,500) in 2012.[22] A former Minister of Finance exclaimed, "There isn't a single private company in Greece with that kind of average pay."[23] It may well be that public sector workers were once paid less than those in the private sector. But that is certainly not the case any more.

All this might be justifiable if the public sector employees were working longer hours than those in the private sector. The U.S. Bureau of Labor Statistics has detailed figures derived from timesheets of all the hours that someone actually works. The survey therefore captures such things as length of vacations and work done at home. Using these figures, Jason Richwine made adjustments so that similar jobs and qualifications could be compared. He found that the average employee of the U.S. federal government works 2.2 hours a week less than his or her equivalent in the private sector—a difference of slightly more than 5 percent. Over a full year—incorporating time taken out of work for sickness as well as holidays and hours per day—a federal employee works the equivalent of three weeks a year less than other people. It's a difference of just over 6 percent.

Richwine found that state and local government employees were working even fewer hours than the federal government workers were. It is true that teachers work fewer hours than others because of school holidays, but Richwine excluded teachers from his calculations.

It would not be fair to say that public sector workers enjoy special privileges always and everywhere. But in many cases and many places, public sector workers get better pension terms, have higher pay, work less, have more sick days off, and are less likely to lose their jobs (see Figure 10.4). The people who pay for this situation consist of everybody else. The public sector often takes advantage of the rest of the population.

2. The public sector tends to be inefficient, wasteful, and overstaffed, resulting in higher costs.

Britain led a global wave of privatization of nationalized industries between 1980 and 2000. One of these was of British Gas Corporation. It had 91,500 employees and, before privatization, some people claimed it was overstaffed and inefficient.[24] Was it?

Well, four years after privatization, it had 12,000 fewer employees. Within another four years, it had shed a further 12,000 employees. There seems to have been no suggestion that customer service deteriorated. If anything, the opposite took place. So, in retrospect it seems that, as a public sector operation, it had

Figure 10.4
GOVERNMENT EMPLOYEES USE MORE SICK DAYS
AVERAGE DAYS OFF SICK IN 2010 IN BRITAIN

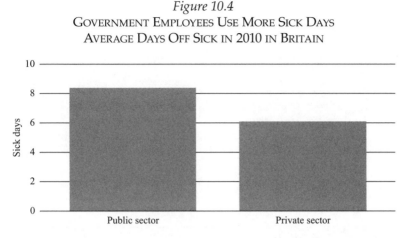

SOURCE: Confederation of British Industry, "Healthy Returns? Absence and Workplace Health Survey 2011," CBI, May 2011, http://www.cbi.org.uk/media/955604/2011.05-healthy_returns_-_absence_and_workplace_health_survey_2011.pdf.

NOTE: The median annual cost of days off sick in the public sector was 46 percent higher than in the private sector (£1,040 compared with £710). The cost for taxpayers of the extra sick days was £5 billion. At an exchange rate of 1 pound = 1.42 U.S. dollars, the median annual cost of days off sick in the public sector was $1,467 compared with $1,008, and the annual cost to taxpayers was $7 billion.

24,000 more employees than were needed to run the business—an excess of 26 percent. It was inefficient and heavily overstaffed. The public, through charges and taxes, had to pick up the bill. (See Figure 10.5.)

The electricity-generating companies in Britain employed 26,700 people when they were nationalized industries.[25] After three years in the private sector, the number of employees had been reduced to 10,400—a decrease of 61 percent. It appears that the business had been extravagantly overstaffed.

When gas and electricity were nationalized industries, strikes took place occasionally, causing disruption and inconvenience to the public and businesses. When they were in the public sector, the unions were strong and could threaten to turn the lights off or keep the country in the cold. Once the state monopolies were broken up, the power of the unions to make such threats diminished. The number of strikes has dwindled to practically zero.

In some countries, it goes beyond employing excessive staff members to do the business of the organization. In the United States,

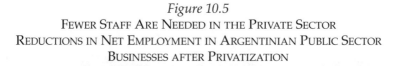

Figure 10.5
FEWER STAFF ARE NEEDED IN THE PRIVATE SECTOR
REDUCTIONS IN NET EMPLOYMENT IN ARGENTINIAN PUBLIC SECTOR
BUSINESSES AFTER PRIVATIZATION

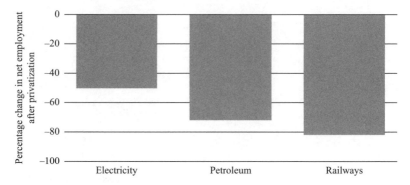

SOURCE: Sunita Kikeri and John Nellis, "An Assessment of Privatization," *World Bank Observer* 19 (2004): 87–118.

NOTE: Overstaffing in the public sectors of developing countries can be on an astonishing scale. In the study of privatizations around the world that is the source of this figure, researchers remarked, "A number of highly protected and deeply politicized enterprises have seen huge declines in net employment."

Britain, and Spain, for example, public sector unions are so strong that the taxpayer is obliged to finance full-time union employees too. They are not helping provide the service in question at all. But they are certainly adding to the costs.[26]

"Los liberados"
The "free" or "liberated." Nickname for union officials in Spanish companies and in government who receive a salary but work full time for the union.

There are two kinds of privatization. One kind creates a market of competing companies. The other involves just contracting out work to private companies. One drawback of contracting out work is that a contract might be awarded to a company or official who has paid a bribe. When in Italy, I was told that there had been scandals of this sort in the south of the country involving health care contracts.

One scandal involved providing prostitutes in an attempt to make sure that the contract was given to a particular company.

But let's ask why governments contract out work at all. They know they will be criticized by the public sector trade unions. One often finds that governments do not explain why they are contracting out, but the answer is simple. Governments contract out almost always because their budgets are under pressure and they find it is the only way they can afford to do what they want to do. They keep quiet about this—the real reason—to avoid inflaming any conflict with the public sector unions. Saving money was the reason the regional government in Valencia contracted out the construction and operation of a hospital in Alzira (see Chapter 3). Valencia got cheaper hospital service and better results.

Saving money is also the main reason the operation of many prisons in the United States and elsewhere has been contracted out. Has money actually been saved? Adrian Moore looked at 14 studies of the subject.[27] Two found that the contractors cost about the same as the public sector. The other 12 found savings of between 5 and 28 percent. Did privatization damage the way these prisons were run? Not according to six studies comparing their quality. In fact, one way in which costs have been reduced is by minimizing the number of violent incidents. That has been achieved in some cases by improving conditions such as by providing prisoners with more opportunities for work, education, and recreation.

Sometimes private sector administration is simply less bureaucratic. One warden in a privately run prison explained that, when he needed some minor piece of office equipment, he did not have to go through some long and complex state purchasing process. He just went out and bought it.[28] In Britain, a time-study was done of the work completed by a social worker on a single case. It was found that only 14 percent of the time was actually spent in the family home, and even that time was used mostly for collecting information to fulfill reporting requirements.[29] (See Figure 10.6.)

Waste and inefficiency can arise in various ways. In October 2002, *The Economist* carried an article about massive improvements that Tony Blair, the prime minister, was promising in Britain's National Health Service (NHS): "Tony Blair talks ecstatically about a new consumer focus—from hospital appointments booked online at times convenient to patients to electronic medical records that can be accessed wherever the patient is."[30] This was going to be a dramatic improvement in efficiency. Patients were going to be able to go to

Figure 10.6
SOCIAL WORKER OR PAPER WORKER?
THE PROPORTION OF TIME SPENT BY A LOCAL GOVERNMENT SOCIAL
WORKER DEALING WITH A SINGLE CASE IN SWINDON, ENGLAND

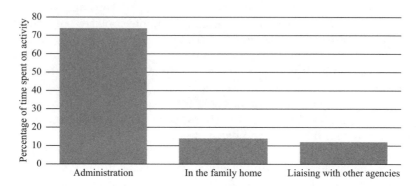

SOURCE: "The Life Programme," Participle website, www.participle.net.

their computers and make appointments. They would be able to see their records online. Doctors anywhere in the country would be able to look up patient records in an instant.

But even at that early stage, *The Economist* sounded a warning note:

> [Tony Blair] is depending on IT [information technology] to deliver the goods. Yet large government IT projects have a habit of going spectacularly wrong. The government thinks it has learned the lessons of past IT disasters. The new Office of Government Commerce has created something it calls the Gateway process, a sensible enough system of appraisal and review, which it believes will cut down the number of "rogue" projects. But it is far from clear that the government understands why IT projects in the public sector are particularly susceptible to failure.[31]

In accordance with *The Economist*'s fears, the project stumbled from one failure to another. Contractors withdrew despite incurring losses of hundreds of millions of pounds. Doctors made criticisms. Costs mounted. I had supper with someone in the information technology business in 2006 who told me that the new NHS computer system was never going to work and that this was common knowledge in the industry. Still, it plowed ahead. More money was spent.

286

Finally in 2011, a House of Commons committee issued a damning report. A month later, the government belatedly brought the project to an end. Some elements of it have survived and have been of use. But the majority of the cost—some £12 billion ($17 billion)—was wasted.[32]

What was the problem?

The Economist, in its 2002 article, had commented: "Big projects are difficult to manage whether public or private. But the most intractable problems arise from attitudes that are distinctively public-sector." It suggested that in the private sector, companies focus on lower costs and improved competitiveness. "But politicians (*vide* Mr Blair), desperate to find quick fixes and unencumbered with any understanding of what technology can and can't do, often expect miracles." Moreover, "'Change management' is never easy, but in the public sector it is especially hard because there is too little competitive pressure pushing it, and there are too many powerful unions holding it back."[33]

Long after the failure of the NHS computer project, a computer magazine obtained records released under the Freedom of Information Act. Its report did not receive much attention, but it was revealing. The records showed that Blair had pressed the NHS to hurry up the project so that the expected benefits could be seen more quickly—by 2005, when a general election was due.[34] This deadline helped contribute to the failure of the project. *The Economist*'s assertion that politically motivated interference was one reason that public sector projects go wrong was vindicated.

"Senior people issue airy instructions—usually in response to a [newspaper] column—but, not understanding management, they do not know how to follow through and ensure things are done."

SOURCE: Dominic Cummings blog, "A Few Responses to Comments, Misconceptions, Etc. about My *Times* Interview," June 20, 2014, http://dominiccummings.wordpress.com/2014/06/20/a-few-responses-to-comments-misconceptions-etc-about-my-times-interview. Cummings, a former U.K. government special adviser also remarked, "Government departments are so dysfunctional that even the great officials who could manage things properly are seldom allowed to by the system."

No one, as far as is known, was fired as a result of the huge waste of money. Certainly neither the head of the NHS nor the prime minister was removed. There were few apparent consequences for anyone in the public sector. This points to another reason the public sector can be wasteful and inefficient: the lack of accountability and clear responsibility that often exists. In the public sector, "the buck doesn't stop here."

In sum, there seems to be a rogues' gallery of reasons for public sector inefficiency and extra cost: more bureaucracy, lack of focus on costs, lack of competitive pressure, powerful unions, politically motivated interference, and lack of accountability.

3. The higher costs of public service lead to higher taxes and public debt.

In France, where public servants are particularly numerous, a magazine expressed widespread exasperation with public services there. Its front cover carried a photo of an empty counter, complete with "Position Closed" sign, where an official should have been attending to members of the public. The headline was "PUBLIC SERVANTS, the pets of power: While the deficit soars out of control, they are twice as numerous as in Germany . . . but where are they hiding?"[35]

It was a cry of frustration at an excess of public servants who, despite their numbers, provide poor service. Everybody has to pay for the self-indulgences and waste. The people who pay include the poor. The poor pay sales or value added tax. In many countries, they pay income tax too. It is wrong that the poor should be taxed to finance the waste and early pensions of the public sector.

4. The public sector tends to create excessive regulations.

Blake Hurst was brought up on a farm in America.[36] At the age of 14, he was put in charge of feeding two steers and planting and harvesting 40 acres of corn. He kept the books for the whole operation. After four years, he had saved enough to pay for his college education.

That was a generation ago. Now, he would not be allowed to do any of this work except the bookkeeping. It is against the regulations.

Blake buys fertilizer from a small-scale supplier. The supplier tells him he has been fined about a third of his annual profit. Why? Because he failed to complete his "Risk Management Plan" correctly despite hiring a consultant to do it for him. The form concerned is so big that it is held in a binder 3 inches thick. The supplier must pay the large fine and refile his plan online. The instructions on how to complete the form are 110 pages long.

288

All the forms, fines, and regulations infuriate Blake and his supplier. But why were they created? Was there a reason?

Let's take the rules that make it difficult for young teenagers to do work on American farms. Yes, there was a reason. They were created to protect children. Hilda Solis, secretary of labor, was one of the people in favor of such rules. She was concerned for the well-being of children. She did not want them to be "robbed of their childhood."[37] She, with the cooperation of others, passed laws and created the regulations. She believed what she was doing was good.

It must be intoxicating to feel that with the stroke of a pen one can improve the world. That is probably an important reason public servants create so many regulations. In France, there are regulations to ensure that two wheelchairs can pass each other on the pavement. Any branch or street sign that gets in the way must be removed.[38] Wheelchair access is required—not just recommended—in more and more places such as hotels, historic houses, hospices, and residential care homes. France has a law protecting the coastline from overdevelopment. One can readily imagine and sympathize with the desire to preserve something natural and beautiful. A law was passed to enforce it. The intention is quite obviously to do good.

Such regulations sometimes come out of a scandal. In Britain, there were concerns that the police were not always maintaining proper standards in their investigations. So they were required to fill in forms showing that interviews had been conducted properly. Politicians were seen to be acting to make the world a better place.

And so the rule books grow. In France, the tax code, the labor regulations, and the planning laws all more than doubled in size between 2002 and 2012 (see Figure 10.7).

Finance ministers doubtless used the tax code to encourage desirable things like investment. The labor code was extended to give further protection to employees. The planning laws were changed to ensure that nothing unpleasant should blot the landscape and that new homes should be more energy efficient.

The French government has the distinction that it counts up the number of its regulations—something that only a centralized country like France can do. It has found that its citizens enjoy the benefit of 400,000 rules.[39] At the current rate of growth, it cannot be long before the count reaches a million. Even then, no doubt, there will be more injustices, depredations, and nuisances to counter. More regulations and forms will have to be created to combat them.

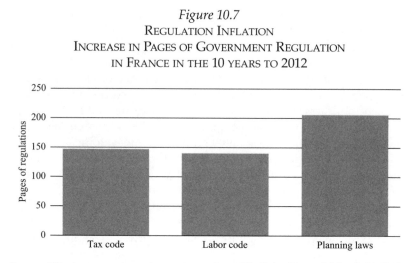

Figure 10.7
REGULATION INFLATION
INCREASE IN PAGES OF GOVERNMENT REGULATION
IN FRANCE IN THE 10 YEARS TO 2012

SOURCE: "Ces bureaucrates qui nous tyrannisent," *Le Point* (France), March 21, 2013.

In most cases, regulations are created to make the world a better place. In other cases, they are created by politicians to please the public. How could things that come from such intentions do any harm?

> "The head of a small company [in France] counted up. Last year he had to reply to 37 [government] questionnaires containing 7,047 questions."
>
> SOURCE: "Ces bureaucrates qui nous tyrannisent," *Le Point* (France), March 21, 2013.

Take the regulations insisting that children should not be used for work on farms. Yes, children are protected from exploitation. They can have childhoods free of remunerative work. But might children not gain satisfaction and life skills from being entrusted with work at a young age? They could earn money and ease the budget of their family if it is poor. They might save, as Blake Hurst did, to finance a college education. Without such work, some children might not be able to afford a college education. Such are the possible unintended consequences that regulators may not always take into account.

Perhaps the regulators might also have done the parents the honor of letting them make the decision.

What about the regulations on fertilizer supplies and the voluminous, complicated "Risk Management Plan"? One consequence is that suppliers have to spend money on consultants or spend their own time filling in the forms. So the financial return on their investment in the business will be lower. This means they are less likely to have money to expand and invest. The money they must spend on a form-filling consultant might have been spent on a new plant or on research and development. The extra cost of fulfilling the regulatory requirements is likely to add to the price of fertilizer and thus the price of food.

Wheelchair access is required for new student accommodations in France. So rooms are made 20 percent bigger, which means the cost is higher and, because there is no extra money, fewer students are able to get student accommodations.[40] Meanwhile, the law protecting the coastline has affected the little town of Plouvien in Brittany.[41] A very short section of the town boundary runs along the inland end of an estuary, miles away from the sea. As a result, almost no building is allowed in Plouvien. This has prevented the construction of a factory that would have provided employment.

"Paper tax"

SOURCE: Phrase coined by a French think tank to describe the burden of filling out forms. The think tank was iFRAP, which stands for *Fondation pour la recherche sur les administrations et les politiques publiques* (Foundation for Research on Administration and Public Policy). Quoted in "Ces bureaucrates qui nous tyrannisent," *Le Point* (France), March 21, 2013.

Planning regulations for building in Britain mean that the cost of obtaining permission to build a house has come to equal the cost of the bricks used in its construction.[42] Housing is therefore more expensive than it otherwise would be, and fewer people can afford homes. The police, meanwhile, have been required to fill in forms answering 1,099 questions when they conduct major crime investigations.[43] According to a report on this subject, "We have armies of people filling in spreadsheets trying to prove their force meets this or that standard. There is one-third of policing that we could cut out." To put it another way, the excessive regulations mean that fewer police officers are available to fight crime.

The unintended consequences of regulations are a kind of undiscovered continent. There are 2.4 times as many companies in France with 49 employees as there are with 50.[44] Why? Because once a company has 50 employees, it is required to introduce profit sharing, to set up three employee worker councils, and to submit plans to the worker councils if ever it wishes to fire anybody. Therefore, small companies are discouraged from growing into middle-size ones, which means lower economic growth than might otherwise have taken place.

"Residents who live near a proposed relief road [bypass road] at Manchester Airport were recently left scratching their heads to be asked in a consultation: 'Is your gender identity the same as the gender you were assigned with at birth?'"

SOURCE: Ross Clark, "Why Councils Ask If You're Transgender When You Call about the Wheelie Bins," *Daily Mail* (London), March 20, 2013, http://www.dailymail.co.uk/news/article-2296107/Why-councils-ask-youre-transgender-wheelie-bins.html.

Contracts with government for support of hospices in Britain can run to hundreds of pages.[45] Dealing with the contracts and making sure all the terms are fulfilled are expensive. Therefore, hospices cannot afford to take in as many people as they otherwise would or else they must save money by giving their elderly customers less care. More subtly, a mentality may be encouraged whereby staff in hospices may come to think of themselves as following a set of rules rather than doing things from an impulse of loving care. As Michael Howard, chairman of Help the Hospices, put it, "hospices began as a response by local people to a lack of dignity and compassion for dying people. . . . We must not allow hospice care, as a humanitarian response to a deeply human issue, to be eroded by inappropriate regulation and red tape."[46]

Regulations affecting companies can be so extensive that only big companies can afford them and survive. That means fewer small companies, less innovation, and less competition. In Manhattan, the number of small finance or insurance companies fell 23 percent between 1998 and 2010.[47]

The examples may seem to some people like a collection of unfortunate events of no great significance. Are regulations so widespread that they make a substantial impact? What is the big picture?

"WHAT INTUITION TEMPTS US TO BELIEVE:
Someone needs to plan, and central planners know best.
WHAT REALITY TAUGHT ME:
No one knows enough to plan a society."

SOURCE: John Stossel, *No They Can't: Why Government Fails—but Individuals Succeed* (New York: Threshold, 2012).

The World Bank examined whether varying levels of state control of the economy and regulation could help explain different rates of economic growth. The answer was "yes"—or, to put it in the bank's more academic way:

> Diverging patterns of reform contribute to explain the puzzling disparities in growth outcomes over the past decade. . . . Our empirical results seem to suggest sizeable benefits from further progress in reforming the regulatory environment and in reducing the role of the state in business activities.[48]

Among the findings, the World Bank concluded that employment protection reduced investment.

John Dawson and John Seater, two economists in North Carolina, have looked at the leading studies of the impact of regulation on growth. They comment, "Almost all these studies conclude that regulation has deleterious effects on economic activity." They themselves studied the effect of regulations in the United States and concluded that extra regulation created since 1949 has reduced economic growth by 2 percent a year.[49] This is an astonishingly large amount. The cumulative effect over time is huge. Dawson and Seater estimate that the economy in 2005 was only 28 percent of what it would have been if the amount of regulation in the United States had remained at 1949 levels. To put it another way, the United States would have been more than three times richer without post-1949 regulation. They comment that this result—which at first seems so remarkable—is in accord with other studies using different methods.

The World Bank has made an index of "ease of doing business," a combination of measures such as the number of days it takes to set up a new enterprise.[50] It is, at least in part, an indication of the

293

burden of regulations. The top-ranked countries for ease of doing business are these:

1. Singapore
2. Hong Kong
3. New Zealand
4. United States
5. Denmark
6. Norway
7. United Kingdom
8. South Korea
9. Georgia
10. Australia

The countries where it is easy to do business have become prosperous or have been growing fast. Some will be surprised to see Georgia, a relatively poor, formerly communist country, on the list. But after it adopted a policy of low regulation, it had one of the fastest growth rates among such countries. It suffered through war with Russia in 2008, but the average growth rate before that, from 2004 to 2007, was 10 percent.[51]

Countries rated badly for ease of doing business tend to have lower per capita incomes. Most tellingly, they have lower incomes than other countries in the same region. Indonesia and the Philippines, for example, have less ease of doing business and their people are poorer than those in Singapore and Malaysia. (See Box 10.3.)

So regulations can do major damage to national economic performance as well as causing other unintended consequences. What should we do about them? Should we abolish them all? Surely not. Some regulations are bound to be beneficial even when all their unintended consequences are included in the equation. But they should probably be minimized. There should be a prejudice against them. Possible unintended consequences should be considered as carefully as benefits. In fact, they should be considered more carefully because they tend to be subtle or indirect whereas the benefits are obvious.

We should probably also guard against the first reaction of politicians, the media, and others when something goes wrong. The first reaction tends to be to create a new rule, but sometimes that is not the best answer. The story about the governors of California and Texas illustrates this (see Box 10.4). Or let's suppose a police officer abuses someone he arrests. People might demand that in the future

Box 10.3
A Tale Of Two Territories

After the Second World War, Hong Kong was a territory with practically nothing. Many people were living in shantytowns. It had a small public sector and few regulations. It had no restrictions or taxes on imports at all.

Meanwhile, France was endowed with centuries of civilization and development. It had a large, centralized government headed by some of the best-educated people in the world—an elite. It created laws and regulations to protect its important industries: farming, car manufacturing, and so on. Under France's leadership, the European Union developed its Common Agricultural Policy to protect farmers from international competition.

How did the two places progress in the following decades?

By 2012, France's gross domestic product (GDP) per capita was $36,785, according to the World Bank, and it ranked 27th in the world. Hong Kong had GDP per capita of $51,170 and ranked 11th. The land of free trade, small public sector, and zero protectionism had overtaken historic France (see Figure B10.3).

Figure B10.3
GDP Per Capita in International Dollars
Reflecting Actual Purchasing Power, 2012

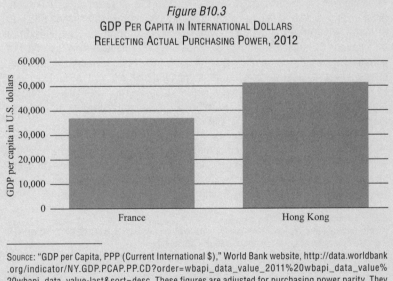

Source: "GDP per Capita, PPP (Current International $)," World Bank website, http://data.worldbank .org/indicator/NY.GDP.PCAP.PP.CD?order=wbapi_data_value_2011%20wbapi_data_value% 20wbapi_data_value-last&sort=desc. These figures are adjusted for purchasing power parity. They represent a standard of living equivalent to what a dollar could buy in the United States.

Note: There will certainly be people who say, "It is not fair to compare France and Hong Kong. Hong Kong has had special advantages. It has been an *entrepôt* for China, for example." I might find this objection more convincing if such people would identify any country with minimal restrictions on trade, commerce, and free enterprise that had done badly and, at the same time, a country with high regulations and restrictions on trade that had done nearly as well. I would also point out that Hong Kong had its own manufacturing and service industries that did not depend on it being an *entrepôt*. Meanwhile, some other islands offshore from great continents have not similarly developed into wonderfully successful economies. Sri Lanka, Malta, Cuba, and Madagascar are examples.

Box 10.4
WHAT DOES A GOVERNOR DO WHEN HE MEETS A COYOTE?

> Richard Fisher, president of the Federal Reserve Bank of Dallas, described what a business friend in Los Angeles told him was the difference between their country's two biggest states:
>
> "The governor of California is jogging with his dog along a nature trail. A coyote jumps out. He attacks the governor's dog and then he bites the governor. The governor starts to intervene but reflects on the movie *Bambi* and then he realizes he should stop because the coyote is only doing what it does naturally. So, instead, he calls Animal Control. Animal Control captures the coyote and bills the state $200 for testing it for diseases and $500 for relocating it. He then calls the veterinarian, who collects the dog and bills the state $200 for testing it for diseases. The governor then goes to the hospital. He spends $3,500 getting checked for diseases from the coyote and getting his bite wound bandaged.
>
> "Of course, being California, the running trail gets shut down for six months while the Fish and Game Department conducts a $100,000 survey to make sure the area is now free of dangerous animals. The governor then spends $50,000 of state funds implementing a 'Coyote Awareness' program. The legislature then spends $2 million to study how to better treat rabies and, in fact, how to permanently eradicate the disease from the world at large. Of course, the government security agent is fired for not stopping the attack, and the state spends $150,000 to train a new protective agent for the governor with special training regarding the nature of coyotes. And then PETA [an animal rights group] contests the relocation and files a $5 million suit against the state.
>
> "The governor of Texas is jogging with his dog along a nature trail. A coyote jumps out and tries to attack him and his dog. The governor shoots the coyote with a state-issued pistol and just keeps on jogging. The governor spent 50 cents on a .38 caliber cartridge and buzzards ate the dead coyote.
>
> "And that, my friends, is why California is broke and Texas is rich."

SOURCE: Richard Fisher, speech at the Cato Institute, Washington, D.C., October 10, 2012, http://www
.cato.org/events/europes-crisis-welfare-state-lessons-united-states.

forms are filled in to provide evidence that prisoners have been well treated. Instead of this, we should perhaps simply demand that the police officer concerned is charged and fired. We are surely all aware that filling in a form does not genuinely prove that a suspect has been well treated anyway.

5. A powerful public sector enables abuses of power.

Lisbeth Salander, a young woman, behaves very abnormally, and a court decides she must have a legal guardian. Her first guardian is kindly but he dies. He is replaced by Nils Bjurman. Bjurman sexually molests Lisbeth and demands she give him oral sex. She resists.

He says, "If you are nice to me, I'll be nice to you. If you make trouble, I can put you away in an institution for the rest of your life."

So she submits and does what he wants.

This is a scene from the best-selling Swedish novel *The Girl with the Dragon Tattoo*, by Stieg Larsson. It is an illustration of how public sector officials have the potential to abuse their power. This power is particularly great because the public sector is frequently a monopoly. The individual cannot switch to a competitor.

Coca-Cola is a powerful and rich company. But if you don't like it for any reason, you can buy Pepsi, fruit juice, or water. If you want public housing, however, there is probably only one place you can go. We have seen (in Chapter 5) how an Australian civil servant abused the power that his government position gave him and how in France such abuse appears widespread.

In the United States, the Internal Revenue Service (IRS) discriminated against organizations that were on the right of American politics.[52] When such organizations applied for an advantageous tax status, they were more likely than left-wing organizations to be subject to delays.

President Obama called the scandal "inexcusable" and remarked, "I will not tolerate this kind of behavior in any agency, but especially in the IRS, given all the power that it has and the reach that it has into all of our lives."[53] That is exactly the point. This scandal was disturbing because of the "power . . . and the reach" of the agency. Staff members at many other government agencies have similar power, including social workers, court officials, social housing officials, customs officials, regulators of industries, doctors in government hospitals, and so on.

The scandalous behavior of the IRS in the United States and the housing official in Australia became public because these two countries are relatively open and people there aspire to behave decently. In some countries, they would not become public at all. These things are difficult to prove even in countries like the United States and Australia. But the fact that they may be exposed probably makes public servants more likely to behave as they should. In less open societies, there is surely much more abuse of public sector power.

"The mystery is over. After a month of waiting, it turns out that an 84-year-old woman in Florida has won the $590 million Powerball lottery. As for how much tax she's going to have to pay, the IRS said it's too early to tell because they don't know whether she's a Republican or Democrat."

SOURCE: Jay Leno, American talk show host, joking about the IRS political favoritism scandal. Quoted in Dan Mitchell, "More Libertarian-Leaning Humor from Jay Leno," International Liberty blog, http://danieljmitchell.wordpress.com/2013/06/23/more-libertarian-leaning-humor-from-jay-leno/?utm_source=twitterfeed&utm_medium=twitter.

When Eastern Europe was under communist rule, if you wanted something from a public servant, you routinely had to give a bribe. Public servants had power in many situations. As one study of bribery noted, "the allocation of economic resources depended primarily on administrative decisions by public officials. Bribes, payoffs, and kickbacks were therefore a way of influencing these decisions."[54] A habit or way of life was established, unfortunately, and became part of the culture. As recently as 2010, it was estimated that bribe giving is more than eight times more common in the former communist countries than in the rest of Europe.[55]

Another abuse of power takes place when public servants cover up their own incompetence. In 2010, there were many warnings about dreadful failings at Morecambe Bay NHS Trust.[56] The Care Quality Commission conducted an inspection over two days and gave the trust a clean bill of health. This finding was completely wrong. It is now believed that between 2001 and 2012, up to 16 babies and two mothers died because of poor care at a maternity unit that was part of the trust. Another nine infants were born with permanent brain damage. When this information emerged, the commission conducted an internal review of what had happened in the original inspection. It was highly critical of the way the inspection was done. But at a meeting at which the chief executive was present, an order was given to delete the review so that it would never be seen by the public. Only because of the bravery of a whistleblower has the truth about this cover-up become known.

6. The public sector's own employees can be intimidated.

This is one of the less obvious ways in which the public service sometimes does not live up to any philanthropic ideal. In England, a terrible scandal took place in Mid Staffordshire National Health

Service Trust between 2005 and 2009. The neglect of patients by staff at Stafford Hospital was so dreadful that between 400 and 1,200 patients died unnecessarily through thirst, starvation, wrong or nonadministration of drugs, and so on (see also Chapter 11).[57] The official inquiry tried to establish why the appalling treatment was not discovered earlier, before so many lives were lost. It found that "an explanation of staff's reluctance to come forward with concerns was that they were scared." Furthermore, "staff lived in an atmosphere of fear . . . promoted by the managerial styles of some senior managers."[58]

The government had set targets for hospitals to attain. So the managers could damage their careers if they failed to meet these targets. This led to bullying and lies. Of course, bullying takes place in the private sector too. But the public sector does not make a bright, cheerful contrast, as some imagine. The fact that it is often a monopoly employer makes its bullying all the more frightening. An employee who is fired by a near-monopoly provider like the NHS does not just lose a job. He or she loses a career.

7. The public sector often provides poor service.

We have referred to quality of service in passing before. But it is a subject by itself.

Hospitals in Valencia, Spain, until very recent times rarely provided an epidural anesthetic to women giving birth (see Chapter 3). Hospital staff members told women it was not recommended or even possible for them to have them. The situation changed when the contract for running a hospital was given to a private company. This hospital offered epidurals. So women started coming from across the region to give birth at this hospital. Then, and only then, did the public sector hospitals start to provide this service too. This is a classic case both of poor service by the public sector organizations and the excuses used to justify it.

Sometimes people do not realize how poor the service is that they are getting from a public sector monopoly. In Argentina, before the water supply was privatized, in many areas a lot of people did not understand how many deaths were being caused by low-quality water. It is estimated that after privatization, the improvement in purity saved the lives of about 500 infants and young children a year.[59] The greatest effect was in the poorest areas.[60]

In Britain, in 1987, it was normal—it simply seemed part of the way of the world—that a quarter of public telephones were out of order.[61] After privatization, the proportion was reduced to 4 percent.

Similarly, it was not uncommon before 1987 to wait weeks to have a telephone line connected to a house or apartment. Officially, the proportion of requests met within eight days was 59 percent. After privatization, the proportion rose to 97 percent.[62]

There are many such examples. The public sector often offers inferior service, sometimes even resulting in loss of life as in Argentina. The public is typically unaware of the poor service because there is no competition and therefore no way of making a comparison.

Those who say they reject the idea that public sector service tends to be inferior sometimes reveal a different view by their actions. Civil service employees in Spain are allowed to choose private or public health care.[63] More than four of five choose private care.

Another revealing phenomenon is that failure by a public sector institution has to be on a major scale to be considered interesting enough to warrant news coverage. A private sector institution that makes even one mistake attracts enormous attention. Why? Surely because poor service is considered unsurprising in the public sector.[64]

* * *

After this list of seven charges against the behavior and performance of the public sector, let me again emphasize the difference between criticizing a system and criticizing the people in it. There are plenty of public sector employees who work hard and go beyond the call of duty. They are all the more admirable for doing their best when they are in circumstances that make providing a good service difficult. But overall, the public sector services tend to be wasteful, inefficient, and expensive. They give themselves special privileges, cause taxes to be higher than they need to be, and provide inferior quality of service. This can damage the education of children and the delivery of health care. It can make the poor poorer and seriously damage economic growth. In view of all this, it makes sense to hand over as many as possible of the public sector's operations to the private sector.

The private sector is sometimes regarded as greedy, ruthless, uncivilized, and unkind. It can exhibit any of these characteristics—like the public sector does. But the advantage of the private sector is that competition creates an incentive to provide good service. If a company fails to provide a good service or product, it is likely to lose business to a rival that does. Companies want to keep a good reputation for the same reason. Supermarkets offer fresh milk and helpful assistants because, if they do not, they will lose out to other supermarkets that do. Historians of human behavior have even argued that commerce has been a factor in the development of civil behavior. In the feudal system, aristocrats had less reason to be polite and helpful than a shopkeeper does. A shopkeeper has a reason to be polite and friendly to everyone: he wishes to keep his customers.

"When governments contract with the private sector, efficiency and innovation do not come about because private firms have some magic pixie dust, unobtainable by the public sector, to sprinkle about. It is competition that creates efficiency and innovation, because competition punishes inefficiency and inertia."

SOURCE: Adrian T. Moore, "Private Prisons: Quality Corrections at a Lower Cost," Policy Study no. 240, Reason Foundation, April 1998, http://reason.org/files/d14ffa18290a9aeb969d1a 6c1a9ff935.pdf.

The private sector service is not better regardless of its setting: a private sector monopoly is no better than a public sector one. It is competition that provides the spur. That is one reason contracting out is the inferior form of privatization. Yes, it can save money. Yes, there is or should be competition between suppliers to get the contract. But the public sector is usually the monopoly lead contractor. In the disastrous NHS computer project, the public sector contracted out to private companies. It was an incompetent monopoly contractor.

There is also the danger in contracting out that private companies may bribe public sector employees. Another problem is that the public sector may be so desperate to save money that it reduces funding to the point that the contractor can only make the work financially viable by providing an inferior service. Then the private sector takes the blame. There have been signs of this happening with Swedish free [charter] schools. For these reasons and more, wherever possible, the public sector should avoid contracting out. What is the alternative?

The best outcomes emerge when there is continuing competition between different companies and perhaps other organizations such as charities, mutual benefit societies, trade unions, churches, and trusts. For example, schools can be run by competing organizations. Pension plans can be compulsory, but the consumer can be given a choice between competing fund managers. Private or charitable hospitals can compete. Funding for their work can be provided by competing private insurance or savings programs.

"No force . . . except the force of competition has ever done anything to keep producers in order."

SOURCE: Sir Ernest Benn, *Why Freedom Works: Passages from Books 1924–53* (London: Benn, 1964).

The principle can be and has been applied in many areas. Competition between providers already exists in health care in the Netherlands, Switzerland, Germany, and Singapore. It exists in schooling in Sweden and, to a smaller degree, in the United States

Box 10.5
HOW TO USE THE PRIVATE SECTOR

DO
- Facilitate competition rather than contracting out, if possible.
- Allow for-profit companies, trusts, churches, trade unions, trade associations, mutual benefit societies, and friendly societies to join in the competition.
- Give all or most of the population a stake in the continuing existence of competition. Let people not government, be the customers.
- Allow public sector entities to compete with the private sector only on a level playing field.
- Create constitutional guarantees of the independence and funding of services paid for by government but provided by the private sector—especially schools.

DON'T
- Overregulate, stifling the variety and competition that drive innovation, ambition, high standards, and choice.
- Create regulations that inhibit competition by creating barriers to entry.

and the United Kingdom. Pensions in Chile, Hong Kong, Australia, and elsewhere incorporate competition between fund managers.[65]

There are still dangers even here, however. As mentioned, governments can create regulations that increase the costs of providers and create barriers to competition, making it expensive for new companies to enter the field. This has already started in welfare in Sweden.[66] Too many regulations can stifle innovation. Another danger is that governments can put a brake on funding so that the standard of service provided by all competitors deteriorates.

There is no sure defense against such things, although in some cases it might help to put some kind of guarantee in the constitution. Otherwise, the best defense can be public opinion, in which case the more people who are dependent on the system the better. If everybody is using, say, compulsory private health insurance, a government might hesitate before cutting the funding.

There is always great scope for human beings to run things badly. There is no foolproof plan. But the record shows that we have a better chance of good service at a reasonable price when private sector competition replaces public sector monopolies (Box 10.5). And nowhere is this more important than in schools and health care, where the education of children and where lives are at stake.

11. "It's Like Putting All Bus Drivers through Astronauts' Training"

The Training and Qualifications Bonanza

It is early evening in Rome. I have had a long day of interviews and now, at last, I am meeting Kishore Jayabalan of the Acton Institute to have supper. I have run out of energy and am happy simply to enjoy his company and that of his friends. It is a warm evening and we go to a little open-air restaurant where we are joined by others. It is a friendly, relaxed occasion—the very image of Italian conviviality. The welfare states of Italy and the world can take a rest. My notepad is closed and my glass is full.

The last person to arrive is a young man called Adriano. We chat and I ask what work he does. He replies that he is a student. He is completing his studies this year. I am astonished. He does not look young enough to be a student. I ask how old he is.

"Twenty-nine," he replies.

"Twenty-nine!" I exclaim. "How can you still be a student at 29?"

"Actually, I am finishing my studies earlier than most. Many of my friends won't finish until they are 30."

"Thirty!" I know it's rude of me to show my surprise, but Adriano isn't offended. If anything, he is bemused. For him, it is normal.

The conversation moves on to other things, but the idea of students continuing until they are 29 or 30 must be sticking in my mind because, as we walk away from the restaurant, I fall into conversation with another of Kishore's friends and ask if he could tell me more about it. He says that it can take five years to get a bachelor's degree. Then one gets a master's degree and finally a doctorate. There is no hurry.

But why do people want to spend these years getting higher and higher academic qualifications when, in most cases, they are not going to be academics?

"To get a job," he replies. It emerges that people spend all their 20s getting higher qualifications to show they are clever. After all those years, it finally enables them to get good jobs at banks or in the government.

"But surely it's crazy!" I exclaim. "Think of the time spent studying subjects completely irrelevant to the work they ultimately do! And ordinary, poorer people have to pay tax to fund this! Also, the working lives of these students are cut short by studying until they are 30 and then probably taking early retirement at 55 or 60! They only work 25 or 30 years out of 75 or 80 years of life. Isn't that ridiculous?"

My companion agrees. He says the government is trying to rein it back. But, from his tone, it sounds like he doesn't expect much to come of that. I subsequently discover that a big effort was made to cut the years of study back in 2000, but it would seem that this effort might not have been altogether successful.[1]

Naturally, most of us assume that training and qualifications are "good things." We all want the surgeon who is about to operate on us to be suitably trained. But can there be too much in the way of training and qualifications? Do these ostensibly good things have a dark side? What could possibly be wrong with them?

1. The motives behind the creation of qualifications are not always pure.

Dick Carpenter has organized the purchase of 50 floral arrangements. Half are from Louisiana and half from neighboring Texas.[2] He has organized 10 florists from Louisiana and 8 florists from Texas to judge these arrangements. The judges are not told which display is from which state or even the purpose of the experiment. Which state comes out better? The displays from Texas are judged to be slightly better than those from Louisiana but Carpenter, being a scrupulous academic, says that the difference is not "statistically significant."

Why has Carpenter done this experiment? What is it all about?

He is testing whether a requirement for florists to be qualified results in higher-quality products. In Louisiana, florists have to be qualified. They have to pass an exam. In Texas, they don't. The answer, according to this little experiment, seems to be that a qualification makes no difference.

If that is right, why does Louisiana legally require new florists to be qualified? Have there been protests by angry consumers demanding that they should be protected from displays made by unqualified florists?

No.

Have Louisiana newspapers and government offices been swamped with customer complaints about inferior displays?

No. The people who demanded a legal requirement for new florists to obtain qualifications were . . . florists. You don't need to be a cynic to suppose that the reason they called for this requirement was probably to reduce competition.

The story of the florists of Louisiana is a gentle introduction to the idea that we should not take it for granted that qualifications always exist for good and honorable reasons. It suggests that requirements for qualifications can, in some cases at least, be excessive and provide no benefit.

In the United States, many occupations require qualifications or "licensing," as Americans call it. In 2003, the Council of State Governments estimated that more than 800 occupations required a license in at least one state.[3] Adam Summers did a survey of them.[4] Some occupations failed what he called "the laugh test." Try these: you are not allowed to be an upholsterer in California without a license. You are not allowed to be an interior decorator there either.

"People of the same trade seldom meet together, even for merriment and diversion, but the conversation ends in a conspiracy against the public, or in some contrivance to raise prices."

SOURCE: Adam Smith, *The Wealth of Nations* (1776).

The fact that you need a license to be an interior decorator is part of the plot of a Woody Allen film, *Blue Jasmine*.[5] Jasmine, played by Cate Blanchett, needs a job and wants to work as an interior decorator. But she is not allowed to. She does not have a license.

Summers found that many occupations required a license in some states but not in others. One might wonder why, if the public needs protection from, say, an unlicensed upholsterer in California, it doesn't need the same protection in Oregon. The difference suggests that this is not a matter of public interest but merely an indication that lobby groups have gotten their way in some states and not in others.

Licenses for floristry, upholstery, and interior decorating may seem merely funny and of no importance. But this introduction is

only to suggest that we should not assume all licensing requirements exist for a good reason. The same can apply in other fields,
and the consequences can be surprisingly serious.

Before the Second World War, black Americans were increasingly successful in becoming plumbers, barbers, and electricians.[6]
Trade unions convinced state legislatures to pass laws that made
it difficult for them to gain licenses. A law proposed in Virginia
provided that only barbers who had been to an approved barbers'
school, had been registered apprentices for 18 months, and had
passed an exam could get a license. But black people could not
even start on this path. There were no licensed barbers' schools
that would admit them.[7] An African-American weekly publication, the *Norfolk Journal and Guide*, denounced the bill in 1929 as a
"pernicious measure, masquerading as a public health effort, but
obviously an organized labor union project drawn in the special
interest of white organized labor."[8]

Licensing rules of this sort were proposed every year from
1928 to 1940. That is why we have good records of what happened. Happily they were defeated each time. But Virginia was
exceptional. By 1941, all the states of America except Virginia and
New York had passed licensing laws obstructing black men who
wanted to become plumbers, barbers, and/or electricians. The
laws exploited the fact that black people tended to be less well
educated and poorer to exclude them from these trades. Simply
by being required to pass written exams and pay for courses, they
were obstructed.

Consequently, in the plumbing trade, there were substantial reductions in black employment. A 1953 investigation discovered that,
of 3,200 licensed plumbers in Maryland, only two were African
American. The purpose of such licensing laws may have been to discriminate against blacks or to reduce competition or both. Whichever it was, it was certainly against the public interest.

If we accept that qualifications are not always created for good
and honorable reasons, we might look afresh at some professions
that are particularly important in welfare states.

At first sight, the medical profession might seem to be one in
which the qualifications would surely not be polluted by selfish
motives. Unfortunately, the history of medical qualifications tells a
different story. Going all the way back to the 15th century, various
kinds of doctors have repeatedly attempted to create monopolies.

Practitioners have variously called themselves surgeons, physicians, or apothecaries. Competition has been unwelcome.

"An average eye exam and eyeglass prescription is 35 percent more expensive in cities with more restrictive optometry regulations."

Source: James F. Cawley, professor in the Department of Prevention and Community Health and in the Department of Physician Assistant Studies at the George Washington University, in email to the author.

In 1902, a doctor distributed leaflets in a poor area of Birmingham, England, announcing that he would see the poor for free. He was inundated with work. To try to reduce the flow, he issued a revised handbill saying that he would now charge the poor threepence per consultation. His motive was obviously philanthropic. But what was the reaction of the General Medical Council? To ban "advertising" such as he had done. The council characterized his behavior as an attempt to take patients away from other medical men. The year before, the council also had banned canvassing for patients. As a historian of the episode has written, "The decisions of 1901 and 1902 were the first occasions on which the powers of the General Medical Council had been openly used to further the pecuniary interests of doctors at the expense of patients."[9]

"When the NHS [National Health Service] was being planned, the BMA's [British Medical Association's] hostility was decisive in ensuring that no role at all was permitted for medical institutes."

Source: David Green, "Medical Care without the State," in *Re-Privatising Welfare: After the Lost Century*, ed. Arthur Seldon (London: Institute of Economic Affairs, 1996). Medical institutes provided price competition to members of the BMA.

There was still competition among doctors over price, however, at this time. The competition annoyed the British Medical Association, which, despite its professional gloss, acted like a trade union trying to keep prices up. The association was politically active, seeking to promote the interests of its members as laws regarding medical practice were developed. Through the General Medical Council and then the government itself, it eventually succeeded in quelling competition. It started to cooperate with the major changes introduced in 1911 and 1946 only in return for government compliance.[10] Competition was almost totally snuffed out. New doctors could not move into an area to compete with the existing ones if provision there was officially considered adequate. Though doctors may have been different from one another in various ways, they were not allowed to compete with each other. Competition, which pushes good performance in so many other parts of life, was eliminated. That remains the position in Britain today.

> "In both the American and English cases, state involvement in the profession's institutions represented a solution to the failure of the profession to eliminate competitors adequately. . . . Unlike the profession, the state had the resources and administrative mechanisms for shaping the medical market in a monopolistic direction."
>
> SOURCE: Jeffrey Lionel Berlant, *Profession and Monopoly: A Study of Medicine in the United States and Britain* (Berkeley: University of California Press, 1975), pp. 303, 305.

Something similar took place in the United States and elsewhere, too. It emerges that even the medical profession, despite the fact that many doctors feel it is a vocation, is capable of seeking to frame regulations for the advantage of practitioners rather than for patients. Bearing this in mind, let's look at medical training.

In the United States, a young person who wishes to become a doctor pursues a college degree for four years. Then he or she goes to medical school for a further four years. Finally he or she does a "residency"—which includes some medical work on a kind of trainee basis—for a further four years. If the budding doctor wants to become a specialist, the training takes even longer. It is not uncommon for people to have reached the age of 30 before they are full doctors, by which point they are burdened with heavy debt unless their parents are rich and have paid for it.

As Clayton Christensen put it, "Counting college, tomorrow's doctors will have spent 10 to 18 of the most productive years of their lives just training for their careers."[11] We will see later that it may be doubted that this decade or more of preparation is truly necessary. But we know for sure that the training and qualification requirements are extremely time-consuming and expensive. This suits the

310

existing practitioners. The drawn-out training keeps down competition and maintains high prices. This raises the prices and taxes paid by others.

"The U.S. system of medical education is like putting all bus drivers through astronauts' training."

Source: Comment repeated among critics of medical training. It is unknown who said it first. Shared with the author in an email by James F. Cawley, professor in the Department of Prevention and Community Health and in the Department of Physician Assistant Studies at the George Washington University.

---

2. Excessive training increases costs.

The academic research into licensing suggests that it increases wages and prices by between 10 and 18 percent.[12] One study found that strict licensing laws increased the wages of clinical laboratory staff by 16 percent. A study that added in the effect of licensing along with nonrecognition of qualifications of one state by another and restrictions on advertising found that the combined effect was to increase wages in more highly paid jobs, such as dentistry, by about 27 percent.[13]

"One of the many sources of high medical costs in the United States is the de facto monopoly of the American Medical Association in the distribution of licences to practice medicine."

Source: Free Exchange blog, *The Economist*, "A Spoonful of Monopoly Helps the Medicine Go Down," September 21, 2007, http://www.economist.com/blogs/freeexchange/2007/09/a_spoonful_of_monopoly_helps_t.

But even that figure may not capture the full effect. The studies compared people of similar knowledge and ability. They did not capture, therefore, the fact that people can spend months or years studying areas that are not necessary for the work that they will do. A doctor may study genetics without any improvement in the quality of his work if his actual work does not involve genetics. The cost of the extra training, which is an extra barrier to entry to the profession and causes a higher price, is not captured.

> "The American Medical Association . . . renders important services to its members and to the medical profession as a whole. However, it is also a labor union and, in our judgment, has been one of the most successful. . . . For decades it kept down the number of physicians, kept up the costs of medical care, and prevented competition . . . all, of course, in the name of helping the patient. . . . The leaders of medicine have been sincere in their belief that restricting entry into medicine would help the patient. By this time, we are familiar with the capacity that all of us have to believe that what is in our interest is in the social interest."
>
> SOURCE: Milton Friedman and Rose Friedman, *Free to Choose: A Personal Statement* (New York: Harcourt Brace Jovanovich, 1980), p. 231.

The large number of eternal students in Italy means that ordinary people there have to pay more in taxes. Excessive training and qualifications increase wages and thus the prices of the professions and trades concerned. People are made poorer because they have to pay for this. And specifically in the services that are often part of welfare states—education and health care—everybody has to pay more.

Some people may be thinking, "Very well. So some prices may be somewhat higher, but at least the demanding qualifications mean we can be sure the quality of our services is good." Is that right?

3. Excessive training can reduce the quality of services.

It is a date unknown sometime between 2005 and 2009. We are in the accident and emergency department of Stafford Hospital in Stafford, England. A stream of people is coming in. Most have minor injuries, but some have a life-threatening condition—perhaps feeling chest pain and about to suffer a heart attack. Which ones are which?

A triage nurse is supposed to see each patient and rush through anyone who is in imminent danger. But no triage nurse is present. The receptionist—who has no medical training—is deciding from a distance whether anyone appears to be in a bad enough condition for her to call someone.[14]

In a ward in the same hospital, a woman presses a buzzer for a nurse.[15] The woman wants to relieve herself, but she is not able to get out of bed. Nobody comes. She buzzes again and again. Still nobody comes. She calls out. Eventually, a nurse arrives. But it is too late. The nurse belatedly moves the woman onto a commode and goes away. Now the woman is left on the commode for half

312

an hour. She wants to go back to bed. But again, nobody comes. Finally she tries to make it by herself from the commode to the bed. She falls onto the floor. A concerned visitor nearby goes searching for a nurse. She can't find one.

Elsewhere in the hospital, many of the patients are developing bedsores. They should be turned regularly so that the pressure on particular parts of their bodies is relieved. But this does not happen frequently enough.

All of these incidents are described in the official government report into the hundreds of unnecessary deaths and incidents of bad care that took place at this hospital over four years (see also Chapter 10 of this book).[16]

What was the root cause of the problem? The chairman of the inquiry unveiled his first report at a press conference in 2010. At that conference he said, "A chronic shortage of staff, particularly nursing staff, was largely responsible for the substandard care."[17]

Why was there a shortage of staff? In fact, why is there often a shortage of staff in the British National Health Service?

The immediate and obvious reason is that the government was trying to save money. Another reason may be the huge amounts of money spent on administrators rather than on frontline medical staff. But there is another reason worth considering: nurses are more expensive than they used to be.

In the 1950s and 1960s, a nurse was like an apprentice. She started straight from school at age 17. She did three years of training at a college attached to a hospital, but most of her time was spent working on the wards. She was junior, but she was a useful member of the team from the beginning. For the hospital, her work was relatively cheap. So she could be more affordable. That, in turn, meant it was less likely that there would be a shortage of nurses.

"America presently suffers from a severe shortage of nurses of every type. The American Hospital Association reported in July 2007 that U.S. hospitals faced a shortage of 116,000 nurses."

SOURCE: Clayton M. Christensen et al., *The Innovator's Prescription: A Disruptive Solution For Health Care* (New York: McGraw-Hill, 2009), p. 357.

Then came demands that nursing should be more prestigious and should be recognized as a profession. The training was transformed into a three-year degree course. Practical work was still done, but there was far less of it. Subjects like sociology were added that were not directly relevant. In the 1950s and 1960s, a trainee who started at 17 was a registered nurse at 20. Now the average age at which an individual becomes a fully registered nurse is 29.[18] Even by that age, she or he has done precious little nursing work. But she or he has already cost £40,000 ($56,800)[19] in tuition fees and more in financial aid and other costs (these figures date back to 2007 and are surely higher now).[20] It has even been suggested that the total cost of a trained nurse could be £100,000 ($142,000).[21] Finally, after all that time and cost, it is quite possible that the new nurse will leave the profession. In an ideal world, perhaps, every nurse would have a degree in sociology and many other desirable qualifications. But it means more expense. This helps to lead to the situation in which a receptionist is doing triage in the emergency department and nobody comes when an elderly patient calls "nurse."

Higher requirements for training and qualifications mean fewer practitioners. In health care, fewer practitioners mean less attention for patients, which amounts to lower-quality care.

Morris Kleiner compared how various trades and professions have developed in different U.S. states. He found that the requirements for a qualification reduced the growth rate of these occupations by 20 percent.[22] Excessive and unnecessary qualifications in all cases reduce the number of practitioners. Where the requirements to become a doctor or nurse are excessive, there will be fewer of them.

Training and qualification requirements can also damage education. In a number of countries and most states in the United States, people are not permitted to teach without an officially recognized qualification. Some may think, "Well, that sounds reasonable. I would like my child to be taught by someone who is qualified." But the certification rule means, as Andrew Coulson has pointed out, that "Bill Gates could not teach computer science." In fact, Einstein could not teach physics if he were alive today, and Churchill and Caesar could not teach history. Maybe they would be no good as teachers. But most principals would be willing to give them a try.

There is also the problem that the teacher training is sometimes of dubious value. "The ed school establishment is more concerned with politics—both academic and ideological—than with learning," according to Rita Kramer, who visited many "ed schools" and wrote a book about what she found.[23] Teacher-training schools have one particular well-known blot on their records. For decades they taught a disastrously bad method of teaching children how to read (see Chapter 4). This took place in France, America, Britain, and elsewhere. The training resulted in lower-quality teaching than would have taken place without it.

So there are several ways in which training—or excessive requirements for training—can damage the quality of services.

4. Monopoly control over training and qualifications reduces competition and innovation.

Typically one institution—the government or an organization approved by the government—decides what qualifications are needed in medicine and teaching. This can lead to a lack of flexibility and innovation in the kinds of training and qualifications. It can inhibit the creation of new kinds of jobs.

> "The licensing of occupations is a continually expanding frontier, ever upgrading old trades and new services to the mantle of professional status, and always justified in service of the public good. On and on it rolls, 'professionalizing' the workforce as it goes with layers of new regulation and board certification, all the way systematically redistributing rents from those outside the licensing system to those inside . . . inhibiting experimentation in new business models and stifling innovation."
>
> SOURCE: Jason Potts, an economist at the Queensland University of Technology, quoted in Dick M. Carpenter II, "Blooming Nonsense," *Regulation* 34 (Spring 2011): 47, http://object.cato.org/sites/cato.org/files/serials/files/regulation/2011/4/regv34n1-8.pdf.

Take physician assistants in the United States (see Figure 11.1). The category was invented because physician assistants take a shorter time to train than full doctors do, but they are able to do at least 73 percent of what general practitioners do, and they do it just as well.[24] The training takes two and a half years instead of seven.[25] The benefit of this job category has been shown by the way demand for physician assistants has subsequently grown. Their numbers have increased from 13,000 to 83,000 in three decades.[26] It seems likely that other categories of medical staff would also have been created if not for the monopoly control over qualifications and the lack of incentive for the profession or government to create new rules or qualifications.

Figure 11.1
FULFILLING A NEED
NUMBER OF PHYSICIAN ASSISTANTS IN THE UNITED STATES

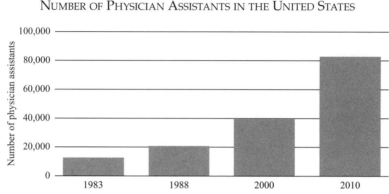

SOURCES: Victoria Stagg Elliott, "Number of Physician Assistants Doubles over Past Decade," amednews.com, American Medical Association, September 27, 2011, http://www.amednews.com/article/20110927/business/309279997/8 for 2000 and 2010 figures; Carol Kleiman, "Physician Assistants Taking a Larger Care Role," *Chicago Tribune*, September 11, 1988, http://articles.chicagotribune.com/1988-09-11/news/8801290433_1_physician-assistants-order-laboratory-tests-patients-medical-histories, for 1983 and 1988 figures.

5. Training and qualification requirements can keep the poor from improving their lives or getting a job at all.

A wide variety of people find it more difficult to get jobs because of licensing laws. Would-be florists in Louisiana have to spend money on training and an exam. Training and qualification requirements stopped black Americans from becoming plumbers and hairdressers before the Second World War. Young people who might be excellent nurses find that they must navigate a degree course and years of training before they are allowed to contribute.

Tough licensing laws can make it difficult for those in the lower half of society to get jobs. Jestina Clayton grew up in a village in Sierra Leone where all girls learned African hair braiding. She was an expert. It was a job she could do well in the United States. Except that, when she went to Utah, she found that she needed a cosmetology license to do hair braiding. Getting the license required two years of schooling on completely irrelevant subjects at

316

a cost of $16,000.[27] The licensing requirement prevented her from working.

Many government schools have failed to teach children to read and write well (see Chapter 4), so millions of people in the advanced world have been left functionally illiterate. In this situation, it is verging on the inhumane to insist on written exams and licensing requirements for jobs or trades for which they are not absolutely necessary.

If this were a matter of a few professions here and there, it might not be so important. But the requirement for qualifications has grown alarmingly. During the 1950s, about 4.5 percent of the workforce in America had to get a license to do their jobs. That figure had risen to 29.0 percent by 2008.[28] That year in the United States there were more than twice as many people whose job was affected by licensing requirements than there were members of a union[29] (see Figure 11.2).

What can be done to reduce the damage inflicted by unnecessary or excessive requirements for training and qualifications?

Figure 11.2
YOU CAN'T DO THAT WITHOUT A LICENSE!
PROPORTION OF THE U.S. WORKFORCE NEEDING
A LICENSE TO DO THEIR JOBS

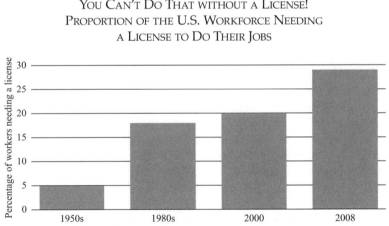

SOURCE: Morris M. Kleiner and Alan B. Krueger, "Analyzing the Extent and Influence of Occupational Licensing on the Labor Market," *Journal of Labor Economics* 31 (2013): S173–S202.

NOTE: These statistics are not all exactly comparable with each other, but they appear to be the best available.

In many cases, like floristry, there should be no requirement for any qualifications at all. But training and qualifications are obviously important in medicine, for example. What can be done here?

One idea comes from an unexpected place. We're in Liverpool in 1870, and there is criticism of accountants who do poor work. A group of accountants agree to band together as the Incorporated Society of Liverpool Accountants to try to establish themselves as well-qualified, honest professionals. Later the same year, a similar institute starts in London. The two institutes and several others decide to join together. Members are required to demonstrate their knowledge and expertise. The combined institute naturally circulates the idea that, if you want a good accountant, you had better make sure he—it is certainly a "he" at this time—is a member of what is soon known as the Institute of Chartered Accountants in England and Wales. This seems perfectly reasonable and sensible.

The institute grows in power and importance, and toward the end of the century, it is close to establishing itself as the sole body through which someone can qualify as an accountant—in other words, it is close to making itself a monopoly. But just before this happens, it faces opposition. Some of the resistance comes from men who have recently returned to Britain after fighting in the Boer War. As with other wars, the Boer War has helped make ordinary people aware of their own abilities and realize they are no less capable than men with advantages of birth and position. Men of this sort who have previously worked in accountancy are annoyed by the suggestion that only those who have the money and higher education that enable them to become members of the Institute of Chartered Accountants should be recognized as professionals.

On November 30, 1904, one of these men, Henry Lewis, convenes a meeting with seven colleagues at Balfour House in London.[30] Henry Lewis is a formidable character—"a born fighter . . . brusque, overbearing often to the point of rudeness." The eight men create the London Association of Accountants. They aim to combat the attempts of the "older established bodies to render the accountancy profession a closed one . . . shutting out many capable and qualified men." They set their own standards for membership. They do not require people to pay to be "articled" to a firm of accountants, a system which costs between 50 and 200 guineas (about \$75 to \$300).[31] New members do not need to have family connections to enable them to get "articles." They do not need to have had higher education. They only need to have expertise and experience as accountants. Women are also admitted.

The fight for recognition takes years. The Institute of Chartered Accountants hoped for the "obliteration" of this and other upstart bodies. But in the 1930s, the London Association of Accountants, by now joined with other bodies to become the Association of Chartered Certified Accountants (ACCA), is fully recognized. Bringing the story up to date, the ACCA now has 178,000 members and is so successful that it has become an international organization with students from 181 countries. It has won a British government award for "enterprise in international trade."

Because of the struggle of these eight men joined by others of a similar kind, there are now six bodies in Britain that can grant qualifications in accountancy. There are also other bodies offering accreditation in related fields such as bookkeeping.

The lesson of this is that if there are rival bodies with different criteria for saying "you are qualified," you can create qualifications that are varied and that suit different people. Rivalry between authorizing bodies means that they are more likely to be enterprising and innovative.

The conclusion, I suggest, is that monopoly licensing should not be permitted.

Unfortunately, it is no easy matter to abolish an established licensing requirement or to give permission to new licensing bodies. In Florida, the government wanted to pass legislation removing licensing requirements for 20 trades including hair-braiding, teaching ballroom dancing, and interior decorating. At first it seemed easy. The legislators were generally in favor of the change. But the interior decorators and others lobbied hard. Some of their arguments were ludicrous. It was claimed that unlicensed interior designers might use fabrics that would spread disease and cause the deaths of 88,000 people a year.[32] One claimed that clashing color schemes might adversely affect "salivation." Yet they won.

The people who cared most about the continuation of such licenses—practitioners who gained financially—lobbied hardest. If the evidently ridiculous arguments of decorators can win, imagine how much more difficult it would be to prevail against organizations of teachers or doctors. They would certainly claim that

Box 11.1
TWO YEARS OF LAW SCHOOL IS PLENTY

"This is probably controversial to say, but what the heck . . . law schools would probably be wise to think about being two years instead of three years."[a]

U.S. President Barack Obama said that to an audience at Binghamton University in New York in August 2013. It is unusual for a politician to suggest that training might be excessive. Obama once taught constitutional law, so he is in a good position to know whether excessive time is spent obtaining legal qualifications.

The *Economist* article in which Obama was quoted asserts that law schools sprang up in the 19th century in two forms: elite universities teaching the subject for three years and night schools that catered to the sons of immigrants. The "snootier" institutions "convinced the American Bar Association to accredit only schools that required a costly three years' worth of courses." The article also claims that the average 2013 graduate will be $140,000 in debt, "according to one estimate."

---

[a] "For Many, Two Years Is Plenty," *The Economist*, August 31, 2013, http://www.economist.com /news/united-states/21584392-president-suggests-scrapping-last-year-law-school-many-two -years-plenty.

infringement on their monopolies would damage children or put lives at risk. Nevertheless, such battles must be fought if the damage done by monopoly authorizing bodies is to be reduced. (See Box 11.1.)

* * *

The issue of training and qualification profoundly affects welfare states. The eternal students of Italy, Germany, and elsewhere are subsidized by taxpayers, many of whom are poor. Excessive requirements for qualifying medical professionals and teachers increase costs for taxpayers and reduce the quantity and quality of the welfare services they provide. The required qualifications trap less well-educated people in unemployment or in lower-skill jobs than they could otherwise do. So they damage social mobility and cohesion. Monopoly control over qualifications can also damage innovation and progress in medical care and education.

It may be difficult to make progress, but the goal should be to achieve something like this:

- Many licensing requirements—especially in the United States—should be abolished altogether.
- Governments should ensure that they are not directly responsible for licensing. Instead, they should confine themselves to recognizing privately created licensing bodies.
- Governments should allow and encourage rival licensing bodies.
- Because practitioners who are already licensed have little incentive to create new bodies, governments should allow consumers of services such as hospitals and schools to establish licensing bodies.
- Eternal students should not be indulged at public expense. As in Switzerland, students should choose vocational or purely academic study at the age of 17 or 18, leading to an exam at 20 or 21.
- Most study beyond that age should be financed by students doing productive and useful work in the field.
- Public subsidies for further study should be granted only to a small proportion of people for, say, another two or three years.
- There should be no opportunity to retake years in which a student has failed to meet the required standard.

There are doubtless other measures that could be taken. But progress depends on a wider understanding that excessive requirements for training and qualification cause damage and that the people who are hurt include patients, students, taxpayers, and low-paid workers.

12. Democracy Is Like a Drunk Husband

The Trouble with Representative Democracies

The scandals surrounding Publius Clodius Pulcher were remarkable even by Roman standards. Among many other things, he was accused of incest with all his sisters. There were four or five of them; historians are not completely sure which. But the biggest scandal involved a special religious ceremony reserved exclusively for women—the Bona Dea. No men were allowed. On this occasion, the ceremony took place at the home of Julius Caesar himself. It was hosted by Caesar's wife, Pompeia. Clodius went to the ceremony disguised as a woman. Some said he wanted to seduce Pompeia, although there was no proof of it. In any event, he was discovered and tried for sacrilege. Caesar divorced Pompeia partly because of this incident. When it was suggested to Caesar that his wife had surely not been seduced by Clodius, he made the famous reply, "Caesar's wife must be above suspicion."[1]

Clodius was highly ambitious. Despite all the scandals surrounding him, he sought high office. He was a patrician—a member of the high aristocracy. But he broke all the rules, getting himself adopted into a plebeian family so that he could achieve power as a tribune of the plebs.[2] He succeeded at this, and in 58 BC, he tried to increase his popularity by offering people free corn.[3] "Corn" here means grain from which people could make a kind of gruel.[4] For some years previously, corn had been sold to the less well off at a subsidized price. But Clodius took it a step further by making it free. To put it cynically—and in Clodius's case, a drop of cynicism seems a minimum—he bought popularity with taxpayers' money.

He was not around long enough to see the results. Along with so many other ambitious Romans, he was murdered. But the policy remained. No one dared remove it. It became ruinously expensive and unsustainable. The rural poor, who were already moving into Rome, arrived in even greater numbers. The policy was subject to fraud. Many people who were not genuinely poor collected free corn, including well-to-do officials and high-ranking military officers. The numbers claiming the corn dole swelled to 350,000, an extraordinary figure considering the population of Rome was only about 600,000, excluding foreigners and slaves.

"In the mid-eighteenth century, 'democracy' was a word . . . associated primarily with the ancient world and had negative connotations: democracies were conceived to be unstable, warlike, and prone to mutate into despotisms."

SOURCE: From the publisher's description of Joanna Innes and Mark Philp, ed., *Re-imagining Democracy in the Age of Revolutions: America, France, Britain, Ireland 1750–1850* (Oxford: Oxford University Press, 2013), http://ukcatalogue.oup.com/product/9780199669158.do.

As one historian puts it, once the dole was established, "The proletariat claimed this as a right which no politician who needed their votes could refuse."[5] The Republic, the semidemocratic government of ancient Rome, could not deal with the problem. Only when Caesar became dictator was the government able to make major inroads into the huge cost. Caesar halved the number entitled to it, saying he was making a different kind of provision by obtaining new colonies for the surplus city population.[6] But not even Caesar tried to abolish it.

The dole remained a feature of Roman life for centuries. You can still see remnants of it today. On the site of the forum in Rome there remain some parts of Trajan's Market, a building that was once so massive it was described at the time as a wonder of the world. It was from here that the dole was administered.

Some Romans were opposed to the dole and even suggested it reflected a decline in the greatness of Rome. Juvenal famously remarked, "The people that once bestowed commands, consulships, legions and all else, now meddles no more and eagerly longs for just two things: bread and circuses."[7] The "bread" he refers to is the corn dole. This corn dole started with Clodius, a politician seeking popularity and power.

The parallels with modern times are striking. Food stamps in the United States are the contemporary corn dole. They and many other provisions of welfare states have, like the corn dole, proved hard or impossible to remove by any politician wishing to hold onto power. No government minister in Britain has ever dared call for the abolition of the National Health Service, for example, any more than Caesar dared abolish the corn dole. No politician would dare suggest that parents should be charged fees for the schooling of their children in France, Germany, or any of the countries where "free" education has become normal.

In democracies, welfare states are like one-way ratchets. "Free" things are promised and given by politicians seeking or holding onto power. Almost never are they removed. It does happen occasionally, but it takes years of effort and usually decades of abuse, expense, and scandal before a problem becomes so widely recognized that even modest reform takes place. Benefits for the incapacitated were increased substantially in Britain in the 1970s. The numbers claiming the benefits soared beyond any idea of how many could genuinely be incapacitated. But the problem began to be tackled seriously only around 2009 or 2010, more than three decades later.

"It has been said that democracy is the worst form of government except all those other forms which have been tried from time to time."

SOURCE: Sir Winston Churchill, former British prime minister, in the House of Commons, recorded in Hansard, HC Deb, November 11,1947, vol. 444, col. 207.

Most of us are committed to democracy, me included. But that should not stop us from admitting that it is not perfect. Democracy is like a drunk husband—self-indulgent, stupid, and possessing a tendency to knock things over and break them. Like a loyal wife, we continue to love democracy. But, also like a loyal wife, we have a right to name its faults:

1. Politicians in democracies get elected by promising "free" services and benefits, ignoring the long-term effects.

"The government consists of a gang of men exactly like you and me. . . . Their principal device . . . is to search out groups who pant or pine for something they can't get, and to promise to give it to them. Nine times out of ten that promise is worth nothing. The tenth time is made good by looting A to satisfy B."

SOURCE: H. L. Mencken, American journalist and satirist (1880–1956).

---

2. Politicians get elected and receive sponsorship by favoring interest groups at the expense of the general public. Advantages are concentrated in the hands of these interest groups—such as trade

unions or businesses—while bad effects are diffused among everyone else. This is known as "the tyranny of the minority."

3. Politicians seeking power encourage the poorer half of society to believe they can become better off by taxing the rich. This may be modestly true in the short term but can make them worse off in the long term. Politicians readily blame the rich for problems because they know the rich have few votes. The rich increasingly tend to be regarded as having no right to consideration. This is a prime example of "the tyranny of the majority."

"A democracy is a state which recognizes the subjection of the minority to majority, that is, an organization for the systematic use of violence by one class against the other, by one part of the population against another."

SOURCE: Vladimir Lenin, *The State and Revolution*, 1917.

---

4. Representative democracy is a blunt instrument. Politicians and parties seek election offering a mix of policies. The electorate might approve of their policies A and B and not C, D, or E. But, once in power, governments claim they have a "mandate" to introduce any or all of them. They are also in a position to impose new policies F and G, which were not mentioned in their manifestos at all.

Half of EU citizens do not have confidence in the democracy of their country. Slightly more than half do not have confidence in the democracy of the European Union.

SOURCE: *Public Opinion in the European Union*, Standard Eurobarometer 78, Autumn 2012, pp. 52, 54, http://ec.europa.eu/public_opinion/archives/eb/eb78/eb78_publ_en.pdf.

---

5. Politicians make deals with each other behind the scenes. They support some of each other's policies even though they do not genuinely agree with them. A deal is made so that each politician can get through what he or she wants. In America, this is known as "logrolling."[8] In the European Union, it is routine.

6. "Checks and balances" and "pork-barrel"[9] politics can make good government almost impossible. The "checks and balances" may be divisions of power—between the House of

Representatives and the Senate in the United States for example—or overlapping authority between national and regional governments. In Australia, the states are responsible for health care but the national government provides the cash. In a sense, the states have responsibility without the power to fulfill it while the national government has power without the responsibility. Pork-barrel politics interferes with good government when a law can be passed only if it is adjusted or distorted to suit the short-term interests of a particular locality. Even the constitution can interfere with good government when it is applied in a way that its creators never imagined.

"What he got is a God-awful mess because that is all you can get past Congress!"

Source: Terry Moe, political science professor at Stanford University, speaking to the author about Obamacare. Moe was talking about the Affordable Care Act (Obamacare), but the individual act is not as significant as the difficulty of getting coherent policy into law.

---

7. There is a fundamental internal contradiction in representative democracy: a politician is meant to represent the wishes and interests of the electorate but he or she is also meant to have individual ideas about what should be done. In the midst of this contradiction, politicians can often pick and choose, sometimes representing the electorate and sometimes themselves. To put it another way, elected representatives can choose not to be representative.
8. Politicians often feel under pressure to talk and act on the basis of what people are supposed to think rather than what they genuinely think. From time to time, there is a difference.[10]
9. Politicians tend to come from a self-regarding, well-educated elite. They tend to become frustrated with the behavior of ordinary people and feel that it is their prerogative to boss them around.

"While democracy means a government accountable to the electorate, our rulers now make us accountable to them."

Source: Kenneth Minogue conversation with Edwin Feulner, former president of the Heritage Foundation, as reported by economist John Blundell in an email to the author. Minogue (1930–2013) was professor emeritus of political science at the London School of Economics and Political Science.

---

10. Electorates are highly susceptible to "magic thinking," whereby they expect an end to be achieved simply because a politician says it is his policy to achieve it. A politician may say he intends to raise wages for the low-paid, for example, even though he has no plan that will actually achieve this goal.[11] Politicians are attracted to magical thinking, too, because they know it will please voters and increase their chances of getting elected. Phrases such as "Yes we can!" and "the Third Way" may be considered by some as examples of magical thinking.

11. Voters have little reason to consider the pros and cons of any issue in any depth because the only power they can exercise is to vote for a party. This is one reason why they are so susceptible to the magical thinking previously described. You could almost say they have been infantilized.

Benito Arruñad: "The government treats people like babies!"
James Bartholomew: "Maybe they are babies."
Benito Arruñad: "They want to be!"

Source: Author's conversation with Benito Arruñada, professor of business organization at Pompeu Fabra University, Barcelona. The conversation was about how governments trick people, how easy they are to trick, and how people may even partly want everything decided for them.

---

12. Because democracies ostensibly reflect the will of the people, individuals and the public generally feel less entitled to object to ever-greater intrusions and instruction by government. So we arrive at a kind of democratic totalitarianism.

"Democracy encourages the fantasy despot in us all. Had we but cash enough, and power, what wrong would we not put right. . . . Fantasy does corrupt, and this particular one has eroded the basic assumption that a man's property is his own business."

Source: Kenneth Minogue, *The Egalitarian Conceit: False and True Equalities* (London: Centre for Policy Studies, 1989), http://www.cps.org.uk/publications/reports/the-egalitarian-conceit.

Criticisms such as these have been made since democracy first appeared. In ancient Greece, Plato caustically remarked, "In politics we presume that everyone who knows how to get votes knows how to administer a city or a state. When we are ill . . . we do not ask for the handsomest physician, or the most eloquent one."[12]

Frédéric Bastiat, the 19th-century French economist, said, "The state is that great fictitious entity by which everyone seeks to live at the expense of everyone else."[13] You could say that the sentence is the appeal of the welfare state in a nutshell.

More recently, Thomas Sowell, the American economist, commented, "The first lesson in economics is scarcity. There is never enough of anything to satisfy all those who want it. The first lesson in politics is to disregard the first lesson of economics."[14]

The flaws of democracy have been particularly dangerous in relation to welfare states. All 12 of the flaws listed have played a part. Neither politicians nor the electorate have had an incentive to think things through. Both have been subject to magical thinking. Politicians have gotten elected by offering things to the population for free— ignoring long-term effects or unintended consequences. And so on.

The way that democracies come to demand that the state should put every problem right regardless of expense or other consequences was brilliantly described by Bastiat:

> Sir, I do not have the honor of knowing you, but I will bet ten to one that for the last six months you have been constructing utopias; and if you have been doing so, I will bet ten to one that you are making the state responsible for bringing them into existence. And you, Madam, I am certain that in your heart of hearts you would like to cure all the suffering of humanity and that you would not be in the slightest put out if the state just wanted to help in this.
>
> But alas! The unfortunate being, like Figaro, does not know whom to listen to nor which way to turn. The hundred thousand voices of the press and the tribune are all calling out to this being at once: "Organize work and the workers. Root out selfishness. Repress the insolence and tyranny of capital. Carry out experiments on manure and eggs. Crisscross the country with railways. Educate the young. Succor the elderly. Lend money interest free to those who want it. Encourage art and train musicians and dancers for us. Prohibit trade and at the same time create a merchant navy. Enlighten, develop, expand, fortify, spiritualize and sanctify the souls of peoples [etc.]"
>
> "Oh, Sirs, have a little patience," the state replies pitifully. "I will try to satisfy you, but I need some resources to do this. I have prepared some projects relating to five or six bright, new taxes that are the most benign the world has ever seen. You will see how pleased you will be to pay them."[15]

Bastiat was satirizing the tendency of democracies to call upon the state to make everything perfect in 1848 when welfare states had hardly gotten into first gear. Since then, we have seen an explosion of demands on governments to provide. I suspect quite a few items on Bastiat's list were meant to be extreme or absurd. Some are now normal parts of welfare states: "succor the elderly," for example.[16]

"What if there are limits to what governments can do?"

Source: Jason L. Riley, *Please Stop Helping Us: How Liberals Make It Harder for Blacks to Succeed* (New York: Encounter, 2014).

There will always be more childcare that people want, more care for the elderly, more expensive medicines, more teachers, more nurses, bigger pensions, and so on. That, in short, is why in America, for example, government spending has gone from a mere 7 percent of gross domestic product (GDP) in 1900 to 41 percent in 2011.[17] The rise in spending has been continuously upward apart from the spikes caused by the two world wars. It seemed for a while as though a plateau had been reached in the 1980s and 1990s around 35 percent of GDP. But that has turned out to be merely a base camp from which spending has made a further assault on a new peacetime peak.

France was ahead of America. Following its revolutions in 1789 and 1870, the government was already spending 11 percent of GDP by 1872.[18] The rise since then has continued relentlessly so that France has maintained its lead. French government spending reached a new record of 57 percent of GDP in 2012 (see Figure 12.1).

In Britain, the 20th century began with government spending at an even higher level than France: 14 percent.[19] It soared to 48 percent in the mid-1970s but then fell back for a couple of decades before recovering to 45 percent in 2011–12.[20]

Looking at the big picture, government spending as a proportion of GDP in these three countries rose six times, five times, and three times, respectively, over 112, 141, and 112 years. It has been typical of advanced countries to triple their spending or more over the past century. More than all of the increase in spending has been focused on welfare. Other kinds of spending have been reduced to make way. Defense expenditures in Britain, for example, fell from 3.7 to

330

Figure 12.1
MARIANNE SPENDS MORE AND MORE
FRENCH GOVERNMENT EXPENDITURE AS A PERCENTAGE OF GDP

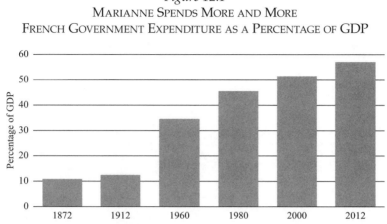

SOURCES: 1872–2000: "Les dépenses publiques depuis un siècle," Vie Publique website, June 12, 2013, http://www.vie-publique.fr/decouverte-institutions/finances -publiques/approfondissements/depenses-publiques-depuis-siecle.html; 2012: "Total Government Expenditure," Eurostat, http://epp.eurostat.ec.europa.eu/tgm/table.do ?tab=table&init=1&plugin=1&language=en&pcode=tec00023.

NOTE: These figures omit the spending spikes during the two world wars.

2.9 percent of GDP between 1900 and 2010.[21] In the United States, defense spending fell from 10.1 percent of GDP in 1960 to 5.6 percent in 2012.[22]

Welfare state spending accounts for 69 percent of the budget in Germany and 71 percent in France[23] (see Figure 12.2). Comparable figures are not easily available for all countries, but four major advanced countries—France, Germany, Italy, and Japan—all allocate remarkably similar proportions to welfare—between 66 percent and 71 percent. Even this is probably an underestimate because other areas of spending such as "General Public Services" often include elements of welfare state expenditure.

Between 1980 and 2012, nearly all of the 35 countries studied by the Organisation for Economic Co-operation and Development (OECD) increased their social spending as a proportion of GDP.[24] The fastest increases were in those countries that previously had the smallest social provision. Japan's social spending doubled. Greece's more than doubled. Portugal's rose two and half times. Turkey's

Figure 12.2
HOW MUCH IS SPENT ON THE WELFARE STATE?
MINIMUM PERCENTAGE OF GOVERNMENT SPENDING DEVOTED TO
"SOCIAL PROTECTION" AND THE WELFARE STATE MORE BROADLY
INCLUDING HEALTH CARE, EDUCATION, AND HOUSING, 2011

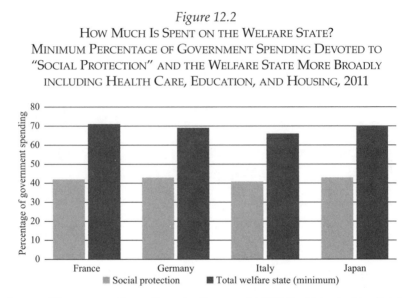

SOURCE: "Government Expenditure by Function," OECD.StatExtracts, http://stats
.oecd.org/Index.aspx?DatasetCode=SNA_TABLE11.

tripled. In democratic states, there is a kind of irresistible drive toward high welfare spending.

There were only two exceptions. One was the Netherlands. It changed course as described in Chapter 2. The other was Sweden.

It is striking that Sweden, the country often regarded as the ultimate welfare state, is one of the few countries to have cut social spending over the past 30 years. How did this happen?

In the 1980s, it was business as usual. Swedish welfare spending was high and rising. At both the beginning and the end of the decade, Sweden was spending more on welfare than any other country studied by the OECD.[25] Then came the recession of the early 1990s. Demand for welfare spending continued increasing, but tax receipts fell. Sweden found that raising the money needed for more welfare spending had gone from hard to impossible. The budget deficit soared to 10 percent.[26] There were only two options: go bust or cut back.[27]

So Sweden cut back (see Figure 12.3). Welfare benefits were reduced and conditions for getting them were made tougher. These and other economic measures were taken to bring the welfare budget back to sustainability. The shock of this crisis also led to some

Figure 12.3
THE SWEDISH WELFARE STATE HITS THE CEILING
PUBLIC SOCIAL EXPENDITURES IN SWEDEN AS A PERCENTAGE OF GDP

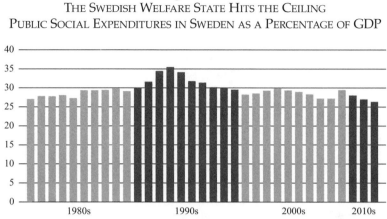

SOURCE: Willem Adema, Pauline Fron, and Maxime Ladaique, "Is the European Welfare State Really More Expensive?," OECD Social, Employment and Migration Working Papers no. 124, October 2011, p. 41.

modest rethinking about how welfare should be delivered and to some measures against unwelcome unintended consequences—such as abuse of the system.

It might be tempting to conclude from Sweden's example, "You see! Democracies can be sensible and draw back from disaster. They can reform their welfare states."

Indeed they can. But what we can see in Sweden is that, even in a particularly mature and level-headed democracy, the electorate needed to go right to the edge of a cliff before deciding to turn back. And subsequently, 19 years after that moment, welfare spending in Sweden, while significantly down from its peak, remains well above average.

Let's take another country where reforms and obstacles have been implemented. The United States, in the 1990s, had a crisis of conscience about welfare spending. There was publicity about the cost, the unemployment that had been created, and the fraud. The growing welfare dependency seemed contrary to the centuries-old national culture of rugged self-reliance. This culminated in President Clinton's signing the Personal Responsibility and Work Opportunity Reconciliation Act of 1996, which enabled and encouraged states to move away from cash entitlements toward workfare. It looked as if a nation was offended by the idea of people getting used to living on welfare and was acting to stop it. The pioneering spirit of the United States seemed to rise up in revolt. Major reforms took place and many people were taken off welfare rolls.

But within a decade, there was a slide back toward more welfare spending. The numbers receiving food stamps soared, partly because the eligibility criteria were loosened. The time during which people could receive unemployment benefits was increased. The semicompulsory health care insurance scheme known as "Obamacare" was introduced.

Sweden and the United States illustrate typical patterns: a country perceives there is a welfare state problem and pulls back. But the first flaw of democracy—the way politicians get elected is by promising "generous" things—sooner or later reasserts itself. So despite occasional retreats, a Utopian idea of the welfare state is never defeated. It rallies and then makes further advances. The tendency is for more and more to be spent until, as in Sweden, the money simply runs out. It is arguable that Greece and Spain faced their recent financial crises, which necessitated sudden, painful cutbacks, because of welfare state spending.

"It is a kind of insanity, this uncontrollable inflation of the state. . . . Regulations pile higher and new benefits accumulate. . . . In Sigmund Freud's *Civilisation and Its Discontents*, he pictures the mind as an ancient city, where nothing is ever demolished but new buildings are continually added. He would have recognised the sick, social democratic states of the twenty-first century, bulging with ever more good intentions, incapable of shedding those past their sell-by date."

SOURCE: Marc Sidwell, "The Long View: Behind the Debt Ceiling Madness Lurks the Insanity of an Uncontrollable State," *City A.M.* (London), October 11, 2013, http://www.cityam.com/article/1381452052/long-view-behind-debt-ceiling-madness-lurks-insanity-uncontrollable-state.

Welfare states in democracies resemble people who can't swim paddling out into the sea. To begin with they are fine. They walk through the shallow water. Gradually, progress gets more difficult, but it is still possible. The water gets higher and higher up their bodies—past their knees, then their chests. Occasionally, one turns back, saying, "This is silly. I'm getting into danger!" But most continue into the sea, because the dynamic of politicians trying to get elected leads to more promises and bigger welfare states. Eventually, the water rises up over the mouths of one or two of them and they are in imminent danger of drowning. Suddenly, they have to be rescued—like Sweden or Greece. But does anyone say, "This is crazy! We need to get back well within our depth—where we were only up to our knees"? No. They keep flirting with the maximum depth at which survival is possible.

But well before they are at this maximum depth, so much money needs to be raised to pay for the welfare states that it is no longer a matter of the government acting as Robin Hood, taking from the rich and giving to the poor. That does not raise enough. So cash is taken from those on average wages and then it is taken from the poor. Effectively, money is taken from the poor and then given back to them after a deduction has been granted to bureaucrats, who have charged them for the administration of the programs and sometimes added in instructions on where they must live, which doctor they should see, what school their children must attend, and what training course they must take.

One of the problems in representative democracies is that those who point out the drawbacks of big welfare states tend to get a hearing only when things are going badly wrong or disaster is afoot. It is hard to persuade people otherwise that a big welfare state has plenty of bad, unintended consequences. Such arguments count for little against the rallying cry of a politician who declares, "It is wrong that in this great nation of ours anyone should go without decent childcare/decent care in old age [or whatever it might be]." Of course, it is always assumed that what the state provides will be "decent" or "high quality" regardless of any previous experience that suggests it will be nothing of the kind. Potential undesirable consequences are ignored or dismissed.

This, at least, is the tendency. Is it an absolute rule? Is every single country that goes toward democracy, from Sweden to India and Brazil to China, bound to end up with a welfare state that keeps growing until the harm is overwhelmingly obvious or the money runs out? Is there any way of stopping the self-harming tendency of democratic countries?

Frankly, it is hard to be confident that there is. Maybe we are headed for a world where—quite unnecessarily—mass unemployment is permanent, where education fails often and badly, where health care is not as good as it could be and millions die needless, early deaths. Maybe it will be a world where the spirit of independence, self-reliance, and freedom continues to fade away, a large minority of children never learn to read, and many people feel alienated from society.

Of course, it is conceivable that the downside of massive welfare states will become better recognized. The generation that believed that more welfare must always be better welfare may be replaced by another that perceives that things are not so simple. Unfortunately, I am doubtful that this will happen—at least within representative democracies. We tend to take this form of democracy for granted as the natural, normal one. In point of fact, it has not existed for very long. It first took shape in the modern world in 17th-century Britain, as it emerged from a war between king and parliament. The parliament, up to that point, had not been powerful. For a long while, it had been merely a way through which powerful landowners could make their voices heard by the monarch. But after the English Civil War, it became much more than that. If this is, indeed, the origin or model for modern parliamentary or representative democracy, let us recognize where it came from: it was a modification of a medieval system originally created for a feudal society. Viewed this way, it seems absurd to assume that it is ideal for modern times.

In America, the democratic system was influenced by both the British and Roman examples. But again, it was formed in circumstances very different from those of the present. The same applies to other democracies, except for some such as Japan where a new democratic system was recently and suddenly accepted. But even in these cases, the constitutions were designed to mimic the representative democracies that derived from 17th-century or 18th-century models. In those times, of course, it took days or even weeks for information to travel from one part of a country to another. Representative democracy was the only democracy practicable.

But we have seen that representative democracy has a plethora of faults. Is there any better form of democracy? In particular, is there any form that would manage a welfare state better?

If one looks around the world, there are two kinds of states that have successfully resisted the siren call of "more welfare." One consists of countries that are not full democracies: dictatorships, oligarchies, or semidemocracies. In modern times, they have included the communist countries of Europe and Asia; Hong Kong when it was a colony; and Singapore, which is a democracy but where the same party has been in power for a generation and has made life very difficult for the opposition. Most of us would not want a democracy with limits. We want government by clear consent.

The other kind of democracy that has kept a lid on welfare takes a different shape. Here is a flavor of how it works in one country.

In May 2013, the smallest region of this country had to make a deci-sion about a proposed railway project costing the equivalent of $7.5 million.[28] As with all such projects, you can imagine that some argued that it would be good for the economy and for access to the rest of the country while others maintained it would cause too much damage.

In most advanced countries, the decision would have been made by a small group of politicians or civil servants. Such decisions are sometimes made by people who have never even been to the place concerned. They are following the orders of their political party or the rules of a system. But in this region, the decision was made by the local population of 15,717 souls.

The voters assembled in the town square. Following ancient tra-dition, men showed they were entitled to vote by carrying a sword. Women carried a voting card. The motion—whether or not to accept the railway project—was made and the individuals voted by raising their hands. This is "direct" democracy.

The decision, incidentally, was to approve the railway project. The region in question was the smallest canton in Switzerland, Appen-zell Innerrhoden.

Not all referenda in Switzerland take place in town squares. The Appenzell Innerrhoden system is a rare, charming relic of old tradi-tions. Most votes, of course, are done in the same way as votes in representative democracies.

Switzerland has national, cantonal, and local referenda. They take place about three or four times a year. Typically, there are two or three national issues, two cantonal, and two local. The total number of issues varies between three and seven, but it all depends on how many petitions have succeeded in obtaining the required number of signatures. Once the signatures are obtained, it can take as many as three years for a national issue to reach the ballot box. First, it is studied and debated by the parliament.

Switzerland's form of democracy is more thorough-going and complete than any other in the world. Switzerland also has a welfare state that is generally smaller and suffers fewer unintended conse-quences than elsewhere. Of course there are criticisms that could be made, but Switzerland gets more things right in welfare than most other countries. One consequence is that unemployment there is sig-nificantly below average, for example.

Switzerland's social spending is lower than average. It absorbs 18.5 percent of GDP compared with the average 22.1 percent, accord-ing to the OECD definition. Switzerland also has lower-than-average total government spending (34.1 percent versus 42.0 percent) and therefore needs to take less in taxes (28.5 percent versus 33.8 percent).[29] This has been achieved despite the fact that Switzerland is surrounded by countries that mostly have above-average spending. The lower welfare spending and taxation are probably part of the reason Switzerland has achieved higher growth than other countries and has made its citizens into some of the most prosperous in the world apart from those in oil-rich and very small countries.[30]

You could argue that the fact that Switzerland has direct democracy and a welfare state under better control could be just a coincidence. It is a sample of only one, so it is not conclusive. Is there any supporting evidence?

Some. There are 26 cantons in Switzerland, and each has its own rules. Each allows referenda to a different degree. So academics have been able to study how the amount of democracy in each of these cantons has affected the way it has been governed. It makes for a bigger sample size. At least three studies have found that the cantons with higher levels of direct democracy spend less on welfare than the rest.[31] These papers also looked at truly local governments—towns and villages—as well as cantons. So the sample size was bigger still and the results more robust. The most recent of these studies found that the correlation between direct democracy and lower welfare spending was "highly statistically significant."[32] Those in the most democratic cantons were also happier. (See Box 12.1.)

The governments of some cantons are obliged to have referenda to approve or reject major spending proposals. A couple of academics studied these cantons and compared them to the others.[33] They found that those with mandatory spending referenda spent 19 percent less. It's a huge difference.

It is ironic. Some politicians and civil servants dismiss direct democracy, arguing that they, with their superior education and intellect, are sure to be better than ordinary people at running a country. Yet the evidence from Switzerland is the opposite. Ordinary people appear to be better and more sober in the exercise of power—when they have it—than are elected, elite representatives (Box 12.2). One Swiss study goes so far as to suggest that the "representatives" in "representative democracies" frequently do not represent. In Switzerland, 39 percent of referenda, over a period of 140 years, turned down the proposals of politicians.[34]

So is direct democracy the answer? It appears to overcome at least 7 of the 12 problems of representative democracy listed

Box 12. 1
DO REFERENDA MAKE PEOPLE HAPPIER?

Professor Bruno Frey of the University of Zurich found a clear correlation between democracy and happiness. He used measures of the amount of democracy in cantons and the level of happiness people in them reported.[a] The canton of Basel Land had the highest democracy rating of 5.69 of 6.00 and was notably happier than the canton of Geneva, with the lowest democracy rating of only 1.75. All the results were adjusted for demographic variables such as age and income. After such adjustments and a barrage of statistical tests, the results were found to be robust. Direct democracy really does appear to make people happier.

How big is the effect?

It was found to be as powerful as moving someone up from a low income to the next level up (out of five). It applies to everybody, too. The happiness effect of direct democracy reaches people of all social and educational classes.

What causes it?

One possible cause is that people get better government or, perhaps, government more in accordance with their views. But another and, it turns out, more significant cause is that people gain a sense of well-being from the feeling that they have the capacity to influence events. It is true that people may not always vote, but they do so in big numbers when an issue is particularly important or is one on which they have strong views. Having a little power and a truly democratic decision makes people feel better.

---

[a] Bruno Frey and Alois Stutzer, "Happiness, Economy and Institutions," *Economic Journal* 110 (2000): 918–38.

earlier—numbers 1, 4, 5, 7, 8, 9, and 11—and to moderate another 3 or 4 of them. Unfortunately, there are a couple of reasons to hesitate. Although Switzerland has one of the lowest rates of expenditure on its welfare state, it has not wholly resisted the international trend. The proportion spent on "public social expenditure" rose by a third between 1980 and 2012.[35] Its total expenditure, including nonwelfare spending, as a proportion of GDP has been stable in recent years, but the current level of 34.1 percent is still up on the 27.9 percent of 1970.[36] This is a country that has resisted the trend toward massive welfare states better than others, but it has not blocked it entirely.

Box 12.2
BETTER A REFERENDUM THAN A POLITICIAN'S GIFT

Would you trust people to vote on whether they should have six weeks' vacation a year?

On March 11, 2012, the Swiss voted on the proposition that everyone should be legally entitled to six weeks of vacation a year. It is the sort of promise that a politician might use to gain popularity—as though he or she were making a gift. But when the Swiss had a referendum on the issue, evidently they seriously considered the drawbacks as well as the attractions. They voted the idea down by 1,531,986 votes to 771,717.[a]

---

[a] "Bundesratsbeschluss über das Ergebnis der Volksabstimmung vom 11 März 2012," p. 6624, http://www.admin.ch/opc/de/federal-gazette/2012/6623.pdf.

A second worry is what we could call "the California problem." California is the most prominent American state where referenda are a regular part of political life. Unfortunately, it is far from being a model of sensible, controlled government. On the contrary, the state increased welfare expenditures to the point at which it got itself into a financial crisis and was obliged to cut spending suddenly. As one report put it, California "thrashed" its welfare programs.[37] The state's budget crisis of 2008–12 even has its own Wikipedia entry.[38]

However, it can be argued that California has a system of direct democracy that is particularly badly designed. A San Francisco resident on November 6, 2013, had to face votes on 7 city issues and 11 state issues.[39] There were separate documents for the city and the state. One was 147 pages long and the other was 144. Voting conscientiously on so many referenda would be a massive undertaking, requiring days of reading and study. Only well-educated retirees could attempt it. Moreover, California has all these votes on one day in the year.

Things are much easier for a voter in Switzerland, who has far fewer ballots to consider at any one time. The Swiss voter is more likely to want to and be able to look at the issues and vote. The exact design of direct democracy matters.

If we accept that direct democracy has something to offer, is there any other or additional strategy that a country might adopt to keep its welfare state under control?

One possibility is to create a binding obligation on governments to limit the level of debt. In Poland, a national debt limit of 60 percent of GDP was introduced in 1997.[40] Despite all Poland's problems, this may well have helped it avoid getting anywhere near the sort of debt crisis experienced in Greece and, to a lesser extent, in Italy and Spain. Poland enshrined the idea that no political party should be able—during its few years in government—to burden future generations with heavy debt.

Singapore has a similar but different law: a self-imposed obligation to maintain a balanced budget.[41] Each administration must balance the budget over its five-year period in office. It is only allowed to break this rule in exceptional circumstances and even then it must write to the president to ask permission. Whether such a rigorous system of budget discipline will be maintained if or when Singapore becomes a more fully free and democratic nation remains to be seen. But the rule has certainly served Singapore well, leading to great stability. Singapore has been more successful than any other advanced country in not imposing a debt burden on the next generation.

Other countries have made similar moves: Germany and Switzerland have introduced or enhanced their constitutions—in 2009 and 1999, respectively—to oblige governments to balance their budgets, as variously defined. Countries that have imposed these rules on themselves certainly appear to have done better than the rest.

A third possible strategy is to "go local." When all voters in a locality have to bear the costs as well as feel the benefits of decisions, they probably make better decisions. It seems to work for Switzerland. Local pride and a sense of identity are very strong there. I was once in Sils Maria, a little village 6 miles from the world-famous skiing resort of St Moritz. I asked if they had any mementos for sale relating to St Moritz.

"No," replied the shopkeeper firmly. "We have mementos of Sils Maria."

There is no sure-fire answer to "the problem of democracy." But there do appear to be things that can be done to improve matters. A well-designed direct democracy, constitutional limits on budget deficits or debt, and "going local" have all shown that they can help.

13. And the Winner Is … ~~Communism~~ ~~Capitalism~~ Welfare Statism!

Summary

A great battle of ideas was played out in the 20th century between communism and capitalism. Revolutions were followed by wars, famines, terror, and millions of deaths. The communist cause was advanced by the Russian Revolution, the take-over of Eastern Europe, and communist revolutions and civil wars in China, Korea, Vietnam, and Cambodia. Millions died from starvation in the Soviet Union and China. In Russia, Korea, Vietnam, and elsewhere, the United States and other capitalist countries tried to resist communism. The Berlin Wall was a physical symbol of the divide between two ideas of how societies should be. As a child, I remember the tension and fear when the United States and the USSR squared up to each other during the Cuban missile crisis. The world waited nervously to see whether a nuclear war would erupt, potentially resulting in the deaths of many more millions.

But then the conflict ebbed. A critical mass of people in the communist countries became disillusioned by the economic underperformance and political oppression. In China in the 1980s, Deng Xiaoping led the country toward capitalism. In 1989, the Berlin Wall came down and all of Eastern Europe forsook communism. Communism was discredited. But capitalism did not completely win, either. In much of the world, a constrained version of capitalism was tolerated without being loved. As memories of the poverty and terror resulting from communism faded, capitalism became subject to more distrust and criticism. And while all this was going on, quietly running past both of these concepts—without a single shot fired—was the ultimate victor of the turmoil of the 20th century: the welfare state.

It was as if two loud, clever politicians contended for leadership of the world but, in the end people chose the quiet, boring one at the back. As a political or economic idea, it has not even got a name. What shall we call it? Welfare statism?

There was no great theoretician who came up with the idea or argued for it. No political thinker is famous for saying what a marvelous thing it is or could be. Welfare statism has no Karl Marx or Adam Smith. The father of the idea—if anyone deserves the title—was a vain, crusty, rather cynical old conservative: Otto von Bismarck. He thought a welfare state—or his modest, early version of it—would be a good way to keep the common people from revolting. He thought of it as a sop to the masses—a bone to be thrown on the floor for dogs to chew on.

From such an inglorious beginning, state welfare grew and conquered the world.

"He who does not work shall not eat."

Source: Vladimir Lenin (clearly not a welfare statist), *The State and Revolution* (1917).

Welfare statism won because it was not an obvious failure like communism and because it appeared kinder than capitalism. Historians have barely noticed it. Sociologists are only beginning to catch up. But welfare states have been established in every advanced democratic country in the world. If you say this to people, they tend to be surprised. They have not thought of the world this way. But there are no exceptions. Welfare states cover the globe more extensively than any empire ever has. It is a fundamental change in the nature of world civilization. Nor is it merely something half way between capitalism and communism. In communist countries, unemployment benefits were small on the basis that work was compulsory. Housing was a reward for a job, not compensation for being poor. Lenin said, "He who does not work shall not eat"—hardly the words of a welfare statist. No, the welfare states of the world are a distinct form.

What has been their effect?

In 1934, Oxford University Press started publishing an ambitious series of books covering English history from the earliest beginnings. The original volumes went up to 1914. Then an additional, 15th volume was commissioned covering 1914 to 1945. It was written by one of the leading historians of the time, Professor A. J. P. Taylor. The opening words were striking:

> Until August 1914, a sensible, law-abiding Englishman could pass through life and hardly notice the existence of the state, beyond the post office and the policeman. He could live where he liked and as he liked. He had no official number or identity card. He could travel abroad or leave his country for ever without a passport or any sort of official permission. He could exchange his money for any other currency without restriction or limit. He could buy goods from any country in the world on the same terms as he bought goods at home. For that matter, a foreigner could spend his life in this country without permit and without informing the police. . . .
>
> [During the First World War] the state established a hold over its citizens which, though relaxed in peacetime, was never to be removed and which the Second World War was again to increase. The history of the English state and of the English people merged for the first time.[1]

Like most traditional historians, Taylor noted the impact of the world wars but underestimated the quieter, less spectacular progress of the welfare state. Yet the picture he paints of a citizen before 1914 with untrammelled freedom and independence from state interference is, to modern eyes, almost incomprehensible.

The freedom Taylor describes might have been dismissed by Marx as "bourgeois"—only affordable by the rich. But the poor exercised some of this freedom, too. Think of the millions who poured across from Ireland, Great Britain, Italy, Poland, Germany, and elsewhere to the United States in the 19th and early 20th centuries. They, too, were free and unconstrained by state control or paperwork. They took risks and were obliged to work to survive. They had freedom and responsibility for themselves. What a huge contrast to how we live now.

"The Great Switch"

SOURCE: Phrase used by Jacques Barzun to describe "the reversal of liberalism into its opposite." Liberals originally believed in minimal government but came to favor welfare benefits and thus big government. Jacques Barzun, *From Dawn to Decadence: 500 Years of Western Cultural Life* (London: HarperCollins, 2000), p. 688.

Take Kate. She was born in a government hospital. Not long after birth, she was visited by a government health visitor.[2] If her mother wanted—or was obliged—to work, Kate was deposited in day care, a nursery, or a school run or paid for by the government. Then she went to government schools run in accordance with rules, regulations, and guidance laid down by the government. The government specified or approved the nature and timing of her exams. This was followed by a university or technical college mostly financed by the government and under its control. Kate paid part of the cost of the course with a loan from the state, to be repaid during her adult life.

When Kate finished her education but was unemployed, the government gave her money on certain terms and conditions. When she had a child but no husband, she was given an apartment by the government. Now that she has got a job, she is taxed by the government. She is obliged to make compulsory contributions to government social insurance, much of which goes to pay the pensions of her grandparents' generation. When she becomes ill, she goes to a state-approved doctor who is paid, one way or another, by the government and who works in accordance with government rules and targets. She probably has a government identity card. She obviously needs a passport to travel, and it is scanned at ports of entry, enabling her government to have a record of when she comes and goes.

"This is the main danger that today threatens civilization: the nationalization of life."

SOURCE: José Ortega y Gasset, *La rebelión de las masas* (1930).

While in government housing, Kate has to qualify for and continue to qualify for the apartment. Official forms have to be filled in. If she starts a business, she will be required to hire and fire staff in accordance with thousands of pages of government rules. She will be obliged to pay social insurance to the government for each employee and to pay tax on any profit her company might make. She would need government permission to start a school, build a home, or create a hospital. She would need to obtain a government-approved license to pursue a wide variety of occupations including, in many countries, teaching.

When she becomes older, Kate will receive a government pension. She may have to prove that she has made the required contributions.

346

If she moves abroad, her country of origin may, in some cases, reduce this pension. If she becomes frail, she may be admitted to a government-financed and government-regulated home. She is quite likely to die in a government hospital and to be cremated in a government crematorium.

All—or nearly all—of the interventions in her life are for her own good. The idea is to protect her from harm. But one effect of all this state-organized, compulsory welfare is that it guides and controls her at every stage. This imaginary woman is monitored, guided, nudged, and provided for "from the cradle to the grave." Financial incentives are imposed on her to push her to do what the government approves of or not to do what it disapproves of. Governments effectively prescribe how she ought to live. The process is limiting and controlling—almost domineering. There is something of Big Brother about it.[3] Orwell may have turned out to be a better forecaster of present times than Marx. But, of course, Orwell was not forecasting. He was warning.

In raising all the money needed to run welfare states and in trying to care for people and guide our behavior, welfare states have caused myriad unintended consequences. They have downgraded the concepts of individual freedom and property rights. Welfare states have given so much in some situations while taking so much in others and have set so many conditions that, inevitably, the ideal of liberty—once so important in the advanced world—has declined. As for property, it has become something to be redistributed rather than respected.

Other effects have been less abstract. In the 19th century, there were outbreaks of widespread unemployment from time to time, but they did not last. People priced themselves into work or moved to find it. Now we have great countries where an unemployment rate of 10 percent is considered normal. In Spain, unemployment reached 27 percent in 2013.[4] Among the young and certain racial groups, unemployment is usually considerably higher than for the rest of the population. With few exceptions, welfare states have made mass unemployment permanent, and that misfortune, in turn, has caused a pandemic of unhappiness.

Even the high official unemployment figures of recent times understate the full extent of the problem. Many people described as incapacitated, disabled, or in "early retirement" should more accurately be described as unemployed. Tens of millions of people around the world have been left living on welfare benefits, creating the bizarre paradox of societies that are richer than ever yet that have more people out of work and more still who are dependent on government handouts.

It has become particularly difficult for those with a low educational level or who are truly disabled or from a racial minority to get work. State schooling has left a large minority of people unable to read and write properly. This deficit has reduced their ability to earn or has led to their being unemployed. The widespread inadequacy of state education has been one of the most shameful aspects of welfare states. It has helped to create a division between the elite at the top and the poorly educated unemployed at the bottom. It is, perhaps, the greatest cause of modern inequality. This is a terrible irony: welfare states that were intended to help the poor instead have sealed many of them in a state of hopelessness.

Welfare states have also had a tendency to increase the amount of single parenting and the number of couples who break up. This has caused millions more children to endure the unhappiness of an unstable home. It has made many women more vulnerable and many men less socialized and satisfied.

There has been a large amount of fraud in the claiming of welfare benefits. Welfare states have given rise to persistently high taxes that have encouraged fraud and substantial hidden economies. High levels of social insurance have similarly encouraged hidden economies.

"In their efforts to cure specific evils, legislators have continually caused collateral evils they never looked for. . . . Though their production is explicable enough after it has occurred, it is never anticipated."

SOURCE: Herbert Spencer, "Over-Legislation," *Westminster Review*, July 1853, available at Library of Economics and Liberty website, http://www.econlib.org/library/LFBooks/Spencer/spnMvS7.html.

Government housing has created ghettos of crime and fear. The illusion has been fostered that every effort is being made to house the poor whereas, in reality, their needs would be more effectively met simply by allowing more housing to be built. Government controls on housing have raised the cost for everyone, but the most devastating effect has been on the poor. They have often been denied the homeownership that could improve their financial security and their sense of being part of society. Housing welfare benefits have trapped many poor people out of work, because by getting a job they would lose those benefits.

Welfare states take care of many frail, elderly people, who then have often become extremely miserable through being looked after by strangers, away from their homes or relatives. Their children have often ceased to feel they have any responsibility for them and have neglected them. This—and the boom in single parenting and in institutional care for infants—is part of a "defamilization" that many welfare states have brought about, causing people to be both less happy and less connected to society. Children, mothers, and fathers all have become more isolated.

As Emile Durkheim, one of the founders of sociology, wrote, "The more weakened the groups to which [a man] belongs, the less he depends on them, the more he consequently depends only on himself and recognises no other rules of conduct than what are founded on his private interests."[5] In Stockholm now, 60 percent of all dwellings are occupied by someone who lives alone.[6]

Welfare states are administered by bureaucracies that may mean well but cannot help appearing to those who must apply to them as faceless authorities telling them what to do—pagan gods to be appeased with forms and applications. Inevitably, in some cases, the bureaucracies are inefficient and slow, leading to a sense of frustration and powerlessness among those who depend on them.

Welfare states divide us into authorities and supplicants. We ask for government housing. We try to get our children into good government schools instead of terrible ones. We plead with overworked nurses to make sure our elderly mothers are given the food and water they need. It is not as if the bureaucrats—or exhausted nurses or much-criticized teachers—are made happy by the arrangement. They feel stressed by the complaints and limited by the many rules they must submit to. Supplicants and authorities—it is a civilization in which personal dignity and responsibility are in retreat.

"Cupcake compliance"

SOURCE: Phrase in a headline above an article about how the U.S. government insisted that "food sold at school fundraising bake sales must, with some exceptions, conform to federal standards." See George F. Will, "Cupcake Compliance Illustrates Washington's Quest to Control Everything," *National Post* (United States), August 21, 2014, http://fullcomment.nationalpost.com/2014/08/21/george-f-will-cupcake-compliance-illustrates-washingtons-quest-to-control-everything.

There are times and occasions when governments—for all that they may be democratic—act with a dogmatism reminiscent of fascist or communist regimes. Some welfare states decree which school a child must attend. They order that children with learning difficulties must be in classes alongside the brightest children regardless of the impact on the clever ones. Some forbid homeschooling, making it explicit that the family has been usurped by the state. There are places where children have literally been taken by police from their homes to prevent homeschooling.[7] The logic of a welfare state can lead to such totalitarianism's being considered right and proper. (See Box 13.1.)

The large number of people of working age who live on welfare benefits could be working and adding to economic output. Instead, taxes must be levied to pay for them and for other aspects of the welfare state. The resulting high rates discourage work, enterprise, and saving—all of which contribute to economic growth. Many studies

Box 13.1
BASTIAT ON THE WELFARE STATE

Classical liberal theorist Frédéric Bastiat (1801–50) saw the welfare state as merely the extension of the greed of men.

"For today, as in the past, each person more or less wants to profit from the work of others. We do not dare display this sentiment: we even hide it from ourselves, and then what do we do? We design an intermediary, we address ourselves to the state, and each class in turn comes forward to say to it, 'You who can take things straightforwardly and honestly, take something from the general public and we will share it.' Alas! The state has a very ready tendency to follow this diabolical advice as it is made up of ministers and civil servants, in short, men, who like all men are filled with the desire and are always quick to seize the opportunity to see their wealth and influence increase. The state is therefore quick to understand the profit it can make from the role that the general public has entrusted to it. It will be the arbiter and master of every destiny. It will take a great deal; therefore a great deal will remain to it. It will increase the number of its agents and widen the circle of its attributions. It will end by achieving crushing proportions."[a]

[a] Frédéric Bastiat, *"The Law," "The State," and other Political Writings 1843–1850—The Collected Works of Frédéric Bastiat,* general ed. by Jacques de Guenin and tr. from the French by Jane Willems and Michel Willems (Indianapolis, IN: Liberty Fund, 2012).

give evidence of the relation between taxation and diminished growth. Meanwhile, the bureaucrats who administer welfare states could otherwise have contributed to actual production or services.

Regulations and licensing add to the downward pressure that welfare states apply to economic growth. The growth rate of the advanced world has slowed in recent years. The root cause could well be our enveloping welfare states and regulations. The advanced world could have enjoyed far more economic growth and prosperity without welfare states.

It is the poor who have been hurt most. They are the ones going to the inferior schools and receiving a second-rate education. They are the ones whose families are most frequently fractured by the perverse incentives that some welfare states have created. They are more likely to be on welfare benefits, so they are the ones most tempted to lie and cheat to continue to qualify for them. They are the ones most likely to be unemployed. All these things have been profoundly damaging to their happiness.

"If you want to predict how happy someone is, or how long she will live, . . . you should find out about her social relationships. . . . Even people who think they don't want a lot of social contact still benefit from it."

Source: Quoted in Jonathan Haidt, *The Happiness Hypothesis: Putting Ancient Wisdom to the Test of Modern Science* (London: Arrow, 2006).

All human beings like to feel they are worthwhile—that they have a role in life. If you take away a person's work, you take away what most powerfully creates a sense of purpose and place in society. The unemployed often feel worthless. Nor does anybody genuinely feel proud and happy about being dishonest. Lives are poorer, too, if people cannot read and their knowledge and experience of culture are cramped. These are lives that have been downgraded by welfare states.

The better-off half of society, while less damaged, has not escaped unscathed. Most have sent their children to schools of a lower quality than they would otherwise have had. Their housing has been more limited than it could have been, their health care is of lower quality, and their income after tax has been smaller. At the top end, they find they are often taxed aggressively as though they were to blame for all the ills of the world. It is as if anger is being taken out on them. They feel defensive. Unsurprisingly, they try to find ways—legal and illegal—to avoid the heavy taxes. Their honesty has been undermined, too. They do not feel good about themselves when they knowingly avoid taxes. As with welfare benefits, the temptation has been too big for too long. The idea that one should always be honest has come to seem impossibly idealistic—even foolish.

The better-off often watch the same television programs that have been dumbed down to reach those who have been failed by their schools. They see how births outside marriage have become normal. They would consider it unkind to condemn the behavior of those who are poorer than themselves. So judgment of such behavior is suspended and affects how they themselves live, too. The sense that adults have a duty to give their children a stable family upbringing has thus been gradually undermined across society, even though it has affected the poor much more than the rich. The concept of right and wrong has withered and become focused on just a few kinds of behavior such as racist comments. Few would now dare say that it is "wrong" for a husband or wife to divorce and go off with someone else, leaving a broken family.

The ideals of philanthropy and charity still exist, but they are not as important as before. Charitable giving in Britain is a fraction of what it was a century ago. Personal virtue has been contracted out to the welfare state. Indeed, some people appear to believe they have asserted their virtue merely by voting for a party that favors more state welfare.

Welfare states have helped create a grievance culture. There is almost competition to be one of the downtrodden who can demand "support" from the welfare state. Even people who are relatively well off have decided to get into the act. There has been talk of the "squeezed middle"—people who cannot claim to be low paid, unemployed, female, discriminated against, or disabled but who realize that the only way to preserve their interests is by joining the ranks of clamoring "victims." This is often now the way to stake a claim on the beneficence of the all-powerful welfare state. (See Box 13.2.)

"Social programs that undermine the work ethic and displace fathers keep poor people poor."

SOURCE: Jason L. Riley, *Please Stop Helping Us: How Liberals Make It Harder for Blacks to Succeed* (New York: Encounter, 2014). The book argues that programs ostensibly designed to help blacks have actually harmed them.

Box 13.2
THE SERVILE MIND—A MODERN MINDSET

Kenneth Minogue (1930–2013), professor emeritus of political science at the London School of Economics and Political Science, wrote a book about how the modern world was changing the mentality of people. He titled it *The Servile Mind*.[a]

Furthermore, he described a demeaning "competitiveness about grievances" in modern political discourse:

Politicians, agitators and lobbyists … have articulated modern societies as a collection of suffering classes, technically called "minorities." The political consequences of this status are such that minorities now constitute the vast majority of our population: women, racial groups, the handicapped, the inhabitants of the Third World, the aged, the mentally handicapped and many others are exploiters of egalitarian sentiments and claimants of advantages to be supplied by the government and enshrined in law. In this way, egalitarianism entrenches a form of mean-spirited competitiveness about grievances at the heart of the political process.[b]

---

[a] Kenneth Minogue, *The Servile Mind: How Democracy Erodes the Moral Life* (New York: Encounter, 2010).
[b] Minogue, writing in a pamphlet on egalitarianism for the Centre for Policy Studies, reported in an email to the author by John Blundell.

The other side of the coin is that the concepts of self-reliance, duty, responsibility, courage, and independence all have dwindled. What use are they when a call to the welfare state may bring benefits that do not need to be worked for but only demanded? But the psychology of victimhood makes no one happy. It is like becoming a permanent teenager—confused, angry, and outraged.

Overall, the picture of our world that emerges is of a diminished civilization, one that is less dynamic and impressive than it would otherwise have been, populated by citizens who are less admirable and less content.

Some might react to this critique by saying, "But at least welfare states have provided for the poor, cared for the ill, and educated everyone. They have helped those who fall on hard times. And even people who are not poor have felt a sense of security." There is truth in this and, insofar as it is true, it is good. But there are three ways in which this is less than a justification.

First, there are the unintended consequences described previously that have been so remarkably bad. Second, we should not compare the provision of welfare states against zero. We should compare them against what would otherwise have been provided by individuals for themselves, by families, mutual organizations, insurance, friendly societies, local government, and charities. Third, we should bear in mind how often welfare states have not provided the services they promised. A large proportion of people have not been properly educated. They are functionally illiterate. The ill have not always been cared for. Some have died waiting for operations or for lack of up-to-date drugs. Some have not even been cared for properly in the hospital. Some have been allocated miserable housing in which they are terrified.

There is a tendency to apply a double standard. Private or independent provision of welfare is judged by its imperfections. A welfare state is judged by its aspirations. Both should be judged on their performance and outcomes, shouldn't they?

Despite all this, let us remember some things that are good and some reasons for hope. Let's recall that the modern world is built on the history, culture, and economic growth of previous centuries. "There is a great deal of ruin in a nation," as Adam Smith said. Major cultural and financial wealth has been established and remains. One might even regard welfare states as a kind of self-harming drug that only the richest countries can afford.

Also, human beings are capable of seeing what has gone wrong and of reacting. We take a long time to understand and even longer to do anything. But we humans are capable—eventually and after enough disasters—of doing the right thing.

What is the "right thing"?

An absolutely minimal welfare state would probably achieve the best possible outcome. But even if democratic societies are not willing to be so radical, there are plenty of things that could make welfare states better. The detailed prescriptions are in each of the previous chapters of this book. But some themes keep cropping up:

- The more that government monopoly power can be broken down, the better.
- Competition between private providers leads to better results at a lower cost.
- Contracting out by governments is not as good as putting purchasing power in the hands of consumers.

- Monopoly power in professions, trades, and services is undesirable. Monopoly power of any kind tends to lead to inefficiency, waste, arrogance, poor service, and rationing.
- Democratic power is better when more truly and precisely democratic with referenda and local power. People also feel better for having the ability to take part in deciding how the country is run.
- We should give up the idea of government as a giant insurance and pension company—a role in which it has proved incompetent and untrustworthy. We could move toward personal savings accounts with each of us having assets of which we are the legal owners. Such accounts can certainly be used for health care and pensions and may also play a role for unemployment benefits or education. People do not readily waste their own money. Such savings can be backed up with insurance.
- We should try to stop welfare states from placing themselves in opposition to the family. Couples have often been discriminated against compared with single parents with respect to welfare benefits and the allocation of housing. Family-provided care of children and of the elderly has been discriminated against in favor of care by strangers.
- Welfare states should, above all, think about what can go wrong when they are being "generous." Politicians delight in the idea that they are changing the world. Rarely do they stop to consider how their measures may have perverse consequences. If welfare benefits are high and easy to obtain, for example, one should consider whether more people might decide not to seek work seriously. There is no need to be cynical about human nature. We just should not treat people as though they were saints. Political discourse sometimes takes place in a parallel world where no one was ever influenced by money.
- Measures such as these might help lead toward better welfare states. They might even lead to happier and more fulfilled people with greater wealth, better education, and improved health care. But there is one problem with such a program that cannot be wished away: the issue of freedom. Welfare states envelop us—particularly the poorest—in a system of government-imposed rules, regulations, programs, insurance policies, and so on. It is not just the chore of filling in the forms

or the expense of paying social insurance and suchlike. There is a loss of personal independence and choice, the idea that, "My life is my own. I go where I like, and, provided I do not commit a crime, I do what I like."

Yes, we may be able to make better welfare states. It is certainly possible that unemployment can be reduced and housing improved, that more children may have their natural fathers with them and more of the elderly may be in close touch with their families. There can be a reduction in dishonesty and a greater sense of responsibility. It is certainly possible, though not inevitable, that better welfare states will be created. This would be of huge benefit to the happiness of mankind. Yet we must admit that freedom will not be as great as it once was. Minor things can be done to salvage some freedom—such as allowing people to opt out of this or that government-approved action. But overall, some diminution of personal freedom is the unavoidable price we pay for welfare states.

Appendix 1. Ten Tips for Better Welfare States

1. Make housing cheaper by allowing supply to increase through an improved planning system. Public housing is a failed policy and is already being downgraded around the world.
2. Enable everyone to choose between competing private schools.
3. Create compulsory health savings accounts and health insurance provided by competing organizations. Allow patients to choose between competing doctors and hospitals.
4. Prefer social insurance to means-tested benefits. Allow private companies and mutual societies to offer it.
5. Make means-tested benefits a last resort, set at significantly lower levels than social insurance benefits. Both means-tested and social insurance benefits should be backed up by active demands that beneficiaries work, coupled with the provision of help in getting work.
6. Minimize benefits or accommodations given to single parents that are not also given to married parents.
7. Make financial support for care for the elderly as even-handed as possible between those in institutions and those cared for by their children.
8. Replace unfunded government pensions with compulsory, individual, funded plans.
9. Introduce regular referenda for national, regional, and local issues.
10. Introduce constitutional limits on budget deficits and total debt.

Appendix 2. Best and Worst Welfare States

Unemployment

Best: South Korea, Switzerland, Singapore, Japan, and Austria have consistently had the lowest rates over the past decade. Germany has significantly reduced its rate since 2005.

Worst: The countries with the highest, persistent mass unemployment in the recent past have been France, Italy, Spain, Greece, and Poland.

Hidden Unemployed

Best: The highest rates of working-age men employed or seeking work are in Singapore, Switzerland, New Zealand, and Japan.[1] (The figure for men is used to exclude varying cultural factors that influence employment rates for women in different countries.)

Worst: In Sweden, over 10 percent of the working age population claim disability benefits. The lowest rates of working-age males employed or seeking work are in Belgium, France, and Poland.

Health Care

Best: Japan, the United States, Switzerland, and Germany have some of the best results, but U.S. health care is very expensive. Singaporean health care, for which comparable results are not available, appears to be an outstandingly good value.

Worst: The United Kingdom, Ireland, and Denmark appear to have the worst outcomes.

Education

Best: Rates of functional illiteracy in Shanghai, China; Hong Kong; South Korea; Ireland; Japan; and Singapore are less bad than elsewhere. However, this may reflect the cultures of East Asia rather than its education systems. In all the East Asian countries, parents supplement the government education with large amounts of "shadow" private education.

Worst: The highest functional illiteracy figures among advanced countries are those for Sweden, Greece, Austria, Italy, and France.[2]

Single Parenting

Best: Greece, Spain, Italy, and Poland have the lowest rates among those countries surveyed.

Worst: The United States has the highest rate, followed by Ireland, New Zealand, Canada, and the United Kingdom.

Crime

Best: Japan, Italy, Portugal, Spain, and Austria have relatively low levels of assaults and threats. Switzerland, the United States, and Japan have relatively small underground economies.

Worst: The worst countries are England and Wales, Ireland, New Zealand, the Netherlands, and the United States (for assaults and threats). Note the overlap with countries that have high rates of single parenting. Italy, Greece, and Poland have the largest underground economies. These are all countries where a great deal of money is taken out of legitimate wages to pay for the pensions of those already retired.

Pensions

Best: New Zealand, the Netherlands, and Sweden have the lowest proportions of old people who are poor compared with the general population. The Netherlands, Australia, and South Korea have the lowest government pension costs as a proportion of gross domestic product (GDP). The Netherlands, Canada, and Sweden have the lowest unfunded public sector pension liabilities. Singapore would be on top in the latter two measures if it had been included in the relevant surveys. Overall, Singapore and the Netherlands come out best.

Worst: Ireland and Australia have a high proportion of relatively poor old people. Italy, France, and Greece have the highest government pension costs as a proportion of GDP. France and Finland have the biggest unfunded public sector pension liabilities. Overall, the overhanging liabilities of France, Italy, Greece, and Finland suggest that they have had the least successful pension systems.

Income

Best: Singapore, the United States, and Switzerland have easily the highest levels of average per capita income.[3] These are all countries where the overall cost of their welfare states, including social security contributions, is below average or, in the case of Singapore, where deductions from pay go into personal accounts with real assets.

Worst: Greece, Portugal, and Spain.

Note that this summary excludes less advanced countries.

Appendix 3. Groundhog Day—But Not Everywhere

Themes and Contrasts

Around the welfare states of the world, the same problems and phenomena appear again and again. But there are also huge contrasts.

Every country that is economically advanced and democratic has a welfare state. There are no exceptions.

Many governments have a problem paying for pensions that are not funded. Only a few have avoided the trap, notably Singapore.

Many countries have semipermanent high levels of unemployment. But there are exceptions such as Switzerland and Singapore.

Most countries have more births outside marriage than in previous generations. In Sweden, well over half of the children are born out of wedlock and, in Iceland, two of three. But in Japan only one of 50 is and, in South Korea, one in 66.

Social housing is a big feature of the welfare states of Austria, France, and the Netherlands. But it is minor in Norway and Germany.

All welfare states have government schooling but, in some East Asian countries, massive private education systems have grown up alongside.

All the welfare states of the advanced world have some government health care. But some, like Australia and France, have big private health care sectors, too.

Many welfare states embraced care for the elderly in institutions but then found it was getting too expensive and have started encouraging more of the elderly to stay at home. In Spain and Portugal, it is commonplace for widowed elderly parents to live with their children as in earlier generations. In other countries, like Denmark, it has almost completely died out.

Appendix 4. Welfare Jargon Explained

Here are some terms you do not hear very often over a drink in a bar. Some are so unintuitive that even after hearing them many times, you may struggle to recall what they mean. "Rent-seeking" has nothing to do with rent. "Moral hazard" looks like a misspelled street sign. There are unnecessary, pretentious words like "eudemonic." And just very occasionally when you are least expecting it, there are phrases that are useful or even witty.

ACTIVE LABOR MARKET PROGRAM A government effort to get the unemployed into work through initiatives such as training, workfare, and sanctions for not seeking work. Distinct from "passive" labor market programs, where governments hand out money to the unemployed without doing very much to encourage or help them to find work.

ACTIVITIES OF DAILY LIVING Activities that people need to be able to do to live independently. If you need help with them, you are deemed to be in need of long-term care. The activities include bathing, eating, dressing, walking across a room, and getting into and out of bed. See also *instrumental activities of daily living*.

THE ALZIRA MODEL System of health care pioneered in Alzira, Spain. The regional government pays a company a sum based on the population of an area to provide both hospitals and primary health care.

BARRIERS TO ENTRY Obstacles that make it more difficult for new companies to compete in a business or for individuals to work in a particular craft or profession. For companies, barriers include onerous government regulations that cost new, small companies a disproportionate amount. For individuals, excessive government requirements for qualifications (licensing) can hinder them from entering trades or professions. In both case, reduced competition means that those already in the market can charge higher prices for inferior performance.

365

BEVERIDGE SYSTEM Welfare benefits system designed by Sir William Beveridge in a British coalition government paper in 1942. It is distinct from the *Bismarckian system* in that everyone is meant to pay the same contribution and to be entitled to the same benefits. In Britain, the welfare system has moved far away from Beveridge's concept. Means-tested social assistance, which Beveridge intended to be of small importance, has come to dominate.

BISMARCKIAN SYSTEM Welfare system based on social insurance and pioneered by Otto von Bismarck in Germany. In contrast to the *Beveridge system*, contributions vary according to the income of the payer. The benefits vary similarly.

BROKEN WINDOW FALLACY See *seen and unseen*.

CHAPUZAS Ad hoc small jobs paid for in cash (Spain).

COMPETITION EFFECT Competition between workers for jobs is said to lower wages and thus increase the number of jobs created, reducing unemployment. Some argue that competition is encouraged if outsiders (the unemployed) are given a subsidy to make them better able to compete with insiders (those already working).

CORPORATIST WELFARE STATE A welfare state in which corporate bodies such as trade unions, business associations, and the church (usually the Catholic Church) play a significant role.[1]

COUNTERFACTUAL How things might have turned out if something had been different, such as a government policy. For example, someone might say, "Many would starve if it were not for food stamps." But a thorough counterfactual considers whether people would act differently in such circumstances. Some might work longer hours to earn more money. Some might buy cheaper food or spend less on other things. Government money saved on food stamps might mean lower taxes and thus higher net incomes for those who work. Other people might create charities to offer food for free, and so on.

CROSS-SECTIONAL STUDY A study of lots of people at one moment in time. (Compare with *longitudinal study*.)

DEADWEIGHT EFFECT or **DEADWEIGHT COST** Some of the cost of a government program may be "wasted" because much of what it is intended to achieve would take place anyway.

DECOMMODIFICATION The idea that people are made into commodities by the requirement of capitalism that they work to earn money is known as "commodification." It is argued that they can be released from this oppression by a welfare state that makes them just as well off without working. They are thus "decommodified." Unfortunately, in countries where this has been tried, so many people have taken up the offer to be decommodified that a shortage of money to pay them has emerged. Consequently, governments have adopted *active labor market programs* and insisted that they work after all. Possibly they have been "recommodified."[2]

DEFAMILIZATION The process by which families become less mutually dependent and connected. It has been encouraged by welfare state subsidies and services such as financial support specifically to single parents, free or heavily subsidized childcare provided only by strangers, and free or subsidized care for the elderly—again, only if it is provided by strangers. It is perceived as a "good thing" by some—particularly in parts of Scandinavia—but as undesirable by others, particularly in Mediterranean countries such as Spain, Italy, and Greece.

DIAGNOSTIC-RELATED GROUP Classification of medical cases for the purpose of payment to hospitals or clinics. This is considered better than paying hospitals simply for medical procedures, which can lead to excessive use of the procedures and high cost. Payment by diagnostic-related group means hospitals have an incentive to be economical and innovative in their treatment. See also *diagnostic treatment combination*.

DIAGNOSTIC TREATMENT COMBINATION A more sophisticated version of a *diagnostic-related group*, introduced in the Netherlands in 2005. Each kind of medical case is defined more exactly and an assessment is made of what would be the normal procedures for dealing with it.

DISPLACEMENT EFFECT Sometimes governments provide subsidies to companies to employ particular kinds of workers such as the young or old. This can increase employment of that kind of person but reduce employment of other kinds of people. The overall net gain in employment might be little or nothing.

DOING BETTER FOR FAMILIES Title of a publication by the Organisation for Economic Co-operation and Development. When politicians and think tanks say they are going to "do better for families," they usually mean that taxpayers' money will replace the need for families to look after their own. The title might be more accurately rephrased as "Doing Away with Families."

DROPOUT FACTORIES High schools in the United States in which more than 60 percent of students leave before completing their studies.

EFFECTIVE MARGINAL TAX RATE Measure of how worthwhile it is for someone to work longer hours or get a promotion or a pay rise. It is the rate of tax plus the welfare benefit withdrawal rate if someone has a small increase in earnings. So if someone would lose 30p in tax and 55p in benefits for an extra pound earned, the effective marginal tax rate would be 0.85. A high rate for low earners is sometimes called the "poverty trap."

ENDOGENOUS Coming from within. Compare with *exogenous*.

EUDEMONIC Making people feel good or happy.

EXCEPTIONALISM The idea that something, usually a country, is special in a way that makes it unlike others. So "American exceptionalism" is the belief that the United States is unique in having certain (good!) characteristics.

EXOGENOUS Coming from outside. Compare with *endogenous*.

EXPRESS FIRING Spanish expression meaning firing someone quickly without argument but at a high cost. In Spain, the alternative is "justified" firing. The employer pays less compensation to the worker when a firing is "justified." However, the courts, at least up until 2012, were reluctant to accept any layoffs as "justified." So rather than waste time and money, some companies would just pay the extra cost of "express firing."

FAMILY POLICY In reality, most measures given this name consist of policies that tend to make the traditional family redundant. They are aimed primarily at getting women to take full-time, paid employment. The taxes used to finance this inevitably come, on balance, from families in which a woman looks after her children at home or works part time.

THE FATAL CONCEIT Title of a book by Friedrich Hayek. He criticizes the idea that an elite group of clever people in government can successfully organize the affairs of the whole population.

FUNCTIONAL ILLITERACY A level of illiteracy that does not amount to total illiteracy but means a person is unable to make use of simple written information such as understanding a poster advertising a pop concert.

GATEKEEPERS General practitioners are called "gatekeepers" when only they can grant patients access to a specialist. Patients are prohibited from approaching specialists directly.

HLM French public housing. The initials stand for *Habitations à loyer modéré* (literally "housing at a moderate rent").

HUD Housing and Urban Development. U.S. federal government department created by President Lyndon Johnson. It directs public and subsidized housing in the United States.

INSTRUMENTAL ACTIVITIES OF DAILY LIVING Activities that help people to live independently, such as using a telephone, taking medication, handling money, shopping, and preparing meals. The ability to do these things is important but not as fundamental as the ability to do *activities of daily living*.

LOS LIBERADOS Trade unionists in Spain who do nothing but union work while on the payroll of a company. They are free (or "liberated") not to work for the company.

LIBERAL "Left wing" in North America, "right wing" in continental Europe, and confusion in Britain.

LOCKING-IN EFFECT or **RETENTION EFFECT** Reduction in the likelihood that a worker will seek another—possibly better—job as a result of receiving a government wage subsidy in his or her existing job.

LONGITUDINAL STUDIES Repeated observations of the same people or items over a period of time, sometimes stretching into decades. These studies are commonly regarded as superior to *cross-sectional studies*, but they obviously take longer and are usually more expensive.

MEANS-TESTED BENEFITS Welfare benefits that are dependent on the "means" (income and/or wealth) of the claimant. Similar to *social assistance* and *needs-based benefits*.

META-ANALYSIS Study combining the results of previous studies. The hope is that this produces a particularly authoritative result.

But there is a risk that the academics who do it may find pretexts to rule out studies they do not like to get the result they prefer.

MORAL HAZARD Danger that people may act in an undesirable way because government policy has reduced the costs or risks of such behavior. For example, a young woman may be encouraged to become pregnant outside marriage if the government provides single mothers with free accommodations and benefits.[3] See also *perverse incentives* and *unintended consequences*.

MULTIVARIATE ANALYSIS Any statistical method that helps evaluate the relative impact of a number of different variables on a given result. For example, it might establish whether loneliness is more highly correlated with living alone, being old, or being a man.

NAMAPO Japanese word used on the Internet meaning "welfare" but with a pejorative overtone. Struck from the list of top 10 buzz-words in Japan "for fear that it promoted discrimination against the poor."[4] Supposedly derived from *seikatsu hogo*, meaning "welfare."

NATIONAL INSURANCE Social insurance in Britain.

NEEDS-BASED BENEFITS Benefits based on a person's needs rather than on his or her entitlement through, say, unemployment insurance. The phrase captures the way in which someone who has more "needs"—as a result of having, say, more children—gets higher benefits under this system. Similar to *means-tested benefits* and *social assistance*.

OBASUTEYAMA Legendary Japanese mountain where eldest sons, who were responsible for their aged parents, left them to die of star-vation and exposure. Can be translated as "Granny-dump Mountain." The word has been used to describe public residential care in Japan and reflects disapproval of families that have resorted to such care.

PARTICIPATION TAX RATE A measure of how worthwhile it is for someone on welfare benefits to work at all. It is calculated as tax plus welfare benefits forgone as a proportion of gross earnings. So if someone earns £300 a week gross but their taxes and welfare benefits forgone amount to £270, then the participation tax rate is 0.9. The equation is (tax + benefits foregone) ÷ gross earnings. See also *replacement rate* and *effective marginal tax rate*.

PERVERSE INCENTIVE An incentive or reward that unintention-ally encourages behavior or results that are undesirable or even the opposite of what was intended. See also *moral hazard* and *unintended consequences*.[5]

PREFERENCE FALSIFICATION The way people declare different views in public from the ones they express when they know they are going to be anonymous.[6]

THE PRODUCER INTEREST or **PRODUCER CAPTURE** The phenomenon of people who provide a service coming to think of their own interest rather than that of the consumer or the taxpayer they are supposed to serve. This can damage the quality, or can raise the cost of the service they provide, or both. For example, teachers or police officers who try to get shorter working hours and early retirement for themselves may increase the cost of education or policing.

PUBLIC CHOICE THEORY The idea that governments often do not act for the good of the people or in accordance with democratic ideals. For example, a politician might accede to the wishes of a lobby group, because it would bring more support than it would lose him or her. Civil servants and administrators may pursue ideas and interests that involve increasing the size of their departments. The same people might be benevolent but make rules or laws on the basis of inadequate information. Their decisions can be biased by a desire to feel active or important.

PUBLIC HOUSING American term for what is called *social housing* in the United Kingdom.

PUBLIC SCHOOLS In Britain: private, fee-charging schools. In the United States, schools paid for by state governments. In this book, I have tried not to use the term at all to avoid confusion, but with regard to the United States, I occasionally use the American meaning of the term.

RAMPING Practice in Australian hospital emergency departments of requiring ambulances to wait outside hospitals (presumably, in some cases, on a ramp) with their patients because there is not sufficient capacity to admit them without breaching a government target for the maximum permissible wait between admission and being seen by a doctor.

REGULATORY CAPTURE Influence over regulations by an interested party to gain advantages. For example, taxi drivers or doctors may influence the regulations concerning their own trade or profession and use this power to reduce competition.

RENTS Advantage or extra income derived by self-interested manipulation of a job, industry, or system. Where there is perfect competition, it should be hard to obtain such rents.

RENT-SEEKING Gaining an advantage—financial or otherwise—by manipulating a system rather than creating new wealth or a better system. For example, nurses might demand higher qualifications for future nurses to increase their own prestige or to limit the number of entrants to the profession, ensuring higher pay and greater job security for themselves.

REPLACEMENT RATE A measure of how worthwhile it is for someone to work rather than living on benefits. It is the net amount that someone would receive in welfare benefits compared with what he or she would get in work after tax. So if someone who got £220 per week in benefits would receive £250 after tax in work, the replacement rate would be 0.88. It is similar to the *participation tax rate*, but the equation is arranged differently so one gets a slightly different result. The equation is this: benefits ÷ (gross earnings − tax).

RESIDENTIAL HOME OR CARE HOME Place for elderly people to live, which is not, in fact, their home. Services such as meals are prepared and some personal care and activities may be provided.

RETENTION EFFECT See *locking-in effect*.

SCREENING EFFECT The way that subsidized, short-term employment may enable an employer to discover whether an unemployed person is productive enough to employ long term.

"SEEN AND UNSEEN" The effects of actions can be divided into those that are obvious (seen) and those that are not (unseen). The French economist Frédéric Bastiat gave the example of a boy who broke his father's window. A glazier was paid 6 francs to replace it. The seen effect is that work was created for the glazier and that he got income. The unseen effect is that otherwise the father would have used that money to buy a book or to get his shoes repaired. The cobbler or the bookseller would have benefited. Overall, no economic benefit is obtained through the breaking of the window. This is sometimes known as the *broken window fallacy*.[7]

SELECTION BIAS The way a study may be misleading because the people who are selected for it—or who select themselves—affect the result. For example, a study might show that married people are less likely to be seriously depressed than are single people. But it could be that people who are not seriously depressed "select" themselves to be married. Superior studies attempt to deal with this problem.

SHADOW EDUCATION Private education that supplements government-provided education. It is widespread in Asia and exists in many other countries, too. The term includes private tutors and *Kumon* after-school centers.

"SIT-DOWN MONEY" Australian native term for welfare benefits.

SOCIAL ASSISTANCE Phrase used in continental Europe and, in earlier years, in Britain. Welfare benefits given when entitlement to unemployment insurance benefits has run out. The amount depends on the means and needs of the claimant. Very similar to *means-tested benefits* and *needs-based benefits*.

SOCIAL HOUSING British term for what Americans call *public housing*.

SOCIAL INSURANCE Compulsory government insurance that covers unemployment or disability. In many European countries, it also covers health care.

SOCIAL TRANSFERS Welfare benefits and services. Money is "transferred" from some to others. The phrase is used by academics and some think tanks to make it sound like an innocuous business. Note how there is no mention of tax.

SUBSTITUTION EFFECT The way in which government incentives to an employer to take on workers with a particular ability can cause the employer to reduce the hiring of workers with a different ability. Similar to *displacement effect*.

THE THIRD SECTOR Charities and other voluntary organizations.

THREAT EFFECT Incentive to search for work created when continuation of unemployment benefits is dependent on something such as participation in a workfare program.

THE TRAGEDY OF THE COMMONS The way assets can be abused if everyone owns them rather than just one person or company. Fishing stocks, for example, may get run down if everyone is allowed to fish in an area whereas, if a company owns the area, it would have a long-term interest in preserving the stocks.

TRANSITION EFFECT Gain in the employability of a long-term unemployed person that comes from doing work in, for example, workfare or public works.

UNINTENDED CONSEQUENCES Results of a policy that are far away from what the politicians or civil servants wanted. All policies—but particularly ones thought of as kind and beneficent—should be vetted for their possible unintended consequences. See also *perverse incentives* and *moral hazard*.

WAGE EFFECT The way a government subsidy for wages may be channeled into higher wages rather than into higher employment.

WORKFARE Government schemes in which unemployed people are required to work in return for their welfare benefits. The work may be for government departments, for charities, or for commercial companies.

It would be marvelous if some of these concepts could be described by phrases that are more self-explanatory: instead of "public choice theory," for example, "public corruption theory"? Unfortunately, once these terms are established, they are difficult to budge.

Afterword

Inequality: Do Bigger Welfare States Create More Equal, Happier People?

When I visited the Organisation for Economic Co-operation and Development (OECD) in Paris, I spent two days interviewing experts there on a wide range of subjects. But even by the end of the first day, I had gotten a strong impression that most of the staff had a shared belief in greater equality.

The following day, the press officer who had kindly arranged all the interviews told me that a talk would be given to the staff that morning. It seems that the OECD has visiting speakers, and on this occasion it would be Richard Wilkinson, one of the two authors of *The Spirit Level*. In this book, he argues that the more unequal a country is, the more likely its inhabitants are to suffer in a wide variety of ways. The press officer invited me to join the OECD staff to hear the talk. I won't repeat what Wilkinson said because I went as a guest rather than as a journalist. But he was very persuasive. Chart after chart indicated a correlation between inequality and bad outcomes such as homicides. The case seemed overwhelming. Any neutral who heard his talk would have come away at least three-quarters convinced. Most of the OECD staff members—though perhaps not all—surely welcomed it as authoritative confirmation of what they already believed.

Wilkinson is part of a worldwide intellectual movement focusing on inequality. Thomas Piketty and Emmanuel Saez have argued that the top 1 percent in the United States have greatly increased their share of income since the Second World War. Since then, Piketty has gone on to write *Capital in the Twenty-First Century*, in which he argues that modern capitalism necessarily means that inequality will increase. Joseph E. Stiglitz, a Nobel Prize winner for economics, has written *The Price of Inequality*, in which he argues that the level of inequality in the world is due to the capitalist system's not working as it should.

Each person who writes about inequality has his or her own ideas. But out of it all emerges a kind of logic that goes like this: inequality causes unhappiness; inequality has increased and therefore unhappiness has increased; the way to put this right is by taxing the rich and giving more money to the poor. In short, the people of the advanced world would be happier with bigger welfare states. More simply still: welfare states make people happier.

If this is true, it should affect what we do. So is it? Let's look at Wilkinson's book because it addresses the issue most directly.

The Spirit Level has charts similar to the ones he showed in his talk in Paris. These repeatedly suggest that the more unequal a society is, the more it suffers. Such a society has more health and social problems and more murders. The children experience more conflict, and more people suffer mental illness. There is no actual chart showing levels of happiness plotted against inequality. But it is implicit that all of these various measures together amount to evidence that greater equality causes greater well-being. The evidence is buttressed with arguments from psychology and anthropology suggesting that people are hardwired to be happier in more equal societies. Inequality, it is argued, produces a sense of failure in those at the lower end.

Let's take the correlation between inequality and homicides (see Figure A.1). It is one of many illustrated with a chart. A scattergraph of dots representing countries shows their level of inequality plotted against the incidence of homicides. Superimposed on the dots is a straight line indicating a trend calculated by a computer from the data. The straight line gently rises, suggesting that the more inequality there is, the more homicides take place.

The point is clearly made. And there are plenty of charts like this with measure after measure showing similar results.

At first sight, it looks like game, set, and match. But in statistics, there are certain tests that are done to establish how good correlations are. One standard procedure is to remove "outliers"—individual cases that seem far removed from the others. In the case of homicides, Portugal is an "outlier." The dot representing the United States is so distant from the other countries that it is an "extreme outlier." Peter Saunders tested what would happen to the correlation if the United States was removed but Portugal retained. There was still a correlation.[1] Then he applied a measure of the strength of this correlation, known as "R squared." R^2 indicates in this case how much of the variance in homicide rates can be

Figure A.1
INCOME INEQUALITY AND HOMICIDE

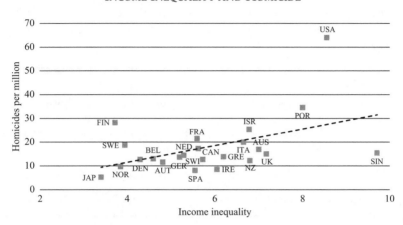

SOURCE: Richard Wilkinson and Kate Pickett, *The Spirit Level* (London: Penguin Books, 2010 ed. with postscript), p. 135.

NOTE: Wilkinson and Pickett state on p. 18 that they use the ratio of the income received by the top 20 percent to the income of the bottom 20 percent for international comparisons of income inequality. Their source is the United Nations. AUS = Australia; AUT = Austria; BEL = Belgium; CAN = Canada; DEN = Denmark; FIN = Finland; FRA = France; GER = Germany; GRE = Greece; IRE = Ireland; ISR = Israel; ITA = Italy; JAP = Japan; NED = the Netherlands; NOR = Norway; NZ = New Zealand; POR = Portugal; SIN = Singapore; SPA = Spain; SWE = Sweden; SWI = Switzerland; UK = United Kingdom; USA = United States.

explained by inequality. It was very low—only 0.1, indicating that only 10 percent of the variance in homicides was associated with levels of inequality.

Saunders then tried another calculation of the statistical significance of the correlation called the p-value. A correlation that is really significant would have a p-value of 0.05 or less. The p-value in this case was 0.159. Professional social scientists simply would not regard the correlation as being of statistical significance. In other words, the correlation between inequality and homicides is not established at all. And if there is not a statistically significant correlation, we are a very long way indeed from proving causation.

Many of the other charts in *The Spirit Level* fail to survive these and other standard procedures such as testing for third variables.

A few correlations in *The Spirit Level* do stand up to the routine tests of social science. But very few. One that does stand up is infant mortality.[2] But even in this case we should recall that correlation does not necessarily mean causation. There may be a third factor at work.[3]

"In the United States . . . those who consider themselves left-wingers exhibit a marked distaste for inequality, whereas those who consider themselves right-wingers are not affected by it. This effect is so strong in the United States that only rich left-wingers are negatively affected by inequality."

SOURCE: Swiss economist Bruno Frey summarizing Alberto Alesina, Rafael Di Tella, and Robert MacCulloch, "Inequality and Happiness: Are Europeans and Americans Different?," *Journal of Public Economics* 88 (2004): 2009–42.

Meanwhile, some charts that could have been created relating inequality to certain measures of well-being are notably absent. They would have shown correlations that are actually contrary to the ideas of Wilkinson and Piketty. The more equal a society, the more racial intolerance there is, the greater the incidence of suicides, and the larger the alcohol consumption. These correlations are not particularly big but they are slightly bigger than most of the associations that go the other way, and they are statistically significant.[4] This is not to claim that any causation is involved, let alone proved. But the evidence that inequality improves outcomes for a society, though small, is just as good or better than the other way round.

It appears that the argument that inequality causes bad social effects is not backed by good evidence. Indeed, there is some evidence that the only people whose happiness is truly disturbed by inequality are relatively rich left-wingers, according to Bruno Frey (see quotation). But there is an even more fundamental problem with the theory. The measure of inequality used in *The Spirit Level* is called the Gini coefficient. It is named after Corrado Gini, the Italian statistician and sociologist who devised it. The Gini coefficient figures are usually assumed to be authoritative. But there is reason to doubt them.

Sweden has a low Gini coefficient with respect to income, which means that it is less unequal than most countries. However, there is a Gini coefficient of wealth as well as income, and according to the

Gini figures, Sweden is one of the most *unequal* countries in terms of wealth. This is strange. It seems improbable that a country with notably equal incomes should have dramatically unequal wealth.

One possible explanation is that rich people in Sweden have reacted to high income tax rates there by minimizing their declared income. Where possible, they may receive their income in less taxable ways. If this is true, the Gini coefficient of income for Sweden is unreliable. It is not measuring real income but merely declared and taxable income. It is measuring an illusion, not the reality. (See Box A.1.)

The figures supposedly representing the incomes of the poor are unreliable too. Chapter 1 of this book describes the in-depth research done by Kathryn Edin and Laura Lein in the United States interviewing single mothers about their income. They discovered that the majority of single mothers on benefits in the United States receive income that is not declared and about 40 percent earn money from "unreported" or "underground" work. Of course, this income is not recorded in the Gini coefficient or most other measures of inequality. So the Gini figures for the poor are sure to be wrong. On top of that, the extent to which the figures for the poor are wrong is likely to vary from one country to another. Britain, the United States, and Australia have welfare benefits based mainly on an assessment of "means." The more "means" one appears to have, the less one receives in benefits. People on means-tested benefits in these countries have more incentive to lie about their means than do people

Box A.1

ONE OF THE RICHEST SWEDES EVER BORN

Ruben Rausing created the first packaging company in Sweden. He made wax-coated cartons in the shape of a tetrahedron—a pyramid with a triangular base—hence the ultimate name of the company: Tetra Pak. It became the largest food packaging company in the world and, at his death, Rausing was the richest Swede in the world. But his income and wealth did not appear in the statistics for Sweden. Rausing left Sweden for Rome in 1969 to avoid high taxes.

Hans, one of his three sons, is credited as a key figure in the success of Tetra Pak. In 2011, he was 83rd in the *Forbes* listing of the richest people in the world. But he left Sweden, too, in 1982, and moved to England. Naturally, his large income has also not affected the Gini coefficient of his native country. The inequality of income in a country can appear lower than it otherwise would be as a result of the richest people leaving.

in countries where most welfare recipients receive insurance-based benefits. Therefore, the inequality of Britain, the United States, and Australia might well appear greater than it really is compared with other countries.

As if this were not enough, the Gini coefficient can be influenced by an influx of immigrants. For a long time, Sweden had a very low immigrant population. But then in the 1990s and 2000s, it allowed in more immigrants, who unsurprisingly received low incomes. The Gini coefficient of Sweden soon changed to indicate a more unequal society.[5] So the Gini coefficient can, in part, be merely a reflection of whether a country has accepted poor immigrants in the fairly recent past.[6]

Yet another difficulty is that some measures of inequality fail to take into account noncash benefits such as health insurance and pensions. These may not appear as taxable income even though they have value to the person concerned.[7] Similarly, some studies do not include the value to poorer people of benefits such as food stamps, housing subsidies, and Medicaid.[8]

So the Gini coefficient and other similar measures of inequality are unreliable. Of course it is possible to try to overcome the difficulties with various statistical techniques, and where this is attempted the process should be analyzed closely to see if it is convincing and rigorously conducted. Such attempts have been thin on the ground. Most people are happy just to use the unreliable Gini coefficient.

It seems, therefore, that the idea that unequal societies cause unhappiness is thoroughly unproven. It is based on correlations that do not stand up to normal academic tests. It is also based usually on Gini calculations of inequality, which are unreliable. The evidence for the inequality idea is therefore about as dependable as a grainy zoom-lens photo of the Loch Ness monster taken on a misty day as night falls.

You might reasonably wonder: why have I spent so much time on it? It is because the theory has gained influence and credibility. It is sometimes talked of as a well-established fact. If the idea were justified by evidence, it would be very important. But it isn't.

Is that the end of the matter? No, of course, there will be further attempts to "prove" the idea and they will have to be examined. But let's note that part of this issue that is currently much talked about has now been left hanging in the air: happiness. If equality does not bring it about, what does?

The study of happiness and, of course, its opposite—unhappiness—has been a growth industry in academia. In the

United States, Europe, and elsewhere, surveys have asked people just how happy or how satisfied they are with their lives. One of the biggest of these exercises took place in Britain in 2012 because the government wanted to start measuring and analyzing "general well-being." The sample was particularly large: 165,000 adults aged 16 and over.[9]

The key question was, "Overall, how satisfied are you with your life nowadays?" People were asked to give a number from 0 to 10, where 0 is "not at all" and 10 is "completely."

Three results were dramatically clear: among those who were employed, only a fifth gave an answer below 7. But among the unemployed, more than twice as many (45 percent) did (see Figure A.2). The unemployed were also 3.6 times more likely than those with jobs to give an answer suggesting serious unhappiness.

A second dramatic finding was related to marriage (see Figure A.3). Among married people only 18 percent rated their level of satisfaction below 7. But among the divorced, more than twice as many (39.3 percent) did so. Also more than three times as many of the divorced rated their satisfaction at a very low level, between 4 and 0.

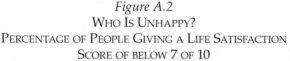

Figure A.2
WHO IS UNHAPPY?
PERCENTAGE OF PEOPLE GIVING A LIFE SATISFACTION
SCORE OF BELOW 7 OF 10

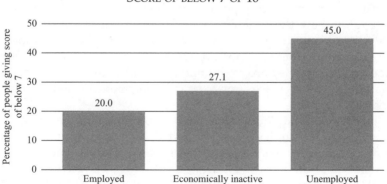

SOURCE: "First ONS Annual Experimental Subjective Well-being Results," U.K. Office for National Statistics, July 24, 2012, http://www.ons.gov.uk/ons/dcp171766 _272294.pdf .

NOTE: The "economically inactive" are people not working but not seeking work.

Figure A.3
WHO ELSE IS UNHAPPY?
PERCENTAGE OF PEOPLE GIVING A LIFE SATISFACTION
SCORE OF BELOW 7 OF 10

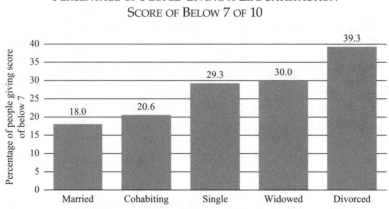

SOURCE: "First ONS Annual Experimental Subjective Well-being Results," U.K. Office for National Statistics, July 24, 2012, http://www.ons.gov.uk/ons/dcp171766_272294.pdf.

A third, powerful contrast emerged between the healthy and the unwell. Among the very healthy, only 2 percent rated their level of satisfaction at between 4 and 0. The number soared to 35.2 percent among those in very bad health.

The numbers I have reported are the bare figures without disentangling how the different factors interact with each other. It is obviously likely that those in very bad health are also unemployed, for example, so there are several factors involved. But I cite the bare figures because they are so dramatic regarding unemployment and marriage. And they are supported by more sophisticated academic analysis.

Bruno Frey and Alois Stuzer, in Switzerland, summarize it this way: "Many . . . studies have . . . found, in many countries and many time periods that personally experiencing unemployment makes people very unhappy."[10] Andrew Clark and Andrew Oswald, in a 1994 study, concluded, "Joblessness depressed well-being more than any other single characteristic, including important negative ones such as divorce and separation."[11] Looking at figures for the United States, Oswald, this time with David Blanchflower, similarly concluded, "Joblessness is associated here with a huge amount of unhappiness," adding, "The other particularly large coefficient is on marriage," which had a positive impact on happiness.[12]

Some may object that asking people whether or not they are happy is only one measure of well-being. It could be misleading. So it is worth trying another measure. If someone commits suicide, it is surely evidence of severe unhappiness.

There are different kinds of studies, and the results vary among them.[13] But among the so-called "individual-level" studies, there seems to be near unanimity in finding a very strong association between unemployment and suicide.[14] Typically, one of them suggests that "those who are unemployed are two or three times more likely to die by suicide than those who are in work."[15] In one extreme case, Barbara Schneider and her colleagues looked at suicides in the Frankfurt-am-Main area of Germany and found that the unemployed were 16 times more likely to die by suicide than the control group and that this was not changed substantially by adjusting the figures to allow for mental illness and personality disorder. In another study, Alfonso Ceccherini-Nelli and Stefan Priebe tried to discover whether it was possible to associate changes in suicide rates in Britain, the United States, France, and Italy with levels of unemployment.[16] They found that "in all four countries, increases in unemployment were associated with higher suicide rates and decreases of unemployment with lower suicide rates."

What about marital status? There appears to be a difference in the reactions of men and women. One study found that divorced or separated women were 50 percent more likely to commit suicide than their married counterparts while the men were almost three times more likely to do so.[17] On top of this, there is the damage to the happiness of the children when parents divorce or separate, as described in Chapter 6 of this book. It is also notable that suicide rates are generally lower in the Mediterranean countries, such as Spain and Italy, where defamilization has not taken place as much as in most other countries.[18] (See Figure A.4.)

From all this evidence, it is clear that unemployment and family breakdown create huge amounts of unhappiness. It also suggests something else. If divorce leads to unhappiness, it might also be the case that living alone—or, more precisely, loneliness—may be an important influence on happiness.

John Cacioppo of the University of Chicago has studied loneliness and living alone, and has discovered some remarkable effects.[19] Loneliness raises blood pressure and levels of stress hormones,

Figure A.4
MALE SUICIDE RATES ACROSS THE WORLD
SUICIDE RATES PER 100,000

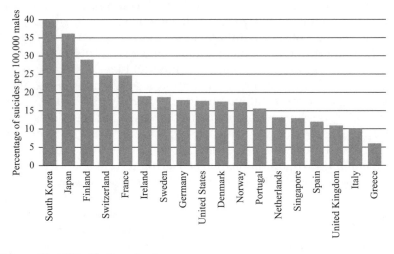

SOURCE: World Health Organization.

NOTE: In most countries, male suicides far exceed female suicides.

leading to a greater risk of illness and death.[20] It damages the quality of sleep so that it restores us less well both physically and mentally. He also found evidence that loneliness increases the risk of suicide.[21] Meanwhile, research in Denmark indicates that individuals between ages 30 and 60 who live alone are more than seven times more likely to say they are not happy than those living with others.[22] (See Box A.2.)

"Western societies have demoted human gregariousness from a necessity to an incidental. . . . The experience of isolation threatens our sense of purpose."

SOURCE: John T. Cacioppo and William Patrick, *Loneliness: Human Nature and the Need for Social Connection* (New York: W. W. Norton, 2008).

I do not want to exaggerate the reliability of this evidence. Compared with unemployment and marital status, the significance of

Box A.2

WHEN ESTHER RANTZEN ADMITTED SHE WAS LONELY . . .

"I am having to face the realities of a life spent largely alone. . . . I can't adjust. From the moment I was born, I have been surrounded by people. Family. School friends. University friends. The teams I worked with. Best of all, my husband, two daughters and a son. . . . My weekdays are still full of activity. But my evenings and weekends are empty.

"You can find widows wherever you look; . . . we come home to an empty house. Statistics tell us that three out of five women over 75 live alone. That's most of us. No wonder so many of us buy a dog or talk to our TVs. . . . But they don't care if the day has been tough or rewarding."[a]

Esther Rantzen admitted that she had called her daughter and told her that God wanted her to move in with her. She confessed she was only thinking of herself—"of walking around an empty flat with no one to talk to."

Of all the articles and books that Rantzen, a British television presenter and journalist, has written in her long career, this article about her loneliness provoked by far the greatest response. Mostly it came from lonely people, particularly widows, "because, alas, we women tend to outlive the men we love. . . . But we don't talk about it because loneliness bears its own stigma. Many correspondents wrote about the 'shame' they felt and how 'brave' and 'honest' I had been, and in their letters they revealed just how much of a taboo there is in admitting you feel lonely."[b]

---

[a] Esther Rantzen, "'I Never Thought I Would Be So Lonely': Esther Rantzen's Aching Emptiness," *Daily Mail* (London), August 8, 2011, http://www.dailymail.co.uk/femail/article-2023581/I-thought-I -lonely-Widowed-Esther-Rantzen-admits-aching-emptiness.html.

[b] Esther Rantzen, "Lonely Britain," *Daily Mail*, October 13, 2011, http://www.dailymail.co.uk/femail /article-2048488/Lonely-Britain-When-Esther-Rantzen-wrote-Mail-aching-loneliness-received -overwhelming-response-heartfelt-understanding.html.

loneliness and living alone (which are not the same) has been studied much less. But it does seem likely that living alone or loneliness reduces levels of happiness.

How is all this information related to a book about welfare states?

In the previous chapters I have argued that all these apparent causes of unhappiness—unemployment, divorce, and living alone— have been made more common by welfare states. The way welfare states have increased unemployment is described in Chapter 3.

Figure A.5
MORE NORDICS THAN MEDITERRANEANS LIVE ALONE
PERCENTAGE OF SINGLE-PERSON HOUSEHOLDS

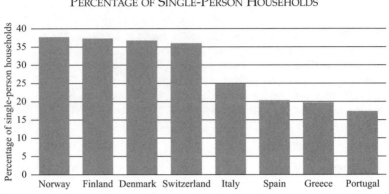

SOURCE: Countries selected from the Organisation for Economic Co-operation and Development Family Database (July 1, 2010, update).

NOTE: Strictly speaking, Portugal is not a Mediterranean country, but I include it with the Mediterranean countries because it has so much in common with them.

The way they have increased divorce and single parenting is outlined in Chapter 6. And the way they have increased the incidence of living alone has been described in the chapters on parenting (Chapter 6 again) and care of the elderly (Chapter 9).

The proportion of people living alone in different countries (see Figure A.5) varies considerably. For example, there is a marked contrast between the Mediterranean countries—Italy, Spain, Greece, and Portugal—and the Nordic countries—Norway, Finland, and Denmark (the figure for Sweden was not given). Living alone is far more common in the Nordic countries than in the Mediterranean countries, and so is suicide.[23]

People ages 25 to 44 are now five times more like to be living alone than they were in 1973.

SOURCE: Report by Wesley Johnson, "Britain 'Becoming Lonelier Place to Live,'" *Telegraph* (London), March 7, 2013, http://www.telegraph.co.uk/news/9916134/Britain-becoming-lonelier -place-to-live.html.

In sum, welfare states have tended to bring about circumstances that have caused unhappiness. There is much better evidence that welfare states cause unhappiness than there is of inequality doing so.

Against this it can be argued that welfare states reduce the fear of unemployment or incapacity and increase happiness in this way. That is possible. But there are other means of mitigating such fears that people have used in the past and could use again now—such as insurance, fraternal societies, and mutual societies. Moreover, as described in the relevant chapters, it is possible to reform welfare states in ways that can reduce their tendency to cause unemployment, broken families, and loneliness. Up until the present moment, however, the increases in unemployment, divorce, and living alone encouraged by welfare states have been massive and have significantly diminished the sum of human happiness.

Acknowledgments

The dedication page at the front of this book mentions some of the people I would like to thank. But there are so many others. I want to thank all who agreed to be interviewed, visited, or photographed or who helped in any way. I cannot name them all, but I will nevertheless mention a random collection of them and pray forgiveness from those I do not thank individually.

In England, I must mention George Currie, who has been a regular visitor to my home. He has helped me with all manner of things, stimulated me with thoughts and information, and brought me good cheer. Martin Durkin should be mentioned because, despite contributing no content whatever, he stiffened my sinews and bolstered morale. Mark Littlewood, director general of the Institute of Economic Affairs, has given me encouragement and support, particularly with regard to launching the book. Peter Saunders gave me advice and information about statistical methods. His book *When Prophecy Fails* is not easy to find, but it is an outstanding critique of *The Spirit Level*, an influential book about inequality.[1] I would love to see him write a critique of Thomas Piketty's *Capital in the Twenty-first Century*. Alan Gibbs kindly made a contribution to the considerable costs of producing the book.

Some people who helped me have views that are very different from mine, but I am still grateful for their input. Peter Whiteford, in Australia, was notable as someone who sees things differently but to whom I am grateful because he gave me the benefit of his considerable knowledge and thoughtfulness.

It was extraordinarily kind of Tharman Shanmugaratnam, the finance minister and deputy prime minister of Singapore, to give me some of his time. I have great respect for his insightfulness and for the welfare systems in Singapore, which are unique and generally far better than those in other advanced countries. I only hope that my remarks about democracy in that country will not mean I am barred from ever visiting again.

In America, I raise a glass of cheer and thanks to the anonymous friendly lady at the Job Center in Madison, Wisconsin, who allowed me to photograph her. Then there were the two joyful girls who let me photograph them near the public housing of the Lower East Side in New York City. I loved it when they mimicked my English accent and laughed with glee.

I am grateful to the schools in and near San Francisco that allowed me to visit, including the American Indian Public Charter School, which has been highly controversial but where I saw the most effective lessons I have ever witnessed. I also visited the Mayo Clinic in Minnesota, where at first I had a wholly inadequate tour but then a staff member took pity on me and agreed to give me an impromptu, fuller, and more informative tour. In Washington, D.C., I enjoyed meeting Anne Montgomery, who is an expert on care for the elderly. I was comforted that the supremely knowledgeable Michael Tanner of the Cato Institute did not think I was completely off the mark in my thoughts on health care around the world. It was a pleasure to have lunch with Robert Lerman of the Urban Institute.

In Holland, it was a delight to meet Dr. Eric Sijbrands, who told me about his innovative efforts to improve care for diabetic patients. In Poland, I had great pleasure interviewing Aleksandra Wiktorow and Zofia Czepulis-Rutkowska in the Blikle café. I also enjoyed meeting Ewelina Nojszewka. And, on the train from Amsterdam to Warsaw, I shared a sleeping compartment with an amiable Polish diplomat—name unknown—who warned me that I would find it difficult talking to Leszek Balcerowicz, the former deputy prime minister. The diplomat was charming but wrong. In fact, one of the happy memories of my trips is of taking an underground train with Balcerowicz after our interview. I was surprised that he traveled by public transport despite being so well known and controversial in Poland. I asked whether he was still unpopular with some people. He drily remarked that he had become less unpopular since he had been out of power.

I visited 11 countries: Sweden, France, Switzerland, Spain, Italy, the Netherlands, Poland, Australia, New Zealand, Singapore, and the United States. It was a great pleasure to travel around the world and meet so many people who kindly gave their time. I thank all of them and sincerely apologize to the many I have not mentioned.

Finally, I would like to thank John Samples and other staff members of the Cato Institute for publishing this American edition of the book. It is an honour to be published by such an impressive organization and I am delighted that, because of the Cato edition, the book will be seen by a much wider audience.

Notes

Front Matter

1. In Sweden 47 percent of households are people living alone. The rate is higher in Stockholm. Eric Klinenberg, "I Want to Be Alone: The Rise and Rise of Solo Living," *Guardian* (London), March 30, 2012, http://www.theguardian.com /lifeandstyle/2012/mar/30/the-rise-of-solo-living.

2. "Employment Situation, First Quarter 2014," Ministry of Manpower, Singapore Government press release, April 30, 2014, http://www.mom.gov.sg/newsroom /Pages/PressReleasesDetail.aspx?listid=561; "OECD Unemployment Increases to 7.6% in February 2014," Organisation for Economic Co-operation and Development press release, April 9, 2014, http://www.oecd.org/std/labour-stats/HUR-Apr14.pdf.

3. OECD, *Health at a Glance 2013: OECD Indicators* (Paris: OECD Publishing, 2013), p. 127, http://www.oecd.org/els/health-systems/Health-at-a-Glance-2013.pdf.

4. F. A. McDougall et al., "Prevalence and Symptomatology of Depression in Older People Living in Institutions in England and Wales," *Age and Ageing* 36 (2007): 562–8, http://ageing.oxfordjournals.org/content/36/5/562.full.

5. "OECD Unemployment Increases to 7.6% in February 2014."

6. Jan van Dijk et al., *Criminal Victimisation in International Perspective* (The Hague: Boom Juridische Uitgevers, 2007), Table 13: Assaults and Threats, One-Year Prevalence Rates 2003-04, http://unicri.it/services/library_documentation /publications/icvs/publications/ICVS2004_05report.pdf. This is an old survey but has the virtue of being an international victimization study, which is likely to be more reliable than police figures compared across countries.

7. *OECD Health Data 2011*, cited in OECD, *Health at a Glance 2011* (Paris: OECD Publishing, 2011), pp. 91, 93, http://www.oecd.org/els/health-systems/49105858.pdf.

8. Franklin Delano Roosevelt, message to Congress on unemployment relief, Washington, D.C., March 21, 1933.

9. See Chapter 6 on parenting.

10. See Chapter 8 on pensions.

11. See Chapter 9 on care for the elderly.

12. See Chapter 11 on training and qualifications.

Chapter 1

1. "Unemployment Statistics during the Great Depression," United States History website, http://www.u-s-history.com/pages/h1528.html.

2. Doris Kearns Goodwin, *Lyndon Johnson and the American Dream* (New York: St. Martin's Press, 1991).

3. Frederic B. M. Hollyday, ed., *Bismarck* (Englewood Cliffs, NJ: Prentice-Hall, 1970); Moritz Busch, *Bismarck: Some Secret Pages of His History*, vol. 2 (Toronto: The Copp, Clark Co., 1898, reprinted by Forgotten Books), p. 257.

4. Busch, *Bismarck: Some Secret Pages*, p. 258.

5. Ibid.

6. Ibid., pp. 258–59. (All quotations in this paragraph.)

7. Ibid., p. 258–59.

8. Ibid., pp. 282–83.

9. Ibid., p. 282–83.

10. The total enrollment in the food stamp program as of January 2014 was 46,542,005. See "Supplemental Nutrition Assistance Program (SNAP)," U.S. Department of Agriculture, Food and Nutrition Service website, http://www.fns.usda.gov/pd/29snapcurrpp.htm.

11. The population of the United States as of December 31, 2013, was 317,292,487, according to the U.S. Census Bureau Population Clock, http://www.census.gov/popclock.

12. "Government Spending Details," Fiscal Year 2014 in $ Billion, usgovernmentspending.com, http://www.usgovernmentspending.com/year_spending_2014USbn_15bs2n_40#usgs302.

13. French unemployment averaged 1.5 percent in the 1950s, 1.7 percent in the 1960s, 3.8 percent in the 1970s, 9.0 percent in the 1980s, and 8.9 percent in the 1990s. See John P. Martin, "The Extent of High Unemployment in OECD Countries," Table 1, in Federal Reserve Bank of Kansas City, *Proceedings of Economic Policy Symposium*, Jackson Hole, WY, January 1994, http://www.kansascityfed.com/publicat/sympos/1994/S94MARTI.PDF. The latest figure for unemployment is the OECD harmonized unemployment figure for April 2014 from OECD.Stat, http://stats.oecd.org/index.aspx?queryid=36324#.

14. France's gross domestic product expenditure on welfare was 12.5 percent in 1960, 15 percent in 1970, 21 percent in 1980, 25 percent in 1990, 29 percent in 2000, and 32.5 percent in 2010. OECD, "Social Spending during the Crisis: Social Expenditure (SOCX) Data Update 2012," 2012, http://www.oecd.org/els/soc/OECD2012SocialSpendingDuringTheCrisis8pages.pdf.

15. Unemployment rose from 4 percent of those of working age to 5 percent. The figure is likely to have risen further in the following years of rising unemployment. See OECD, "Sickness, Disability and Work: Keeping on Track in the Economic Downturn," Figure A2.7, background paper, High-Level Forum, Stockholm, May 14–15, 2009, http://www.oecd.org/employment/emp/42699911.pdf.

16. Walter Galenson and Arnold Zellner, "International Comparison of Unemployment Rates," in *The Measurement and Behavior of Unemployment,* ed. National Bureau of Economic Research (Princeton, NJ: Princeton University Press, 1957), pp. 439–585, http://www.nber.org/chapters/c2649.pdf.

17. See the OECD's harmonized unemployment rates at http://stats.oecd.org/index.aspx?queryid=36324#.

18. OECD, "Trends in Retirement and in Working at Older Ages," in *Pensions at a Glance 2011: Retirement-Income Systems in OECD and G20 Countries* (Paris: OECD Publishing, 2011), pp. 39–47, http://dx.doi.org/10.1787/pension_glance-2011-6-en.

19. "Employment and Labour Markets: Key Tables from OECD," Table 6, OECD iLibrary, http://www.oecd-ilibrary.org/employment/employment-rate-of-older-workers_20752342-table6.

20. OECD, *OECD Employment Outlook 2009: Tackling the Jobs Crisis,* Chapter 4 (Paris: OECD, 2009), http://www.oecd.org/els/employmentpoliciesanddata/45219540.pdf.

21. Michael R. Strain, "A Jobs Agenda for the Right," *National Affairs* 18 (Winter 2014), http://www.nationalaffairs.com/publications/detail/a-jobs-agenda-for-the-right.

22. Ben Gersten, "5 Charts Show Alarming Trend in Number of Americans Collecting Social Security," *Money Morning*, April 10, 2013, http://moneymorning .com/2013/04/10/5-charts-show-alarming-trend-in-number-of-americans-collecting -social-security/. Gersten asserts that the percentage of Americans of working age on social security disability insurance more than tripled from 1.7 percent to 5.8 percent between 1970 and the time when the article was written.

23. Kathryn Edin and Laura Lein, *Making Ends Meet: How Single Mothers Survive Welfare and Low-Wage Work* (New York: Russell Sage Foundation, 1997).

24. For example, in France, welfare expenditure is 56.5 percent of government spending; in Austria, it is 55.1 percent; and in Italy, it is 53.6 percent. See OECD .Stat, "Social Expenditure—Aggregated Data," http://stats.oecd.org/Index.aspx ?DataSetCode=SOCX_AGG.

25. Ibid. This is the OECD figure for 2013, up from 15.5 percent in 1980 and surely far greater than in the 1950s.

26. Barack Obama, *Dreams from My Father: A Story of Race and Inheritance* (New York: Random House, 1995).

27. I first saw the excerpts from *Dreams from My Father* that appear in this section in Paul Tough, "What Does Obama Really Believe In?," *New York Times Magazine*, August 15, 2012.

Chapter 2

1. *Men, Suicide, and Society: Why Disadvantaged Men in Mid-life Die by Suicide* (Surrey, UK: Samaritans, 2012), http://www.samaritans.org/sites/default/files/kcfinder /files/press/Men%20Suicide%20and%20Society%20Research%20Report%20151112 .pdf. Phil's story, one of six case studies, is available at http://www.samaritans.org /caller-case-study-phil.

2. Rafael DiTella, Robert MacCulloch, and Andrew J. Oswald, "The Macroeconomics of Happiness," ZEI working paper B 03-1999, Center for European Integration Studies, University of Bonn, Germany, 1999, p. 5, http://www.econstor.eu /bitstream/10419/39619/1/269376186.pdf.

3. Ibid.

4. David Bell and David Blanchflower, *Youth Unemployment: Déjà Vu?*, IZA discussion paper 4705, Institute for the Study of Labor, Bonn, Germany, 2009, http:// ssrn.com/abstract=1545132.

5. Arthur H. Goldsmith, Jonathan R. Veum, and William Darity Jr., "Unemployment, Joblessness, Psychological Well-Being, and Self-Esteem: Theory and Evidence," *Journal of Socio-Economics* 26 (1997): 133–58; Arthur H. Goldsmith, Jonathan R. Veum, and William Darity Jr., "The Psychological Impact of Unemployment and Joblessness," *Journal of Socio-Economics* 25 (1996): 333–58.

6. T. A. Blakely, S. C. D. Collings, and J. Atkinson, "Unemployment and Suicide: Evidence for a Causal Association?," *Journal of Epidemiology and Community Health* 57 (2003): 594–600, http://jech.bmj.com/content/57/8/594.full. The findings suggest that the unemployed are two to three times more likely to commit suicide even after various controls. "About half of this association might be attributable to confounding by mental illness," according to the report. Even so the association remains,

and I guess that it is possible that the mental illness is itself made worse by being unemployed. Regarding life expectancy, the way that unemployment reduces it is well established in many papers. See M. Harvey Brenner, "Major Factors in the Prediction of National Life Expectancy: GDP and Unemployment," testimony before the U.S. Senate Committee on Environment and Public Works, 112th Congress, 1st session, June 2011, http://www.epw.senate.gov/public/index.cfm?FuseAction=Files .View&FileStore_id=37188bea-2c5f-4100-a767-f264f1a1ced2.

7. I say "at least four" because Figure 2.1 shows four years. However, another source shows six: Walter Galenson and Arnold Zellner, "International Comparison of Unemployment Rates," in National Bureau of Economic Research, *The Measurement and Behavior of Unemployment* (Princeton, NJ: Princeton University Press, 1957), Table 1, available at http://www.nber.org/chapters/c2649.pdf. This is the source for the German figures.

8. Lucrezia Reichlin and Catherine Guillemineau, "Chômage et croissance en France et aux États-Unis: une analyse de longue période," *Observations et diagnostics économiques: revue de l'OFCE* 29 (1989): 161–84, chart at 164, http://www.persee.fr /web/revues/home/prescript/article/ofce_0751-6614_1989_num_29_1_1192.

9. "Labour market," Destatis website, https://www.destatis.de/EN/FactsFigures /Indicators/LongTermSeries/LabourMarket/lrarb003.html.

10. Jerome Fahrer and Alexandra Heath, "The Evolution of Employment and Unemployment in Australia," Reserve Bank of Australia, December 1992, http://www .rba.gov.au/publications/rdp/1992/pdf/rdp9215.pdf.

11. 2012 figures: Switzerland $78,928, Bermuda $84,460, Qatar $93,825, Norway $99,636, Luxembourg $103,925, Monaco $163,026. "GDP per Capita [Current US$]," World Bank website, http://data.worldbank.org/indicator/NY.GDP.PCAP .CD/countries/1W?order=wbapi_data_value_2012%20wbapi_data_value%20 wbapi_data_value-last&sort=asc&display=default.

12. Those workers employed for up to a year must be given a month's notice. Those who have worked for between one and nine years must get two months' notice. Beyond that, it is three months. These minimums are far less than in some countries.

13. There have been union campaigns for a minimum wage, but they have not been successful. A referendum in 2014 rejected its introduction.

14. Jean-Michel Bonvin and Eric Moachon, "Reframing the Issue of Legitimacy in Workfare Policies," in *Workfare and Welfare State Legitimacy,* ed. Helena Blomberg and Nanna Kildal (Helsinki, Finland: NordWel, 2011), pp. 62–95, https://helda.helsinki .fi/bitstream/handle/10138/41875/nordwel1.pdf?sequence=1, at pp. 80–81.

15. "Social Welfare," Migraweb website, http://www.migraweb.ch/en/themen /sociale-sicherheit/sozialhilfe/.

16. Bonvin and Moachon, "Reframing the Issue of Legitimacy in Workfare Policies," pp. 77–78.

17. Nicola Duell, Peter Tergeist, Ursula Bazant, and Sylvie Cimper, "Activation Policies in Switzerland," OECD Social Employment and Migration Working Papers, 2010, OECD, Paris, http://www.oecd.org/berlin/46224109.pdf. "Studies from several countries have shown that strong job-search controls can have a considerable impact on re-employment rates. Switzerland stands out as *one of the countries with the strongest job-search requirements in the OECD. Even at initial registration for placement, Swiss jobseekers are liable to be sanctioned if they cannot present evidence of recent job-search*

actions. During the subsequent monthly face-to-face meeting with their counsellors, jobseekers need to present proof of their job applications during the past period. The approximate number of job-search actions they need to report is often as high as 10 per month. Even during participation in an active measure, job-search efforts (as well as placement efforts by counsellors) need to be continued, albeit to a more limited extent [emphasis added]."

18. It was 8.4 percent in 2012 compared with 16.3 percent for the OECD. See "Employment and Labour Markets: Key Tables from OECD," Table 2: Youth Unemployment Rate, OECD iLibrary, http://www.oecd-ilibrary.org/employment /youth-unemployment-rate_20752342-table2.

19. *The Economist* blog, "Young and Restless: The Ratio of Youth to Adult Unemployment Worsens," December 16, 2010, http://www.economist.com/blogs /dailychart/2010/12/youth_unemployment.

20. At the time I was in Spain, the national minimum wage came out to €640 a month. One source told me that it applies to fewer than 3 percent of workers.

21. For the purposes of this book, 1 euro = 1.10 U.S. dollar (March 2016).

22. In such circumstances, the longer-serving workers were so expensive to fire that they were practically unsackable. This, it is said, has led such workers to not work very hard. If that situation is true, the law will have damaged Spanish productivity.

Inevitably the cost of significant layoffs has been extremely expensive. I say "has been" because while I was in Spain (March 2012), the new government had changed the law. Layoffs became easier to justify. People in Spain were waiting to see if the change would make any difference or if the labor court judges would argue that the change was unconstitutional.

When unemployment soared to 20 percent in 1984, a new law was passed permitting employers to hire people on temporary contracts. See "Spain Un-employment Rate," Index Mundi website, http://www.indexmundi.com/spain /unemployment_rate.html, for unemployment rate and section 1.4 of "Spain: Young People and Temporary Employment in Europe," European Monitoring Centre on Change, December 8, 2013, http://www.eurofound.europa.eu/emcc/erm/studies /tn1304017s/es1304011q.htm for introduction of temporary contracts. Thus lawmakers implicitly acknowledged that the high security of long-term employ-ment had been bought at the expense of individuals who were not employed. The change in law, however, still did not solve the problem. The majority of workers remain on long-term contracts, and those who are on the new short-term contracts are the people who have been fired.

23. Andrés Torres and Enrique Morales, "Las ETT colocan hasta seis veces más desempleados que el antiguo Inem," June 24, 2014, *Teinteresa.es* (Spain), http://www .teinteresa.es/empleo/ETT-colocan-desempleados-antiguo-Inem_0_1162686123 .html.

24. "Consecuenciasderechazarunacolocaciónadecuadaenelparo," *Citapreviainem.es* (Spain), http://www.citapreviainem.es/rechazar-colocacion-adecuada-paro/.

25. Susana Serrano Davey, "Employing Staff in Spain," Andalucia.com, http:// www.andalucia.com/spain/business/employing-staff-spain2.htm.

26. "Spanish Income Tax 2014," SpainAccountants website, http://www.spain accountants.com/it.html; "Rates and Allowances 2014," SpainAccountants website, http://www.spainaccountants.com/rates.html.

27. In Switzerland, the employer pays about 11.45 percent of the wage and the employee about 7.7 percent. The amount of income tax depends on the individual canton but in Geneva, which has relatively high taxes, it is less than 11 percent for someone on a modest income. Federal income tax is well under 1 percent. "Swiss Rental Income Tax Is High," Global Property Guide website, April 8, 2013, http://www.globalpropertyguide.com/Europe/Switzerland/Taxes-and-Costs.

The position could be something like this:

Cost to employer

Wage	€1,500
plus Social security	€171.75
Total	**€1,671.75**

The money in the pocket of the employee could be this:

Received by worker

Wage	€1,500
less	
Social insurance @7.7 percent	(€115.5)
Tax @about 11 percent	(€165)
Net	**€1,219.5**

28. The OECD publishes an index of "employment protection" for each country. Nations with high employment protection tend to have high unemployment— including Spain, France, Greece, and Portugal. But having low protection is not a guarantee of low unemployment.

29. See Table 4.1 in Chapter 4, on education, for rates of functional illiteracy in various countries.

30. Cited in Mark Wilson, "The Negative Effects of Minimum Wage Laws," Cato Institute Policy Analysis no. 701, June 21, 2012, pp. 7–8, http://object.cato.org/sites/cato.org/files/pubs/pdf/PA701.pdf.

31. This could be expressed as a kind of equation: Factors that increase the cost of employing people *or* Factors that reduce the net pay of workers + High minimum wage/welfare benefits supplemented, perhaps, with cash jobs = Unemployment. Or to put it more simply: F + H = U.

32. Jochen Kluve, "*Fördern und Fordern*: The Principle of 'Help and Hassle' in German Labour Market Policy," in *When Hassle Means Help: The International Lessons of Conditional Welfare*, ed. Lawrence Kay and Oliver Marc Hartwich (London: Policy Exchange, 2008), p. 59, http://www.policyexchange.org.uk/images/publications/when%20hassle%20means%20help%20-%20oct%2008.pdf.

33. Ibid.

34. Ibid.

35. Caitlin Kenney, "Germany's Painful Unemployment Fix," *Planet Money* blog, September 23, 2011, http://www.npr.org/blogs/money/2011/09/23/140707524/germanys-painful-unemployment-fix.

36. The summary of the Hartz reforms is derived from Kluve, "*Fördern und Fordern*."

37. "In 2004, small businesses with fewer than ten employees were made exempt from dismissal protection for employees," according to Ryan Bourne, "Economic Lessons from Germany," *Spectator Coffee House* blog, June 12, 2012, http://blogs.spectator .co.uk/coffeehouse/2012/06/economic-lessons-from-germany/.

38. Chile, Israel, and Turkey were the others.

39. Jason DeParle, *American Dream: Three Women, Ten Kids, and a Nation's Drive to End Welfare* (New York: Penguin, 2005).

40. Version sent to me by email by Jennifer Noyes.

41. Jocelyn Bourgon, *A New Synthesis of Public Administration: Serving in the 21st Century* (Montreal: School of Policy Studies, Queen's University, 2011), p. 222.

42. For the fiscal year 2014 the caseload of TANF (Temporary Assistance for Needy Families) single parents was averaging 14,186. Email to the author from Maura Taggart, Division of Family and Economic Security/Bureau of Working Families/Research and Statistics section chief, Wisconsin Department of Children and Families, June 25, 2014. See also "TANF Caseload Data 2014," Office of Family Assistance website, U.S. Department of Health and Human Services, http://www.acf .hhs.gov/programs/ofa/resource/caseload-data-2014.

43. "IMF World Economic Outlook, April 2014," Knoema website, http:// knoema.com/IMFWEO2014Apr/imf-world-economic-outlook-april-2014. See also "Unemployment," Singapore Ministry of Manpower website, http://stats.mom.gov .sg/Pages/Unemployment-Summary-Table.aspx.

44. The applicant gets none of the sense of entitlement that is so common elsewhere. Each case is treated individually, and the applicant is obliged to think in terms of his or her own resources and those of the family. If someone comes in with a sense of entitlement, this attitude is immediately confronted.

There are a few other aspects to the Singapore approach:

- A prized government rental flat is not allocated just because someone is poor and wants to leave the family home. Getting such a flat may be a reward for getting work but not a reward for being unemployed. The whole organization is very conscious that it must avoid creating perverse incentives— rewards for "bad" behavior.
- There is absolutely no minimum wage.
- As in Switzerland and Germany, there is a strong emphasis on vocational education from the age of 16. About 65 percent of students at that age attend polytechnic or technical schools. Only 30 percent go to a university initially, and a further 15 percent go on to a university after attending a polytechnic school.

45. The 4.2 percent rate applies to earnings below $61,538 (£39,000, both at November 2014 exchange rates). From 2012, earnings up to $20,000 are not taxed. The next $10,000 is taxed at 2 percent, according to "Income Tax Rates," Inland Revenue Authority of Singapore website, http://www.iras.gov.sg.

46. Workers are obliged to make payments to the Central Provident Fund at a rate of 20.0 percent, and their employer pays a further 15.5 percent. Employees do not contribute if they earn less than $500 a month. Employers contribute to the fund for employees earning more than $50 a month. The full employer contribution rate of 15.5 percent is payable for all employees under age 35, according to "About the Central Provident Fund," OECD website, http://www.oecd.org/finance/private -pensions/46260911.pdf.

Chapter 3

1. Much of the information about the history of the system came from an interview with Tom Groot and Yvonne Krabbe at Vrije Universiteit Amsterdam.

2. My information came from an interview, but information on the Dekker Commission appears in Kieke G. H. Okma, "Recent Changes in Dutch Health Insurance: Individual Mandate or Social Insurance?" working paper, National Academy of Social Insurance, Washington, D.C., January 2009, http://www.nasi.org/usr_doc/Recent_Changes_in_Dutch_Health_Insurance.pdf. Dekker had been chief executive of Philips Electronics from 1982 to 1986.

3. When I was in the Netherlands in 2011, I was told they were about to bring the numbers down from 30,000 diagnostic trouble codes to 4,400. They were using the list produced by the World Health Organization. The list was based not on the specifications of the specialists but on the diagnosis.

4. And indeed I have obtained and looked at several of the relevant papers and publications: Isabelle Joumard, "Health Care Systems: Getting More Value for Money," Economics Department Policy Note no. 2, OECD, Paris, 2010; Isabelle Joumard, Christophe André, and Chantal Nicq, "Healthcare Systems: Efficiency and Institutions," Economics Department Working Papers no. 769, OECD, Paris, 2010; Valérie Paris, Marion Devaux, and Lihan Wei, "Health Systems Institutional Characteristics: A Survey of 29 OECD Countries," OECD Health Working Papers no. 50, OECD, Paris, 2010; OECD, *Value for Money in Health Spending* (Paris: OECD, 2010).

5. Jeremy Sammut is a research fellow at the Centre for Independent Studies in Sydney. His paper "Why Public Hospitals are Overcrowded" cites a 2007 report that states that more than a third of emergency patients requiring admission to a public hospital waited over eight hours for a bed.

6. American Association of Port Authorities, world port rankings 2011. Tianjin comes third and Rotterdam fourth. See http://aapa.files.cms-plus.com/PDFs/WORLD%20PORT%20RANKINGS%202011.pdf.

7. "Health Expenditure, Total (% of GDP)," World Bank website, http://data.worldbank.org/indicator/SH.XPD.TOTL.ZS?order=wbapi_data_value_2012+wbapi_data_value+wbapi_data_value-last&sort=desc.

8. Readers familiar with American health care may be thinking, "Wait a minute. This sounds like managed care. We have that in the States." Yes, the system does seem to have a lot in common with "managed care." People pay a company that provides health insurance and much of the medical care, too. One of the biggest managed care companies is Kaiser Permanente. I visited its offices in Oakland, California, and found that Kaiser, too, puts a lot of effort into keeping its customers healthy. And for the same reason: that effort saves money.

9. I met Alberto de Rosa, director general of a company that has a stake in private hospitals. He was the first manager of the Ribera Hospital, so he has seen the story from the beginning. I asked whether the innovations of the Ribera and its successors have affected how the public hospitals perform.

"The Ribera Hospital was the first hospital in Valencia to make epidurals available on a routine basis," he told me. "Because of this, many mothers came to the Ribera Hospital to have their babies." The public hospitals elsewhere in the region saw this happening, so to prevent a deluge of pregnant mothers going to the

Ribera, they started offering epidurals too. And now? "Now *all* the hospitals offer epidurals."

The Ribera Hospital also offered private rooms to mothers giving birth. In the public hospitals, women gave birth in wards of two or three. Again, to prevent an exodus to the Ribera, the other hospitals improved what they offered.

It is a classic story of how a little competition can buck up standards. It tells us something about monopolies in public provision. They can be full of people working for the public good yet offer services well below a good standard.

De Rosa put it more bluntly. He said that the public hospitals put the interests of the professionals above those of the patients. The thought is contrary to what many assume. But when hospital professionals stop work at 3 p.m. and decline to offer epidurals to mothers, it is hard to conclude anything else.

10. For long-term growth in private health insurance see David McDaid et al., "Ireland: Health Systems Review," *Health Systems in Transition* 11 (2009): 81, Fig. 3.6, http://www.euro.who.int/__data/assets/pdf_file/0004/85306/E92928.pdf. For material on waiting times, see Elliot Bidgood, "Healthcare Systems: Ireland and 'Universal Health Insurance'—An Emerging Model for the U.K.?," Online report, Civitas, London, December 17, 2013, http://www.civitas.org.uk/nhs/download/IrelandBrief20131.pdf.

11. Can we really expect that this would save money? In addition to the experience of Singapore, which has achieved low-cost health care, researchers have undertaken a number of studies of health savings accounts in the United States. One of the most comprehensive, conducted by RAND, concluded that people with health savings accounts and with insurance policies that require patients to pay out of their own pockets until a certain level of spending is reached spent about 30 percent less on their health care than those with conventional, full-coverage insurance. Did this result in their going without treatment that was important for their health? No. The policy had no adverse effect on their health outcomes. See John C. Goodman, *Priceless: Curing the Healthcare Crisis* (Oakland, CA: Independent Institute, 2012), pp. 161 and 162, citing Amelia M. Haviland et al., "How Do Consumer-Directed Health Plans Affect Vulnerable Populations?," *Forum for Health Economics and Policy* 14 (2011).

12. Goodman, *Priceless*, citing Devon M. Herrick, "Consumer Driven Health Care: The Changing Role of the Patient," National Center for Policy Analysis Policy Report no. 276, May 2005; Devon M. Herrick, "Shopping for Drugs: 2007," National Center for Policy Analysis Policy Report no. 293, November 2006.

Chapter 4

1. Marc Le Bris, *Et vos enfants ne sauront pas lire, ni compter ! La faillite obstinée de l'école française* (Paris: Stock, 2004).

2. Ibid.

3. Michael Gove, UK education secretary, speech to the World Education Forum, January 11, 2012, https://www.gov.uk/government/speeches/michael-gove-to-the-education-world-forum.

4. I was speaking to Schleicher before the PISA 2012 study came out, so he was referring to PISA 2009. In PISA 2012, all the figures were different to a greater or lesser extent. The OECD functional illiteracy rate fell from 18.8 percent to 18.0 percent.

However, reading was not the main focus of the later study, whereas it was the main focus of the 2009 study. So the 2009 results are worth considering also. It is also conceivable, at least, that some countries are learning how to "game" the PISA tests so that they look better. If this has been happening, then the earlier results may be more reliable. The 2009 results were as follows:

Shanghai	4.1%
South Korea	5.8%
Finland	8.1%
Hong Kong	8.3%
Canada	10.3%
Singapore	12.4%
Japan	13.6%
Australia	14.3%
New Zealand	14.3%
Netherlands	14.4%
Norway	14.9%
Poland	15.0%
Denmark	15.2%
Switzerland	16.9%
Sweden	17.5%
Portugal	17.6%
Belgium	17.7%
United States	17.7%
Germany	18.5%
United Kingdom	18.5%
OECD average	**18.8%**
Spain	19.5%
France	19.7%
Italy	21.0%
Greece	21.3%
Czech Republic	23.1%
Turkey	24.5%
Israel	26.6%
Russia	27.4%
Austria	27.5%
Mexico	40.1%

SOURCE: OECD, *PISA 2009 Results, vol. 1: What Students Know and Can Do* (Paris: OECD Publishing, 2010), p. 194.

5. Harriet Sergeant, *Among the Hoods: My Years with a Teenage Gang* (London: Faber and Faber, 2012). Further details appear in Sergeant, *Wasted: The Betrayal of White and Black Caribbean Boys* (London: Centre for Policy Studies, 2009), http://www.cps.org .uk/files/reports/original/111027122608-20091127SocialPolicyWasted.pdf.

6. Sergeant, *Among the Hoods*, p. 8.

7. Ibid., p. 9.

8. Ibid., p. 12.

9. Ibid., p. 10.

10. Ibid., p. 8.

11. All sorts of statistics are bandied about relating to illiteracy and juvenile offenders and prisoners, and some are more dramatic than the ones I have used. See, for example, Statistic Brain, http://www.statisticbrain.com/number-of-american -adults-who-cant-read/. However, often I have not been able to trace the figures to their original sources. The figures I have used come from National Center for Education Statistics, "Literacy behind Prison Walls," October 1994, Table 2.3, http://nces .ed.gov/pubs94/94102.pdf. The figures are clearly based on the National Adult Literacy Survey, which includes various measures and levels of literacy. I have used the so-called quantitative scale. According to this scale, 40 percent of prison inmates are at the lowest level of literacy compared with 22 percent of the general population.

12. Again, some sources cite more dramatic figures. A website in British Home Office archives provides details of the What Works initiative from the first years of this century. The site refers to research by Lipton (1999), http://webarchive.national archives.gov.uk/20100413151441/http:/www.crimereduction.homeoffice.gov.uk /workingoffenders/workingoffenders1.htm.

13. "Literary Statistics," Begin to Read website, www.begintoread.com/research /literacystatistics.html

14. Ibid.

15. Ibid.

16. See Chapter 10 for more on the difficulties of firing teachers in the United States.

17. Mark Bray and Chad Lykins, *Shadow Education: Private Supplementary Tutoring and Its Implications for Policy Makers in Asia* (Manila: Asian Development Bank, 2012), p. 5, http://www.adb.org/sites/default/files/publication/29777/shadow-education. pdf. The actual sentence in this report is this: "In addition, 6.8 percent of junior secondary 3 pupils received tutoring at home, and 15.0 percent followed correspondence courses." It is not clear whether there might be overlap, and if so, how much, between students at the *juku*, students with private tutors, and students taking correspondence courses. The figures come from a 2008 Japanese government report, which is written in Japanese. I am tempted to think, however, that the overlap is unlikely to be very great. Any children following two kinds of shadow education would be extraordinarily exhausted. So it seems likely that a minimum of 80 percent of the children have private supplementary schooling at this age.

18. Ibid.

19. Andrew Coulson, email to the author, November 2012.

20. Michael B. Horn, "What Koreans Wish Obama Understood about Their Schools," EducationNext website, April 9, 2014, http://educationnext.org/koreans -wish-obama-understood-schools/.

21. Bray and Lykins, *Shadow Education*.

22. Ibid.

23. Ibid.

24. There is also supplementary education in other countries but it is less widespread. In Britain, the Sutton Trust, an education charity, did a survey of 11- to 16-year-olds and found that 20 percent of white pupils received some kind of private tuition and 45 percent of south Asian children. "On the Road," *The Economist*, November 16. 2013, http://www.economist.com/news/britain/21589874-ethnic-minority-pupils-are -storming-ahead-thanks-partly-tutors-road.

25. "List of Countries by Foreign-Born Population," Wikipedia, http://en.wikipedia.org/wiki/List_of_countries_by_foreign-born_population_in_2005, citing United Nations figures.

26. Andrew Coulson, director of the Center for Educational Freedom at the Cato Institute in Washington, D.C., argues that, wholly by chance, the Finnish curriculum happens to be more closely aligned with the method of testing in the PISA test than that of other countries. Both concentrate on "everyday" math and science rather than on higher-level skills. See Andrew Coulson, "Being a Policy Specialist," in *Creating Your Path to a Policy Career,* Institute for Humane Studies, George Mason University, Arlington, VA, http://www.theihs.org/academic/wp-content/uploads/2014/08/CreatingYourPathToAPolicyCareer.pdf. Coulson draws attention to the fact that Finland did not do so well in another international assessment, the Trends in International Mathematics and Science Study (TIMSS) test. It came eighth in math at the eighth-grade level, with a score only fractionally higher than those of the United States and England (TIMSS study 2011). Finland scored 514, the United States scored 509, and England scored 507. This compares with 613 for top-scoring Korea. It should also be noted that the Finnish result in the TIMSS study may be higher because many European countries, including Germany, the Netherlands, and France, did not participate. Coulson also notes that "over 200 Finnish mathematics professors signed a letter in 2005 lamenting the poor and declining mathematics skills of their entering freshmen, and warning against generalizations based on misleading PISA results," citing Kari Astala et al., "The PISA Survey Tells Only a Partial Truth of Finnish Children's Mathematical Skills," Matematiikkalehti Solmu website, August 31 2005, http://solmu.math.helsinki.fi/2005/erik/PISAEng.html.

27. Winton appears to be 101 miles away, so it is surprising that this was an alternative for his mother. But this is what I believe he said.

28. For more information on KIPP, see http://www.kipp.org/about-kipp.

29. Karl Weber, ed., *Waiting for "Superman": How We Can Save America's Failing Public Schools,* (New York: Public Affairs, 2010), p. 28.

30. *Waiting for "Superman,"* Hollywood, CA: Paramount Pictures, 2010.

31. Caroline M. Hoxby, Sonali Murarka, and Jenny Kang, "How New York City's Charter Schools Affect Achievement," New York City Charter Schools Evaluation Project, September 2009 report, http://users.nber.org/~schools/charterschoolseval/how_NYC_charter_schools_affect_achievement_sept2009.pdf.

32. Ibid., pp. iv–13.

33. See OECD, *PISA 2009 Results, vol. 4: What Makes a School Successful?* (Paris: OECD Publishing, 2010), pp. 224 and 225, http://www.oecd.org/PISA/PISAproducts/48852721.pdf.

34. The rate of functional illiteracy at the government schools is lower, at 12.3 percent, than at the private schools, at 16.7 percent. There are several reasons for this. The vast majority of all the students covered by the study, including most of those at private schools, were in state schools the year before. The PISA study takes in children who in Japan have just competed to get one of the limited places in the government secondary schools. The most able get the places. Some of those who do not succeed, obviously the less able ones, go to private schools, presumably to be able to continue their education. So the sample of those at private schools is skewed toward the less able. Moreover, the private schools have not at this stage had the children for long enough to make any difference. It should be added that some

elite private schools have students who were able to pass the government test. I am grateful to Miyako Ikeda at the OECD for explaining these circumstances to me. Any misunderstanding is my fault. If the figures from Japan had been included, the average figure for government schools would have been 17.8 percent and that for private schools, 6.5 percent.

35. Andrew J. Coulson, "Comparing Public, Private, and Market Schools: The International Evidence," *Journal of School Choice* 3 (2009): 31–54.

36. Cited in the education chapter of James Bartholomew, *The Welfare State We're In*, rev. ed. (London: Biteback, 2014). One of the papers was "The Relative Effectiveness of Private and Public Schools: Evidence from Two Developing Countries" (1989). The countries in question were Colombia and Tanzania.

37. Ibid.

38. Funding was made available for private schools as well as for government schools to enable different religious denominations to have their own schools. "Overview of the Dutch Secondary Education System," Fulbright Center. But over time, regulation of the schools increased. See Andrew Coulson, "On the Way to School: Why and How to Make a Market in Education," in *Freedom and School Choice in American Education*, ed. Greg Forster and C. Bradley Thompson (New York: Palgrave Macmillan, 2011). The schools' control over the use of their buildings was removed. The government specified how decision-making powers were to be allocated among management, teachers, and parents. A common curriculum was introduced and then extended. Schools were required to teach certain combinations of subjects. Particular tests were specified, and even the way in which teachers instructed. This erosion of independence discouraged the creation of new independent schools. Further, barriers to new schools were erected, such as minimum sizes. As the creation of new schools dwindled, the element of competition was eroded, too.

39. Coulson, "On the Way to School."

40. "Fast Facts on Private School Choice," Friedman Foundation for Educational Choice, June 2014, http://www.edchoice.org/Newsroom/Fast-Facts-on-Private-School-Choice.pdf.

Chapter 5

1. He was appointed prime minister in March 2014.

2. The spelling and French in some of these comments were variable, which makes exact translation difficult. These are the original words in French: *"repaire de malfrats"*; *"ça ressemblait un peu à un camp de concentration (un ancien d'AFN)"* and *"cité tres grande avec 10 batiments, plusieurs dealeurs associé avec les flaments et les iris, tous armée."*

3. For the purposes of this book, 1 euro = 1.10 U.S. dollars (according to the exchange rate in March 2016).

4. Rebecca Tunstall, et al., "The Links between Housing and Poverty: An Evidence Review," Joseph Rowntree Foundation, April 2013, http://www.jrf.org.uk/sites/files/jrf/poverty-housing-options-full.pdf.

5. Stuart Adam, Mike Brewer, and Andrew Shephard, "Financial Work Incentives in Britain: Comparisons over Time and between Family Types," WP06/20, Institute of Fiscal Studies, October 2006, Table 2.1, http://www.ifs.org.uk/wps/wp0620.pdf.

6. In the long term, it depends whether the better incentive to work for those already getting the benefit has a bigger effect on unemployment levels than the reduced incentive to work for those who would become newly entitled to the benefit.

7. There is probably some damage in continental countries. It could come from reducing the mobility of those with favored low rents who are reluctant to move to another part of the town or country to take a better job (or any job).

8. The waiting lists can be very long. In Stockholm they have been as long as eight years. See "Sweden's Housing Queues 'Getting Worse,'" *The Local* (Sweden), March 11, 2013, http://www.thelocal.se/20130311/46672.

9. To those of us in Britain and America who have seen the damage done by rents adjusted for income, the Swedish example might seem like a refreshing example of how this damage might be avoided. But there is some indication that the European Union does not see things this way and has clashed with Sweden because it wants public housing to be made available only for the poor. This is opposed to the Swedish idea that social housing should be available for everybody. See "Worrying Development Concerning Social Housing at EU Level," AK Europa website, November 8, 2012, http://www.akeuropa.eu/en/worrying-development-concerning-social -housing-at-eu-level.html?cmp_id=7&news_id=1432&vID=9.

Similarly in Denmark, "The majority of vacant units are assigned by the respective housing associations on the basis of time on the waiting list and household size. There are no restrictions on who may join a waiting list, apart from a minimum age of 15 years. . . . Municipalities have the right to assign tenants to at least 25 percent of vacant housing-association units. They (and the housing associations) do not necessarily do so on the basis of need. Many local authorities give priority on troubled estates to people working in the local area in order to improve their social composition by introducing residents with jobs." Christine Whitehead and Kathleen Scanlon, *Social Housing in Europe* (London: London School of Economics and Political Science, 2007), http://vbn.aau.dk/files/13671493/SocialHousingInEurope.pdf.

10. Howard Husock, "The Myths of *The Pruitt-Igoe Myth*," *City Journal*, Manhattan Institute, February 17, 2012, http://www.city-journal.org/2012/bc0217hh.html.

11. Whitehead and Scanlon, *Social Housing in Europe*, p. 65.

12. Ibid. Table 4 on page 154 shows that there is an over-representation of single parent households in Swedish public housing, but this is on a relatively minor scale compared with, say, Britain. It shows 9.4 percent of tenants are single-parent households compared with 5.5 percent for all households combined. Of the tenants, 12 percent are couples with children. So in Sweden, there are more couples with children in social housing than there are single parents. In Britain, it is very much the other way around.

13. Associated Press, "Chicago Closes Cabrini-Green Project," *USA Today*, updated December 22, 2010, http://usatoday30.usatoday.com/news/nation/2010-12 -01-cabrini-green_N.htm.

14. Associated Press, "At Fla. Housing Project, Rape Just Another Crime," *NBC News*, July 11 2007, http://www.nbcnews.com/id/19698132/ns/us_news-crime_and _courts/t/fla-housing-project-rape-just-another-crime/#.UY07h7Vtggs.

15. Ibid.

16. Ibid.

17. "Valls: 'C'est une guerre contre la barbarie,'" *Journal du dimanche* (France), March 17, 2013, http://www.lejdd.fr/Politique/Actualite/Manuel-Valls-C-est-une -guerre-contre-la-barbarie-interview-596711.

18. British Crime Survey 2008–2009, cited in "Burglary Risk: How Much Crime Is There?," the *Crime Prevention Website*, http://thecrimepreventionwebsite.com /home-security-assessment/470/burglary-risk/.

19. Amelia Hill, "Council Estate Decline Spawns New Underclass," *Observer* (London), November 30, 2003, http://www.guardian.co.uk/society/2003/nov/30 /housing.uknews.

20. Barbara Sard and Will Fischer, "Preserving Safe, High-Quality Public Housing Should Be a Priority of Federal Housing Policy," Center on Budget and Policy Priorities, Washington, D.C., October 8, 2008, http://www.cbpp.org/files /9-18-08hous.pdf.

21. "Demolished Housing Estates," U.K. Housing Wiki, http://ukhousing.wikia .com/wiki/Category:Demolished_housing_estates.

22. Aline Leclerc and Elodie Ratsimbazafy, "La démolition d'une nouvelle barre s'annonce à la cité des 4000," La Courneuve: urbains sensibles blog, *Le Monde* (Paris), May 22, 2012, http://lacourneuve.blog.lemonde.fr/2012/05/22/la-demolition-dune-nouvelle-barre-sannonce-a-la-cite-des-4000. See also "Cité des 4000," Wikipédia (French), http://fr.wikipedia.org/wiki/Cité_des_4000.

23. Aline Leclerc and Elodie Ratsimbazafy, "Des faits divers et des politiques," La Courneuve: urbains sensibles blog, *Le Monde* (Paris), June 20, 2010, http:// lacourneuve.blog.lemonde.fr/2010/06/20/des-faits-divers-et-des-politiques.

24. See for example "Implosion Capendeguy Beziers," http://www.youtube.com /watch?v=rydT54QYX50.

25. "La barre d'immeuble explosée en 8 secondes," LaDepeche.fr (France), http:// www.ladepeche.fr/article/2008/01/28/429638-la-barre-d-immeuble-explosee-en -8-secondes.html.

26. Hugh Schofield, "Interview Sealed Minister's Fate," *BBC News*, February 25, 2005, http://news.bbc.co.uk/1/hi/world/europe/4299003.stm; "Les 600m2 du couple Gaymard," *Le Parisien*, February 16, 2005, http://www.leparisien.fr/politique/les -600-m-2-du-couple-gaymard-16-02-2005-2005707104.php.

27. Schofield, "Interview Sealed Minister's Fate."

28. Ibid.

29. "Comment expliquer qu'on trouve davantage de ménages aisés dans le parc locatif public que dans le parc locative privé." Interview with Nicolas Lecaussin, *Atlantico* (France), January 27, 2014, http://www.atlantico.fr/decryptage/comment -expliquer-qu-on-trouve-davantage-menages-aises-dans-parc-locatif-public-que -dans-parc-locatif-prive-charles-beigbeder-964545.html. It is said that the assertion was made by Charles Beigbeder, a candidate for mayor of Paris, citing Vincent Bénard. Lecaussin makes the point that affluent families get both rent-controlled housing (HLM) and housing under the auspices of various institutions such as the state railway—all paid for by the public.

30. "Department of Housing: Allegations of Corrupt Conduct in Allocation of Public Housing (Operation Greenway)," Independent Commission Against Corruption (New South Wales, Australia) website, http://www.icac.nsw.gov.au /investigations/past-investigations/investigationdetail/19.

31. See Les Kennedy, "Housing Bribes Official Faces Jail," *Sydney Morning Herald*, September 13, 2007, http://www.smh.com.au/news/national/housing -bribes-official-faces-jail/2007/09/12/1189276810256.html, and "Recommendations for Prosecutions and Updates," Independent Commission against Corruption

(New South Wales, Australia) website, http://www.icac.nsw.gov.au/investigations /past-investigations/article/3119 for more details of the case. Norris was sentenced in 2011 but only given concurrent suspended sentences for his crimes.

32. For the purposes of this book, 1 pound = 1.44 U.S. dollars (according to the exchange rate in March 2016).

33. Figure for 2014; see http://parliamentarystandards.org.uk/payandpensions /Pages/default.aspx. Average earnings were £27,017 (about $38,000) in 2013; see http://www.ons.gov.uk/ons/publications/re-reference-tables.html?edition=tcm% 3A77-332352.

34. James Chapman, "How the Taxpayer Is Funding 6,000 Council Houses for Tenants Who Earn More than £100,000," *Daily Mail* (London), February 6, 2012, http://www.dailymail.co.uk/news/article-2097473/Revealed-6-000-council-house -tenants-earn-100-000.html.

35. Patrick Hennessy, "Council House Tenants Who Sublet Homes to Be Prosecuted," the *Telegraph* (London), December 31, 2011. http://www.telegraph.co.uk /news/politics/8986185/Council-house-tenants-who-sublet-homes-to-be-prosecuted .html.

36. Ibid.

37. According to a "Whitehall analysis" that was leaked to the *Daily Mail* reported in Chapman, "How the Taxpayer Is Funding 6,000 Council Houses." See note 33.

38. Ibid.

39. Howard Husock, "Puffing the Projects," *New York Post*, June 8, 2009, http:// nypost.com/2009/06/08/puffing-the-projects.

40. Alex Morton, *Ending Expensive Social Tenancies: Fairness, Higher Growth, and More Homes* (London: Policy Exchange, 2012), http://www.policyexchange.org.uk /images/publications/ending%20expensive%20social%20tenancies.pdf.

41. Peter King, *Choice and the End of Social Housing* (London: Institute of Economic Affairs, 2006), http://www.iea.org.uk/sites/default/files/publications/files /upldbook327pdf.pdf.

42. Ibid.

43. Douglas Rice, "Sequestration Could Deny Rental Assistance to 140,000 Low-Income Families," Center on Budget and Policy Priorities website, April 2, 2013, http://www.cbpp.org/cms/?fa=view&id=3945. See also "Budget Authority by Program," U.S. Department of Housing and Urban Development, http://portal.hud .gov/hudportal/documents/huddoc?id=2012budgetauthbyprog.pdf, p. 83.

44. "Budget Authority by Program," HUD.

45. Rice, "Sequestration Could Deny Rental Assistance."

46. "Worrying Development Concerning Social Housing at EU Level." See also Florence Martin, "Sweden: Social Housing under "Businesslike Principle,'" in *EU Rethinks Role of Social Housing, Europolitics* supplement, December 16, 2011, p. 23, for further insights into the Swedish system and how the European Union has put pressure on it to change.

47. For 1979, the peak year, there were 5,187,000 dwellings rented from local authorities and 353,000 rented from "private registered providers" (mostly housing associations), giving a combined total of 5,540,000. This represented 31 percent of the total 17,882,000 dwellings in England. By 2012, the number rented from local authorities had fallen to 1,689,000 while the number rented from private registered providers had increased to 2,304,000, giving a combined total of 3,993,000. This represented

17 percent of the total 23,111,000 dwellings in England. Data taken from "Live Tables on Dwelling Stock (including Vacants)," Gov.uk, Table 104, https://www.gov.uk /government/statistical-data-sets/live-tables-on-dwelling-stock-including-vacants.

48. "Facts about Public Housing," CLPHA (Council of Large Public Housing Authorities) website, Washington, D.C., http://www.clpha.org/facts_about_public _housing#_edn3. The figures given here are a fall from 1,329,000 to 1,191,110. This is slightly different from the figures and source quoted earlier in the chapter, but the proportionate change is similar.

49. "Housing Assistance in Australia 2011," Australian Institute of Health and Welfare, June 2011, http://www.aihw.gov.au/WorkArea/DownloadAsset .aspx?id=10737419156. See "Australia: Housing Tenure," .id website, http://profile .id.com.au/australia/tenure, which shows a modest decline in the proportion of Australian social housing in "greater capital cities" between 2006 and 2011.

50. Kathleen Scanlon and Christine Whitehead, *International Trends in Housing Tenure and Mortgage Finance* (London: London School of Economics and Political Science), Table 4, available at http://www.iut.nu/Literature/2004/InternTrends _Whitehead_etal_2004.pdf. A draft paper by Björn Egner, "Housing Policy in Germany, 1945–2010: Continuity and Change," http://www.academia.edu/2963591 /Housing_Policy_in_Germany_1945-2010_Continuity_and_Change, shows the dramatic decline in the volume of social housing constructed, from 450,000 a year at the peak in the 1950s to less than 50,000 a year in the late 1990s. The author says, "Do not quote," so I apologize to him for doing so. If I had unlimited time and resources, I would have tried to find another source.

51. Percentage weightings in the British Retail Price Index. The raw figures can be found by going to "Consumer Price Indices—Series," U.K. Office for National Statistics website, http://www.ons.gov.uk/ons/datasets-and-tables/data-selector .html?table-id=2.5&dataset=mm23, and selecting the category of food.

52. U.S. Bureau of Labor Statistics, "Reflections," in *100 Years of U.S. Consumer Spending: Data for the Nation, New York City, and Boston*, BLS Report 991, U.S. Department of Labor, Washington, D.C., 2006, p. 66, http://www.bls.gov/opub/uscs /reflections.pdf, citing the U.S. Bureau of Labor Statistics consumer expenditure survey. See also Chart 42, p. 69.

53. Food as a percentage of household expenditure was 15 percent and 16 percent for the lowest deciles of income in 2010 in the United Kingdom, compared with an average of 11 percent for the overall population and only 8 percent for the highest-earning decile. So food expenditure is a more significant item for the least well off. See Giles Horsfield, ed., "Family Spending: A Report on the 2010 Living Costs and Food Survey," U.K. Office for National Statistics, 2011, Table 3.3, http://www.ons .gov.uk/ons/rel/family-spending/family-spending/family-spending-2011-edition /family-spending-2011-pdf.pdf.

54. "Communications Market Report," Ofcom, July 2012, p. 350, http:// stakeholders.ofcom.org.uk/binaries/research/cmr/cmr12/CMR_UK_2012.pdf.

55. Percentage weightings in the British Retail Price Index. The raw figures can be found by going to "Consumer Price Indices—Series," U.K. Office for National Statistics website, http://www.ons.gov.uk/ons/datasets-and-tables/data-selector .html?table-id=2.5&dataset=mm23, and selecting the category of housing (CZHF).

56. Oliver Marc Hartwich, "The Cult of Australian Property," *Business Spectator* website (Australia), February 3, 2011, http://www.businessspectator.com.au /article/2011/2/3/australian-news/cult-australian-property.

57. Ibid.

58. "International House Price Database," Federal Reserve Bank of Dallas website, http://www.dallasfed.org/institute/houseprice/index.cfm. Click on "First quarter 2014" to download data and then click RHPI (Real House Price Index) tab. The *Economist* interactive guide to the world's housing markets shows a much more modest rise in the price of U.K. housing of only 100 percent in real terms over an almost identical timescale. There are, of course, many different ways to calculate average housing prices. One could take a single dwelling and see how it changes in value. Or one could take an average of prices and see how they change. The latter could be misleading because the average dwelling might become bigger or smaller over the period in question. I have found the Dallas index more credible. The *Economist* index shows real house prices actually lower in 1997 than in 1975.

Having lived through that time and owned housing, I find this frankly hard to believe. A given dwelling in any part of London, certainly, rose in real terms. In any case, for those who prefer the *Economist* calculation, the increase is still very dramatic and a marked contrast to what happened in Germany. *The Economist* agrees that German prices fell in real terms. The *Economist* data is here: http://www .economist.com/blogs/dailychart/2011/11/global-house-prices. *The Economist* says that prices in Switzerland rose 35.5 percent in real terms. See also Halifax House Price Index at http://www.lloydsbankinggroup.com/media1/economic_insight /halifax_house_price_index_page.asp and click on "Historical house price data."

59. "House Prices Versus Earning," *Monevator*, March 15, 2012, using figures from the Halifax and from national average full-time earnings for men, http://monevator .com/house-price-to-earnings-ratio-2012.

60. Table A32: Household Expenditure by Tenure, 2011, in "Family Spending, 2012 Edition," U.K. Office for National Statistics website, December 4, 2012, http:// www.ons.gov.uk/ons/publications/re-reference-tables.html?newquery=*&newoffse t=50&pageSize=25&edition=tcm%3A77-267317.

61. Different measures of similar things can come up with some markedly different figures. Earlier in the chapter, there is reference to housing accounting for over a quarter of the Retail Price Index (RPI). But in another table produced by the Office for National Statistics, housing, fuel, and power together amount to 22 percent of the expenditure of the lowest decile in Britain in 2011 and 8 percent for the highest. The figures are lower than the weighting in the RPI, but the way that the poor have to spend much more of their income on housing is dramatically made. See U.K. Office of National Statistics, *Family Spending, 2012 edition*, Appendix A, Table A8, http://www.ons.gov.uk/ons/rel/family-spending/family-spending /family-spending-2012-edition/family-spending---list-of-tables-appendix-a --2012-edition.html#tab-List-of-tables--Appendix-A.

62. Unfortunately, I have not gotten the directly comparable figure for Germany. *The Economist* uses OECD and other figures to make a useful chart of house prices measured in different ways. Unfortunately, the measure of housing price compared with earnings is rebased to a supposed long-term average of 100. The raw figures, which would be more useful, are not shown. The fact that the OECD thinks that there is a long-term average to which such figures, implicitly, are likely to return

shows how it has misunderstood what has been happening in different housing markets most strongly affected by planning controls. See http://www.economist .com/blogs/dailychart/2011/11/global-house-prices.

63. Figures from Tobias Just, managing director of the International Real Estate Business School at the University of Regensburg, in an email to the author. The figures are for average apartment prices in euros per square meter compared with "local purchasing power parity." For Germany overall, the cost fell from 0.159 to 0.140. Just included the year-by-year series for Germany overall and some of the major cities. It is fair to say that the picture for the cities is more varied. In four, the cost went up and, in three, it went down. It seems likely that the cost of apartments in the cities rose relative to those elsewhere. But even in Berlin, which saw the biggest increase following the reunification of Germany and the move of the government there from Bonn, the increase was not huge (from 0.165 to 0.19). I am grateful to Oliver Hartwich for putting me in touch with Tobias Just.

64. "House Price to Income Ratio, Germany Compared to Continent," Global Property Guide, http://www.globalpropertyguide.com/Europe/germany/price-gdp-per-cap.

65. Cologne Institute for Economic Research, cited in Hartwich, "The Cult of Australian Property."

66. Hartwich, "The Cult of Australian Property."

67. Alan W. Evans and Oliver Marc Hartwich, *Unaffordable Housing: Fables and Myths* (London: Policy Exchange, 2005), p. 24, citing "European Union, Housing Statistics in the EU 2002," http://www.policyexchange.org.uk/images/publications /unaffordable%20housing%20-%20jun%2005.pdf.

68. From 98.8 square meters to 96.8. Becky Barrow, "The Big Squeeze: Average British Home Has Shrunk by Two Square Metres in Just a Decade Forcing Families to Split Bedrooms and Even Store Their Shopping in Their Car," *Daily Mail* (London), January 7, 2014, http://www.dailymail.co.uk/news/article-2535136/Average-British -family-home-size-shrinks-two-square-metres-decade-increasing-numbers-forced -live-flats.html.

69. *Property Market Report 2011*, U.K. Valuation Office Agency, 2011, http://www .voa.gov.uk/dvs/_downloads/pmr_2011.pdf. In the northwest, the value of un- equipped dairy land in Cheshire was £14,820 and of land for residential develop- ment in Liverpool £1.5 million. In both cases, I have taken the more valuable kind of agricultural land in the area concerned.

70. Patrick Law of Barratt, email to the author, July 14, 2014.

71. Government data on "average valuations of residential building land with outline planning permission: weighted average valuation per hectare," in England, taken from "Live Tables on Dwelling Stock (including Vacants)," Gov.uk., Table 104.

72. In London, the price rose from £1.9 million per hectare to £6.5 million per hectare in the same period, having peaked at £10.5 million in 2008.

73. Kristian Niemietz, "Abundance of Land, Shortage of Housing," Institute of Economic Affairs Discussion Paper no. 38, April 2012, http://www.iea.org.uk/sites /default/files/publications/files/Abundance%20of%20Land%20Shortage%20of%20 Housing.

74. Randall O'Toole, *American Nightmare: How Government Undermines the Dream of Homeownership* (Washington, D.C.: Cato Institute, 2012), Table 9.1.

75. Ibid., p. 148.

76. O'Toole, *American Nightmare*, p. 149. California: Environmental Quality Act 1969, housing unaffordable by 1979. Oregon: legislation 1973, housing unaffordable by 1979. King County, Washington: urban growth boundary in 1985, housing unaffordable by 1989.

77. I have since researched all the figures except one independently and from official sources. They are slightly different from those cited by Bénard but not significantly so. However, the figure that was most difficult to confirm was the increase in the price of land with permission to build over that period. I spent some hours on this and so did a researcher who speaks French better than I do, but without complete success. Bénard writes that such land rose seven times in value. I have no reason to doubt it, but neither have I been able to confirm it. However, I found another source which refers to a 3.6-times increase in real terms over the period 1997–2011: "Augmentation du prix des terrains à bâtir," SeLoger website (France), http://financer.seloger. com/160465/225429/cnt.htm. That figure, with inflation added back in, would mean a rise of 4.4 times given that the general price level rose from 82 to 100, according to OECD statistics. But the official sources show that land with permission to build rose 7.6 percent between 2010 and 2011, so I have taken that off, which brings the increase to 2010 to 4.06 times. I have then quoted this as a percentage rise of 306 percent—or 300 percent to use a round number. This is used as a minimum that is as reliable as possible under the circumstances. The actual figure may be a great deal bigger, as Bénard asserts. We do have official figures from 2007 that show an increase from €51 to €64 per square meter between 2007 and 2011. That increase of 25 percent may look modest at first glance, but it is actually remarkably strong considering that this was a period of worldwide financial crisis and rising unemployment in France. Here are links to some of the statistics available: http://www.statistiques.developpement -durable.gouv.fr/donnees-ligne/r/enquete-prix-terrains-batir-eptb.html;http:// www.statistiques.developpement-durable.gouv.fr/fileadmin/documents/Produits _editoriaux/Publications/Chiffres_et_statistiques/2013/chiffres-stats473-eptb2012 -decembre2013-v2.pdf.

Chapter 6

1. At the time of writing, he is an associate professor at the Research Institute of Industrial Economics in Stockholm and at the University of Lund.

2. Organisation for Economic Co-operation and Development, *Doing Better for Families* (Paris: OECD Publications, 2011), p. 27.

3. Andrea Cianini, researcher in economic sociology at the Department of Social and Economic Sciences of Sapienza University of Rome, interview with the author at the university.

4. "Birth Summary Tables, England and Wales, 2012," U.K. Office for National Statistics website, http://www.ons.gov.uk/ons/publications/re-reference-tables.html ?edition=tcm%3A77-314475.

5. U.S. Census Bureau, *Statistical Abstract of the United States 2012*, Table 1335, http://www.census.gov/compendia/statab/2012/tables/12s1335.pdf. I have combined this with Eurostat figures that do not go so far back but that go further forward, to 2012, "Live Births outside Marriage," Eurostat, http://epp.eurostat.ec.europa.eu /tgm/table.do?tab=table&plugin=1&language=en&pcode=tps00018.

6. These figures from Eurostat are markedly and surprisingly lower than those supplied by the U.S. Census Bureau, *Statistical Abstract of the United States 2012*, Table 1336, http://www.census.gov/compendia/statab/2012/tables/12s1336.pdf. The link to the Eurostat figures is here: http://ec.europa.eu/eurostat/tgm/table.do?tab =table&init=1&plugin=1&pcode=tps00012&language=en. I guess they have different ways of measurement, but they tell the same story of a rally in the rate of marriage in Sweden.

7. Gundi Knies, "Life Satisfaction and Material Well-being of Children in the U.K.," Institute for Social and Economic Research Working Paper no. 2012-15, July 2012, https://www.iser.essex.ac.uk/publications/working-papers/iser/2012-15.pdf.

8. Ibid.

9. Paul R. Amato, "The Impact of Family Formation Change on the Cognitive, Social, and Emotional Well-Being of the Next Generation," *Marriage and Child Wellbeing* 15 (2005): 75–96. It would appear that Amato is referring to studies that generally did not control for socioeconomic status. If so, it is a pity. However in my book *The Welfare State We're In*, rev. ed. (London: Biteback, 2014), the chapter on parenting refers to numerous studies that did control for socioeconomic status and still found that single parenting and divorce are associated with an increased incidence of the same sort of disadvantages. It can also be argued that single parenting generally results in the child's living in a poorer household so, to this extent, the effect of being poorer should be included as an effect of single parenting.

10. Judith S. Wallerstein and Joan B. Kelly, *Surviving the Breakup: How Children and Parents Cope with Divorce* (New York: Basic, 1996 reprint), p. 73.

11. Ibid., p. 73.

12. Amato, "The Impact of Family Formation Change on the Cognitive, Social, and Emotional Well-Being of the Next Generation," p. 79.

13. Harry Benson, Marriage Foundation research director, in an email to the author. Benson wrote that 21 percent marry and stay married and 14 percent remain living together unmarried. One drawback of this study is that it is based on official figures that count parents who jointly register the birth of a child but who live at separate addresses as "cohabiting." Obviously, this may not be cohabiting. There seems to be a lack of authoritative and reliable research on the subject.

14. Amato, "The Impact of Family Formation Change on the Cognitive, Social, and Emotional Well-Being of the Next Generation."

15. Bryan Rodgers and Jan Prior, *Divorce and Separation: The Outcomes for Children* (York: Joseph Rowntree Foundation, 1998), p. 25, cited in Heather Juby and David F. Farrington, "Disentangling the Link between Disrupted Families and Delinquency," *British Journal of Criminology* 41 (2001): 22–40, http://troublesofyouth.pbworks.com/f /Ruby+and+Farrington.pdf.

16. Israel Kolvin et al., "Social and Parenting Factors Affecting Criminal Offence Rates: Findings from the Newcastle Thousand Family Study (1947–80)," *British Journal of Psychiatry* 152 (1988): 80–90, cited in Juby and Farrington, "Disentangling the Link between Disrupted Families and Delinquency."

17. Juby and Farrington, "Disentangling the Link between Disrupted Families and Delinquency." One should add that in this study, the boys who stayed with their mothers and had no stepfather did as well as boys did in intact families.

18. Linda J. Waite and Maggie Gallagher, *The Case for Marriage: Why Married People Are Happier, Healthier, and Better Off Financially* (New York: Doubleday,

2000), p. 77, cited in Kelly Musick and Larry Bumpass, "Re-examining the Case for Marriage: Union Formation and Changes in Well-being," *Journal of Marriage and Family* 72 (2012): 1–18.

19. Cited by John Cairney et al. in the introduction to "Stress, Social Support, and Depression in Single and Married Mothers," *Social Psychiatry and Psychiatric Epidemiology* 38 (2003): 442–49.

20. L. E. Young, S. L. Cunningham, and D. S. Buist, "Lone Mothers Are at Higher Risk for Cardiovascular Disease Compared with Partnered Mothers: Data from the National Health and Nutrition Examination Survey III (NHANES III)," *Health Care for Women International* 26 (2005): 604–21.

21. Hara Estroff Marano, "Debunking the Marriage Myth: It Works for Women Too," *New York Times*, August 4, 1998, http://smartmarriages.com/debunking.html. The article cites research quoted by Linda J. Waite, a professor of sociology. Waite's book *The Case for Marriage* (with Margaret Gallagher) includes research of these issues.

22. Andrew Steptoe, Panayotes Demakakos, and Cesar de Oliveira, "The Psychological Well-Being, Health and Functioning of Older People in England," in *The Dynamics of Ageing: Evidence from the English Longitudinal Study of Ageing 2002–10 (Wave 5)*, ed. James Banks, James Nazroo, and Andrew Steptoe (London: Institute of Fiscal Studies, 2012), Chapter 4, http://www.ifs.org.uk/elsa/report12/ch4.pdf.

23. Marano, "Debunking The Marriage Myth."

24. The story of Jay Belsky is taken from his own account, "The Politicized Science of Day Care: A Personal and Professional Odyssey," *Family Policy Review* 1 (2003): 23–40, http://kidsfirstcanada.org/politicized-science.pdf.

25. Ibid.

26. See Belsky's CV, http://www.psychology.sunysb.edu/attachment/vitae/belsky_cv.pdf.

27. Belsky, "The Politicized Science of Day Care."

28. Ibid.

29. Jenet Jacob Ericson, "The Effects of Day Care on the Socio-emotional Development of Children," FamilyFacts.org Report no. 2, April 2011, http://www.familyfacts.org/reports/2/the-effects-of-day-care-on-the-social-emotional-development-of-children. This report summarizes 30 years of research but concentrates on the NICHD study.

30. Ibid.

31. Ibid.

32. Ibid.

33. Cited in Lance T. Izumi, "Universal School Programs Don't Recognize the Diversity of Needs," *New York Times*, February 25, 2013, http://www.nytimes.com/roomfordebate/2013/02/25/is-public-preschool-a-smart-investment/universal-school-programs-dont-recognize-the-diversity-of-needs.

34. Ericson, "The Effects of Day Care on the Socio-emotional Development of Children."

35. Ibid., p. 19.

36. Jonas Himmelstrand, "Universal Daycare Leaves Sweden's Children Less Educated," *National Post* (Ontario), April 26, 2011, http://fullcomment.nationalpost.com/2011/04/26/jonas-himmelstrand-two-generations-of-universal-daycare-have-left-sweden's-children-less-educated.

37. Penelope Leach, *Children First: What Society Must Do—and Is Not Doing—for Our Children Today* (London: Penguin, 1994).

38. As described by Jonathan Haidt, *The Happiness Hypothesis: Putting Ancient Wisdom to the Test of Modern Science* (London: Arrow, 2006), p. 111.

39. Ibid., p. 114.

40. I know this from personal experience. When I was taken to nursery school by my father, I revolted and struggled against it to such a degree that the headmistress ended up holding my arms and my father my legs as I kicked and screamed. The story may, of course, have gained in drama as my parents told it in later years, but it is clear that I rebelled sufficiently against being left there to make a notable scene. I then spent a lot of time with the cooks in the kitchen because I did not want to accept going to the school. Meanwhile, I have personal knowledge of a little girl who, deposited at a nursery school, refused to join the others and sat outside in the corridor for her first six months there.

41. Described in Haidt, *The Happiness Hypothesis*, p. 114.

42. Leach, *Children First*, pp. 77–78.

43. For the purposes of this book, 1 euro = 1.10 U.S. dollars.

44. In the United States, if a single mother were to marry a man with a job, the rent would more or less double because the rent in public housing is more or less 28 percent of total household earnings. Additionally, the "tax credit" received by the woman—really a wage subsidy—would disappear because she would be assessed on household income, not her own.

45. Figures from interview with Howard Husock, vice president for policy research at the Manhattan Institute.

Chapter 7

1. The information for this match is from "Blackpool 4 Bolton 3: How the Thrilling Matthews Final Unfolded at Wembley," *Mail* online (London), May 11, 2011, http://www.dailymail.co.uk/sport/football/article-1385690/Blackpool-4-Bolton-3-How-Matthews-Final-unfolded-Wembley.html. This is an abridged version of the *Daily Mail*'s original report on the match. See also "1953 FA Cup Final," Wikipedia, http://en.wikipedia.org/wiki/1953_FA_Cup_Final; "The Matthews Final," BBC Sport online, October 1, 2000, http://news.bbc.co.uk/sport1/hi/in_depth/2000/wembley/936013.stm.

2. "Blackpool 4 Bolton 3."

3. Simon Rice, "The Ten Best Acts of Sportsmanship: Lutz Long," *Independent* (London), November 20, 2009, http://www.independent.co.uk/sport/football/news-and-comment/the-ten-best-acts-of-sportsmanship-1823706.html?action=gallery&ino=3. The Wikipedia entry for Luz Long differs slightly from the version in the *Independent* but is more detailed, http://en.wikipedia.org/wiki/Luz_Long. A *Spiegel* online article casts doubt on the idea that the men became friends, but it confirms the help and the congratulations. It adds that Rudolf Hess was angry about the gesture of congratulations. See Michael Wulzinger, "Hitler's 'Battle of the Colors': Doubt Cast on Olympic Friendship between Owens and Long," January 27, 2012, *Spiegel* (Germany), http://www.spiegel.de/international/zeitgeist/hitler-s-battle-of-the-colors-doubt-cast-on-olympic-friendship-between-owens-and-long-a-811582.html.

4. Rice, "The Ten Best Acts of Sportsmanship."

5. "Bradman, Sir Donald," Australian Inspiration, http://www.australianinspiration .com.au/Quotes/Authors/B/BradmanSirDonald.aspx.

6. John Clark, "Foxsports.com.au Takes a Look at the Greatest Sledges in Cricket History as the India Series Approaches," Fox Sports online, December 13, 2011, http://www.foxsports.com.au/cricket/foxsportscomau-takes-a-look-at-the-greatest -sledges-in-cricket-history/story-e6frf3g3-1225975348816#.UhtHQBttimU.

7. Sunil Gavaskar in the Colin Cowdrey lecture at the Marylebone Cricket Club, 2003. Text available at http://www.espncricinfo.com/wctimeline/content /story/129197.html.

8. Shane Warne, "It Seemed My Sledging Had Gone Too Far When McMillan Stormed in Wielding a Gun," *Mail* online (London), August 26, 2013, http://www.dailymail .co.uk/sport/article-63591/It-sledging-gone-far-McMillan-stormed-wielding-gun .html.

9. Gavaskar, Colin Cowdrey lecture.

10. Clark, "Foxsports.com.au Takes a Look at the Greatest Sledges in Cricket History."

11. Jason Epstein, "A-Rod is Not One of History's Greatest Monsters," *National Review* online, August 12, 2013, http://www.nationalreview.com/article/355495 /rod-not-one-historys-greatest-monsters-jason-epstein.

12. Barbara Holland, *Gentlemen's Blood: A History of Dueling from Swords at Dawn to Pistols at Dusk* (New York: Bloomsbury, 2003).

13. Field Marshal Sir William Slim, *Defeat into Victory* (London: Cassell, 1956).

14. Marcus Aurelius, *The Emperor's Handbook: A New Translation of the Meditations*, tr. C. Scot Hicks and David V. Hicks (New York: Scribner's, 2002), IV.33.

15. *The Book of Common Prayer* has gone through a number of versions. I am not sure in which edition these words were first used, but they were in the book by the time of the 1662 edition.

16. In parallel with the way that the words of confession have been revised over the years, so the words of the L'Oréal slogan have been revised. Originally they were "Because I'm worth it." Then they were changed to "Because you're worth it" in the mid-2000s and again, in 2009, to "Because we're worth it." The slogan thus shifted to involve everybody—or at least every woman—in a sense of original worth, as opposed to original sin. L'Oréal also owns a hair and body products line for children called L'Oréal Kids, the slogan for which is "Because we're worth it too."

17. "At the Movies with Margaret and David," ABC, http://www.abc.net.au /atthemovies/txt/s3235006.htm.

18. I wrote a fuller note on this film on the website www.thewelfarestatewerein .com. Please use the search facility to find the entry.

19. *Reducing Re-offending by Ex-prisoners*, U.K. Social Exclusion Unit, July 2002, http://www.bristol.ac.uk/poverty/downloads/keyofficialdocuments/Reducing%20 Reoffending.pdf.

20. Denis Fougère, Francis Kramarz, and Julien Pouget, "Crime and Unemployment in France," March 2003, http://dev3.cepr.org/meets/wkcn/3/3519/papers /Kramarz.pdf.

21. Povilas Lastauskas and Eirini Tatsi, "Spatial Nexus in Crime and Unemployment in Times of Crisis: Evidence from Germany," Cambridge Working Papers in Economics CWPE 1359, December 2013, http://papers.ssrn.com/sol3/papers .cfm?abstract_id=2365267.

22. An Australian study in 1992 (admittedly rather out of date) asserts that cross-sectional and individual-level studies provide good evidence for the link but that studies over time do not. The evidence for studies over time is mixed. The paper tries to make sense of the paradox by suggesting that female work participation rates, given a "patriarchal society," result in greater opportunities for crime because, for example, children are less supervised and women are putting themselves in more vulnerable situations. John Braithwaite, Bruce Chapman, and Cezary A. Kapuscinski, "Unemployment and Crime: Resolving the Paradox," Australian National University, Canberra, April 1992, http://crg.aic.gov.au /reports/50-89.pdf.

23. Fiona Brookman, *Understanding Homicide* (London: Sage, 2005).

24. This seems intuitively true. A boy who makes an insulting gesture at a teacher or someone in the street would seem more likely to commit a burglary than one who doesn't. But I admit I have not tracked down much academic study of this. One reference I can offer, however, is "Violence and Discipline Problems in U.S. Public Schools: 1996–97," National Center for Education Statistics statistical analysis report, March 1998, http://nces.ed.gov/pubs98/98030.pdf.

25. Allen Beck et al., *Survey of State Prison Inmates, 1991*, U.S. Department of Justice Bureau of Justice Studies, March 1993, http://www.bjs.gov/content/pub/pdf /SOSPI91.PDF.

26. Steven D. Levitt and Lance Lochner, "The Determinants of Juvenile Crime," in *Risky Behavior among Youths: An Economic Analysis*, ed. Jonathan Gruber (Chicago: University of Chicago Press, 2001), http://www.nber.org/chapters/c10692.pdf.

27. *Reducing Re-offending by Ex-prisoners*, U.K. Social Exclusion Unit.

28. According to a 1987 survey, "only one quarter were living with both parents." Andrew Bebbington and John Miles, "The Background of Children Who Enter Local Authority Care," *British Journal of Social Work* 19 (1989): 349–68.

29. One useful study of this sort puts it this way: "The influence of family structure is mediated by family processes," which means, in lay language, that broken families come to be associated with higher adolescent crime through the way the parents tend to supervise the children less and, even more, the way the parents tend to have less close relationships with their children. But the study found that when it came to violent crime, even these and other "processes" could not fully account for the lower rate among the children of married, natural parents. See Stephen Demuth and Susan L. Brown, "Family Structure, Family Processes, and Adolescent Delinquency: The Significance of Parental Absence versus Parental Gender," *Journal of Research in Crime and Delinquency* 41 (2004): 58–81, http://ejournal.narotama.ac.id /files/DeMuthandBrownJRCD%5B1%5D.pdf.

30. "The percent of female-headed households raised the level of social interactions for murder, serious crimes generally, burglary (at the 10 percent level), and larceny." Edward L. Glaeser, Bruce Sacerdote, and José A. Scheinkman, "Crime and Social Interactions," *Quarterly Journal of Economics* 111 (1996): 540–41. In this sentence, the term "social interactions" appears to refer to interactions with people who may influence someone toward crime. They are therefore undesirable interactions. The authors quote from another study in which a young criminal says, "That [the gang] is the only thing I'm connected to. That's my family" (note 29).

31. See for example, "Study Links Crime with Literacy Skills," *BBC News* online, November 3,1998, http://news.bbc.co.uk/1/hi/uk/206732.stm; Christina Clark and

George Dugdale, "Literacy Changes Lives: The Role of Literacy in Offending Behaviour," National Literacy Trust, November 2008, p. 7, http://www.literacytrust.org.uk/assets/0000/0422/Literacy_changes_lives__prisons.pdf. It is also worth noting that an American study stated that black and Hispanic prisoners actually had better literacy than those of the same races who were not in prison. Overall, however, the prison population had lower literacy than the overall U.S. population. See "Literacy Behind Bars: Results from the 2003 National Assessment of Adult Literacy Prison Survey," National Center for Education Statistics, May 2007, http://nces.ed.gov/pubsearch/pubsinfo.asp?pubid=2007473.

32. Mark Morgan and Mary Kett, "The Prison Adult Literacy Survey: Results and Implications," Irish Prison Service, June 2003, http://www.epea.org/uploads/media/Adult_Literacy_Survey.pdf.

33. See Chapter 4 on education.

34. Jonathan Haidt, *The Happiness Hypothesis: Putting Ancient Wisdom to the Test of Modern Science* (London: Arrow, 2006).

35. *Bromley Briefings Prison Factfile June 2011*, Prison Reform Trust, June 2011, p. 52.

36. Ibid.

37. As a journalist, I interviewed fraud teams working for the British Customs and Excise and Inland Revenue departments some years ago.

38. Edgar L. Feige and Richard Cebula, "America's Underground Economy: Measuring the Size, Growth, and Determinants of Income Tax Evasion in the U.S.," Munich Personal RePEc Archive Paper no. 29672, January 2011, http://mpra.ub.uni-muenchen.de/29672/1/MPRA_paper_29672.pdf.

39. *The Economist*, July 20, 2013.

40. Ibid.

41. Gary C. Robb, "Police Use of CCTV Surveillance: Constitutional Implications and Proposed Regulations," *University of Michigan Journal of Law Reform* 13 (1979): 571.

42. Tom Reeve, "How Many Cameras in the U.K.? Only 1.85 Million, Claims ACPO Lead on CCTV," *Security News Desk*, March 1, 2011, http://www.securitynewsdesk.com/2011/03/01/how-many-cctv-cameras-in-the-uk. The effectiveness of cameras in reducing crime is a matter of dispute. It has been claimed that they can achieve a 51 percent reduction in crime in parking lots but that the improvement elsewhere is much more modest. See Brandon C. Welsh and David P. Farrington, "Public Area CCTV and Crime Prevention: An Updated Systematic Review and Meta-analysis," *Justice Quarterly* 26 (2009): 716–45. The report's results appear unconvincing. It seems unlikely that so many cameras would be installed if there were not many people in security who have been convinced that they make a significant difference.

43. Geoffery Li, "Private Security and Public Policing," Statistics Canada, December 2008, http://www.statcan.gc.ca/pub/85-002-x/2008010/article/10730-eng.htm.

44. Ronald van Steden and Rick Sarre, "The Growth of Private Security: Trends in the European Union," *Security Journal* 20 (2007): 222–35.

45. "State-by-State and National Crime Estimates by Year(s)," Uniform Crime Reporting Statistics, http://www.bjs.gov/ucrdata/Search/Crime/State/RunCrimeStatebyState.cfm. These data are "offenses known to law enforcement" and are not based on victim studies.

46. One quickly learns that in the business of levels of crime, there is no such thing as a wholly reliable statistic.

47. For more on this, see my book *The Welfare State We're In*, rev. ed. (London: Biteback, 2014).

48. Charles Murray, *Coming Apart: The State of White America 1960–2010* (New York: Crown Forum, 2012).

Chapter 8

1. I later discover that her title is undersecretary of state for social affairs in the chancellery of the president.

2. Organisation for Economic Co-operation and Development, *Pensions at a Glance 2011: Retirement-Income Systems in OECD and G20 Countries* (Paris: OECD Publishing, 2011), table on p. 155, http://www.oecd-ilibrary.org/docserver/download/8111011e .pdf?expires=1417104070&id=id&accname=guest&checksum=471AAB11D6F95A1A 98702650AB5CD443.

3. For the purposes of this book 1 pound = 1.42 U.S. dollars (exchange rate during March 2016).

4. "Poland," OECD Better Life Index, http://www.oecdbetterlifeindex.org /countries/Poland.

5. Friedrich Schneider, Andreas Buehn, and Claudio E. Montenegro, "Shadow Economies All over the World: New Estimates for 162 Countries from 1999 to 2007," World Bank Policy Research Working Paper 5356, July 2010, http://www-wds.world bank.org/servlet/WDSContentServer/WDSP/IB/2010/10/14/000158349_20101014 160704/Rendered/PDF/WPS5356.pdf. See also Jacek Krawczyński, "The Shadow Economy in Poland: How Payment Systems Help Limit the Shadow Economy," presentation given in Warsaw, September 23, 2009, http://www.konferencje.kmbase.pl /downloads/KrawczynskiEN.pdf.

6. Rebecca Christie and Peter Woodifield, "Europe's $39 Trillion Pension Risk Grows as Economy Falters," *Bloomberg Business*, January 11, 2012, http://www .bloomberg.com/news/2012-01-11/europe-s-39-trillion-pension-threat-grows-as -regional-economies-sputter.html.

7. "World Population Ageing 2009," United Nations Department of Economic and Social Affairs, New York, December 2009, http://www.un.org/esa/population /publications/WPA2009/WPA2009_WorkingPaper.pdf.

8. Christie and Woodifield, "Europe's $39 Trillion Pension Risk Grows as Economy Falters."

9. "Paying for the Past, Providing for the Future: Intergenerational Solidarity," OECD Issues Paper, OECD Ministerial Meeting on Social Policy, Paris, May 2–3, 2011, Session 3, http://www.oecd.org/els/public-pensions/47711990.pdf.

10. Ibid.

11. Richard Jackson, *The Global Retirement Crisis: The Threat to World Stability and What to Do about It* (Washington, D.C.: Center for Strategic and International Studies, 2002), p. 24, http://csis.org/files/media/csis/pubs/global_retirement.pdf.

12. Richard Jackson, senior fellow at the Center for Strategic and International Studies. Testimony before the Commission on Security and Cooperation in Europe, June 20, 2011, http://csis.org/files/ts110620_Jackson.pdf.

13. Wataru Suzuki et al., "Intergenerational Inequality Caused by the Social Security System," ESRI Discussion Paper Series no. 281 (English translation of abstract), January 2012, http://www.esri.go.jp/en/archive/e_dis/abstract/e_dis281-e.html. In

this study, "Intergenerational inequality can be represented by the net benefit rate defined as the ratio of the net benefit by the social security system to the lifetime income." I believe that here social security refers to pensions. I am not sure whether lifetime income refers to total earnings or total contributions to the pension system. If it is the latter, the change is very dramatic. But even if it is the former, the point remains that the later generations are going to do badly compared with the earlier generations.

14. "Paying for the Past, Providing for the Future," OECD.

15. Laurent Mauduit, "La privatisation rampante de la Sécurite sociale," *Marianne* (France), March 25, 2013, http://www.marianne.net/La-privatisation-rampante-de -la-Securite-sociale_a227460.html.

16. Cited in Christie and Woodifield, "Europe's $39 Trillion Pension Risk Grows as Economy Falters."

17. Greece is a dramatic example: "Legislation passed in 2010 reduced state pension benefits, imposed penalties for early retirement and increased average retirement age so that workers must now work for at least 40 years, up from 37. Benefits can now no longer exceed 65 percent of final salary (down from 70 percent) and must be based on average career earnings instead of an average over the final five years of service." David Adams, "A Greek Tragedy," *European Pensions*, November/December 2011, http://www.europeanpensions.net/ep/A-Greek-tragedy.php.

18. "Present value" estimates are calculated using a 2 percent discount rate. The Urban Institute website explains the study used a 2 percent real rate "because it's as good a rate of return as one can expect from a private annuity and not far from a long-term real rate of return on a fairly protected mix of government securities." Furthermore, "you don't want a much lower rate of return because you want to take some account of economic growth. So 2 percent real return seems to us to be a reasonable compromise. The Congressional Budget Office has used a 3 percent rate of return for some of its calculations—a bit high, but in the same ballpark" (http:// www.urban.org/retirees/Estimating-Social-Security.cfm#Q2).

19. The rates of income tax are relatively low, especially for the low paid, which makes up for the higher social security payments. See http://www.expat.hsbc .com/1/PA_ES_Content_Mgmt/content/hsbc_expat/pdf/en/global_tax_navigator /going_to_japan.pdf.

20. In South Korea, 28.8 percent of workers are self-employed compared with 7.0 percent in the United States, 12.3 percent in Japan, and 13.9 percent in Britain, "Underground Economy Amounts to 23% of National GDP in Korea," *BusinessKorea*, March 5, 2013, http://www.businesskorea.co.kr/article/767/underground-economy -amounts-23-national-gdp-korea, citing a report by the Hyundai Research Institute.

21. Schneider, Buehn, and Montenegro, "Shadow Economies All over the World."

22. Ibid.

23. Nina Adam, "Southern Europeans Flock to Germany," *Wall Street Journal*, May 7, 2013, http://online.wsj.com/article/SB10001424127887323372504578466836047 2635932.html.

24. Vivienne Walt, "Forget Paris: Stymied by Socialist Policies, the French Start to Quit France," *Time*, May 21, 2013, http://world.time.com/2013/05/21 /forget-paris-stymied-by-socialist-policies-the-french-start-to-quit-france.

25. Kelly Greene and Vipal Monga, "Workers Saving Too Little to Retire," *Wall Street Journal*, March 19, 2013, http://online.wsj.com/article/SB10001424127887323639 60457836882340639860.6.html.

26. Jill Insley, "Half of U.K. Not Saving Enough for Retirement, Says Study," *Guardian* (London), June 7, 2011, quoting figures given by Tom McPhail of Hargreaves Lansdown, http://www.guardian.co.uk/money/2011/jun/07/half-uk-not-saving-retirement.

27. OECD, *Pensions at a Glance 2011*, p. 149.

28. Daniel Borenstein, "Public Employee Pensions Much Higher than Advertised," *Contra Costa Times* (California), May 2, 2011, http://www.contracostatimes.com/daniel-borenstein/ci_17299237?nclick_check=1.

29. Cited in Steven Malanga, "Pension Propaganda: Don't Believe the Public-Sector Unions When They Say That Worker Pensions Are Modest," *City Journal*, Manhattan Institute, Summer 2011, http://www.city-journal.org/html/pension-propaganda-13407.html.

30. The best possible figure for this does not seem to be easily available so I have had to use an estimate. The Census table referred to in this note shows full-time workers' median earnings of $36,378 for females and $47,127 for males. Weighting the average according to the different numbers creates a figure of $42,404 for both genders. That figure was for 2009. Raising it by 4 percent to get to a 2011 figure brings it to $44,098. I am grateful to Christian Wignall for his help with this. See U.S. Census Bureau, *Statistical Abstract of the United States 2012*, Table 650, http://www.census.gov/compendia/statab/2012/tables/12s0650.pdf.

31. Francis J. Lawall and Justin C. Esposito, "Chapter 9 Bankruptcy of Stockton, Calif., Moves Forward', *Mondaq*, May 24, 2013, http://www.mondaq.com/unitedstates/x/241040/Insolvency+Bankruptcy/Chapter+9+Bankruptcy+Of+Stockton+Calif+Moves+Forward.

32. Eduard Ponds, Clara Severinson, and Juan Yermo, "Funding in Public Sector Pension Plans: International Evidence," OECD Working Papers on Finance, Insurance and Private Pensions no. 8, May 2011, http://www.oecd.org/finance/private-pensions/47827915.pdf.

33. James Bloodworth, February 25, 2013, http://www.leftfootforward.org/2013/02/how-best-to-support-an-ageing-population-more-immigration.

34. The Pensions Commission "Turner Report" commented in 2004, "Only high immigration can produce more than a trivial reduction in the projected dependency ratio over the next 50 years." See "20 Bogus Arguments for Mass Immigration," Migration Watch U.K. website, http://www.migrationwatchuk.co.uk/briefingPaper/document/269, item 12 and footnote 13.

35. OECD, *Pensions at a Glance, 2011*, p. 149.

36. Ibid., p. 272

37. Richard Evans, "Holland's Pensions Superiority Called into Question," *Telegraph* (London), May 12, 2013, http://www.telegraph.co.uk/finance/personal-finance/pensions/10050061/Superiority-of-Dutch-pensions-called-into-question.html.

38. Oonagh McDonald, "Holding Back the Flood," *Financial World* (United Kingdom), November 2012.

39. See Central Provident Fund (CPF) website, http://mycpf.cpf.gov.sg/CPF/About-Us/HistoryofCPF.htm.

40. CPF website: http://mycpf.cpf.gov.sg/CPF/About-Us/Intro/Intro. When the worker turns 55, the money goes into a Retirement Account, subject to various provisions and choices.

41. These rates were new for 2014: see CPF website, http://mycpf.cpf.gov.sg /Employers/Gen-Info/cpf-Contri/ContriRa.htm. When I was in Singapore, the rates were slightly different and the highest rate of contribution to the Special Account was 8 percent. The system is being constantly reviewed and revised.

42. Based on the rate of 1 Singapore dollar = 0.74 U.S. dollar (exchange rate during March 2016).

43. See CPF website, http://mycpf.cpf.gov.sg/Members/Gen-Info/Int-Rates.

44. The minimum is S$20,000 (about US$14,790) in the Ordinary Account and the minimum is S$40,000 (US$29,577) in the Special Account: see "Instruments That Can Be Invested under CPFIS," CPF website, http://mycpf.cpf.gov.sg/NR/rdonlyres /DCD118FF-473E-4A5C-8A0F-322687316646/0/INV_InstrumentsunderCPFIS.pdf.

45. In the Ordinary Account, people have a wider choice of investments than in the Special Account. The rules are quite restrictive in terms of allowing people to choose stocks for themselves. See "Instruments That Can Be Invested under CPFIS."

Most of the money that is eligible to be invested in financial instruments such as unit trusts is not invested in this way but remains on deposit. According to an advertisement by the bank OCBC, in 2005, only S$29 billion of a possible S$104 billion was invested in financial instruments, http://www.ocbc.com/assets/PDF /Retirement_How_to_invest_your_CPF_wisely.pdf.

46. Joaquin Vial Ruiz-Tagle and Francisca Castro, "The Chilean Pension System," OECD Ageing Working Paper AWP5.6 1998. http://www.oecd.org/els /public-pensions/2429310.pdf. Ruiz-Tagle was director of the budget and Castro was counsellor, Ministry of Finance, in Chile.

47. While at the OECD, a senior and notably anti-capitalist employee was positively complacent in dismissing Chile as an idea that had flopped.

48. Australia's superannuation system, started in 1992, is also worth considering. In the relatively short time since its creation, the assets rose to $1.5 trillion, equivalent to the national GDP in 2012. See Martin Parkinson, "Future Challenges: Australia's Superannuation System," speech by secretary to the treasury, Association of Superannuation Funds of Australia national conference, Sydney, November 2012, http://www.treasury.gov.au/PublicationsAndMedia/Speeches/2012/Australias -Superannuation-System. It may be significant that Australia's gross savings rate rose from 21 percent to 25 percent between 2005 and 2012. This savings rate was above that of most comparable countries. For example, here are some rates in 2012: France, 18 percent; Germany, 24 percent; United States, 17 percent; United Kingdom, 11 percent, "Gross Savings (% of GDP)," World Bank website, http://data.worldbank.org /indicator/NY.GNS.ICTR.ZS.

49. In New Zealand a person qualifies for a flat-rate benefit, which varies according to living circumstances such as living alone or with a partner, but not according to income. You must also have lived in New Zealand for at least 10 years since you turned 20 and 5 of those years must be since you turned 50, according to "New Zealand Superannuation Overview," Work and Income (New Zealand) website, http:// www.workandincome.govt.nz/individuals/65-years-or-older/superannuation /superanuation-overview.html. The rate for a single person living alone as of April 1, 2014 was NZ$421.76 (about US$289). Rates table is available at http://www .workandincome.govt.nz/manuals-and-procedures/deskfile/nz_superannuation _and_veterans_pension_tables/new_zealand_superannuation_tables.htm.

Chapter 9

1. Leonardo Fusè, *Parents, Children and Their Families: Living Arrangements of Old People in the XIX Century, Sundsvall Region, Sweden* (Umeå: Umeå University, 2008), http://umu.diva-portal.org/smash/get/diva2:141642/FULLTEXT01.

2. Ilona Ostner et al., "Family Policies in Germany," http://www.york.ac.uk /inst/spru/research/nordic/gerpoli.PDF. The report is undated but it appears to have been written in 2003 or 2004.

3. "Current Conditions and Challenges of Japanese Senior Citizens: Aging of the Elderly Population," JARC website, Japan Aging Research Center, Tokyo, August 27, 2008, http://www.jarc.net/int/?cat=23. The figure is 61.7 percent for 2005.

4. Marie-Eve Joël, Sandrine Dufour-Kippelen, and Sanda Samitca, "The Long-Term Care System for the Elderly in Portugal," ENEPRI Research Report no. 84, June 2010, http://www.ceps.eu/book/long-term-care-system-elderly-portugal; Norma K. Raffel and Marshall W. Raffel, "Elderly Care: Similarities and Solutions in Denmark and the United States," *Public Health Reports* 102 (1987): 494–500.

5. Raffel and Raffel, "Elderly Care."

6. It is true that the proportion of elderly living with their children has fallen. "The proportion living alone has increased steadily since 1960, at an estimated rate of about 1 percent a year," Alberto Palloni, "Living Arrangements of Older Persons," *Population Bulletin of the United Nations* 42–3 (2002), http://www.un.org/esa /population/publications/bulletin42_43/palloni.pdf. It is also true that government provision was increased and changed in 2000, although this was scaled back somewhat in 2005 because of the rising cost. Japan introduced a long-term care insurance program, which involves means testing and assessment of the physical and other needs of the elderly person. I suspect the terms are quite strict and so, despite this extra provision, there is still more incentive in Japan than elsewhere for children to take responsibility for their parents. In any case, most of the statistics in this chapter predate the 2000 reform or were produced not very long after it.

It used to be a matter of shame if a family failed to look after its elderly. Scandals of families not looking after their elderly well presumably encouraged the new government provision. But it must surely be difficult to know how widespread the problem truly was. See Mayumi Hayashi, "The Care of Older People in Japan: Myths and Realities of Family 'Care,'" History and Policy website, June 3, 2011, http://www .historyandpolicy.org/papers/policy-paper-121.html.

"The number of elders receiving care at home—compared to institutions—is high. A total of 12.6 percent of the population over the age of 65 received long-term care, of which 2.8 percent in institutions (4 percent OECD average) and 9.8 percent at home (OECD average 7.9 percent) in 2011 (OECD Health Data 2012)." See "Japan: Highlights from *A Good Life in Old Age? Monitoring and Improving Quality in Long-term Care*, OECD Publishing, 2013," OECD website, http://www.oecd.org/els/health -systems/Japan-OECD-EC-Good-Time-in-Old-Age.pdf.

7. Gary V. Engelhardt and Nadia Greenhalgh-Stanley, "Public Long-term Care Insurance and the Housing and Living Arrangements of the Elderly: Evidence from Medicare Home Health Benefits," Care for Retirement Research Working Papers, December 2008, http://crr.bc.edu/working-papers/public-long-term-care -insurance-and-the-housing-and-living-arrangements-of-the-elderly-evidence -from-medicare-home-health-benefits.

8. Pew Research Center, "The Return of the Multigenerational Family Household," Social and Demographic Trends Report, March 18, 2010, http://www.pewsocialtrends.org/2010/03/18/the-return-of-the-multi-generational-family-household. "Multigenerational" here means "at least two adult generations or a grandparent and at least one other generation."

9. For example, the EU treats publicly provided care for the elderly as a human right rather than merely a good thing and suggests that for the poor it should be free or low cost. See "The Future of Health Care and Care for the Elderly: Guaranteeing Accessibility, Quality, and Financial Viability," Europa website, http://europa.eu/legislation_summaries/employment_and_social_policy/disability_and_old_age/c11310_en.htm. That is easy for a supranational organization to say when it does not have to raise the money and appears uninterested in the choice of individual elderly people or the fact that paying for one person's elderly care means taking money from another's. The OECD, to be fair, takes a more realistic approach. However, it tends to take for granted the idea of government care and to call for more regulation and better statistics rather than to review the big picture and ask whether its dream system of highly regulated care by well-qualified people is either affordable or wholly desirable.

10. Survey by the Japanese Ministry of Health, Labour and Welfare's Health and Welfare Bureau for the Elderly. In the survey, 46 percent chose "Receive long-term care at home if there are services that enable me to live at home independently of my family members"; 24 percent chose "Live at home receiving combination of external long-term care services and care by my family"; 4 percent chose "Live at home receiving care by mainly my family." As for those who preferred institutional care, 12 percent chose "Move into fee charging home for the aged or house for the elderly with care to receive long-term care"; 7 percent chose "Stay in special nursing home or other facility for the elderly to receive long-term care"; 2 percent chose "Stay in the hospital to receive long-term care." I do not know what age group was asked this question or what the participants thought of as being "long-term care," which might be somewhat different from what people have in mind in Britain or America or elsewhere. The figures appeared on the slides of a talk given by Masahiko Hayashi, deputy assistant minister for international affairs at the Ministry of Health, Labour and Welfare. The talk was given at the Daiwa Anglo-Japanese Foundation on November 6, 2013.

11. A blog for the *New York Times* refers to a study that says that money influences the decision. Paula Span, "They Don't Want to Live with You Either," New Old Age blog, March 24, 2009, http://newoldage.blogs.nytimes.com/2009/03/24/they-dont-want-to-live-with-you-either/?_php=true&_type=blogs&_r=0. I agree. But the blog does not refer to any research into what the elderly actually want. It is conceivable that some of the elderly do not want to impose on their children but that, in taking that view, they are condemning themselves to lonely isolation. Even if they do not want to live in the same household, they might well like to live close by so that they can see their children and grandchildren easily and often.

12. "Having access to practical help from others was not related to happiness, but levels of loneliness and self-esteem were," John T. Cacioppo and William Patrick, *Loneliness: Human Nature and the Need for Social Connection* (New York: W. W. Norton, 2008), p. 218, referring to evaluations of older people.

13. Ibid., p. 93, citing research covered by *Science* magazine.

14. Ibid., p. 94, citing research by psychologist Dan Russell and colleagues.

15. Joseph E. Gaugler et al., "Predicting Nursing Home Admission in the U.S.: A Meta-analysis," *BMC Geriatrics* 7 (2007): 13.

16. Cacioppo and Patrick, *Loneliness*, p. 94.

17. For example, "An elderly person living alone increased his or her likelihood of institutionalization by 1.79 times compared with an elderly person living with his or her spouse." Ulrike Steinbach, "Social Networks, Institutionalization, and Mortality among Elderly People in the United States," *Journal of Gerontology* 47 (1992): S183–S190.

18. Judith D. Kasper, Liliana E. Pezzin, and J. Bradford Rice, "Stability and Changes in Living Arrangements: Relationship to Nursing Home Admission and Timing of Placement," *Journal of Gerontology: Social Sciences* 65 B:6 (2010): 783–91.

19. All the more so considering that the results are controlled for factors such as income.

20. F. A. McDougall et al., "Prevalence and Symptomatology of Depression in Older People Living in Institutions in England and Wales," *Age and Ageing* 36 (2007): 562–68. This study does not seem to state explicitly that those who are at home are both those living alone and those with family, but it appears to be the case. The main focus of the study is the condition of people in institutions.

21. Christine Smoliner et al., "Malnutrition and Depression in the Institution-alised Elderly," *British Journal of Nutrition* 102 (2009): 1663–67.

22. Ibid.

23. Ibid.

24. Quite bizarrely, the report does not highlight this appalling finding and even reverses the emphasis by saying that 62 percent of inpatients said they "always" got enough help with feeding. Care Quality Commission, *The State of Health Care and Adult Social Care in England: An Overview of Key Themes in Care in 2011/12*, November 2012, HC 763, http://www.cqc.org.uk/sites/default/files/documents/cqc__soc_201112_final_tag.pdf.

25. Chris Smyth, "NHS Care of Elderly: The Scandal Gets Worse," the *Times* (London), October 13, 2011, http://www.thetimes.co.uk/tto/health/news/article3192887.ece.

26. Daniel Martin, "Frail Elderly Patients 'Left to Starve in Hospitals,' Admit More than Two-Thirds of NHS Nurses," *Daily Mail* (London), August 31, 2010, http://www.dailymail.co.uk/health/article-1307250/Frail-elderly-patients-left-hungry-hospitals-admit-thirds-NHS-nurses.html.

27. On looking more closely at the actual report, it seems that a more precise figure for those not treated with proper respect was actually 9 percent rather than 10 (p. 42). The report sometimes uses rounded up numbers and in other places shows more precise numbers. Some things are either not measured or the figures are not revealed. For example, no patient survey figure of whether patients had enough help with feeding in private hospitals is given

28. J. Kayser-Jones et al., "Factors Contributing to Dehydration in Nursing Homes: Inadequate Staffing and Lack of Professional Supervision," *Journal of the American Geriatrics Society* 47 (1999): 1187–94.

29. Sandra F. Simmons, Cathy Alessi, and John F. Schnelle, "An Intervention to Increase Fluid Intake in Nursing Home Residents: Prompting and Preference Compliance," *Journal of the American Geriatrics Society* 49 (2001): 926–33.

30. Lani G. Gallagher, *The High Cost of Poor Care: The Financial Case for Prevention in American Nursing Homes*, National Consumer Voice for Quality Long-term Care, April 2011, http://theconsumervoice.org/uploads/files/issues/The-High-Cost-of-Poor-Care.pdf.

31. Ibid.

32. Ibid., citing Vicky Lyman, "Successful Heel Pressure Ulcer Prevention Program in a Long-term Care Setting," *Journal of Wound Ostomy and Continence Nursing* 36 (2009): 616–21.

33. Daniel R. Levinson, "Medicare Atypical Antipsychotic Drug Claims for Elderly Nursing Home Residents," U.S. Department of Health and Human Services, May 2011, http://oig.hhs.gov/oei/reports/oei-07-08-00150.pdf.

34. Ibid.

35. Sophie Borland, "One in Four Dementia Sufferers Prescribed Dangerous 'Chemical Cosh' Drugs Which Are Only Meant as a Last Resort," *Daily Mail* (London), February 21, 2012, http://www.dailymail.co.uk/health/article-2103979/One-dementia-sufferers-prescribed-dangerous-chemical-cosh-drugs-meant-resort.html.

36. See, for example, Jane Worroll, "'I Used a Spy Camera to Catch a Care Home Thug Beating Up My Mother': How a Daughter's Suspicions Lead to Her Uncovering Harrowing Abuse," *Daily Mail* (London), April 23, 2012, http://www.dailymail.co.uk/news/article-2133673/BBC-One-Panorama-Undercover--Elderly-Care-Ash-Court-residents-daughter-uncovers-harrowing-abuse.html.

37. James Slack and Ryan Kisiel, "Profits before Patients: Care Home Residents Subjected to Horrific Abuse Went to A&E 76 Times in Three Years—But Private Owner Did Nothing," *Daily Mail* (London), August 8, 2012, http://www.dailymail.co.uk/news/article-2184892/Winterbourne-View-abuse-report-Pinned-slapped-doused-water.html.

38. "73 Percent of Councils Still Commission 15 Minute Care Visits," press release, Unison website, June 17, 2013, http://www.unison.org.uk/news/73-of-councils-still-commission-15-minute-care-visits. In theory, this is the minimum, but it is thought that it tends to become the norm.

39. Ibid.

40. "America's Long-Term Care Crisis: Challenges in Financing and Delivery," Bipartisan Policy Center, April 2014, http://bipartisanpolicy.org/wp-content/uploads/2014/03/BPC-Long-Term-Care-Initiative.pdf.

41. Pedro Olivares-Tirado et al., "Predictors of the Highest Long-Term Care Expenditures in Japan," *BMC Health Services Research* 11 (2011): 103, http://www.biomedcentral.com/1472-6963/11/103.

42. Christine de la Maisonneuve and Joaquim Oliveira Martins, "Public Spending on Health and Long-Term Care: A New Set of Projections," OECD Economic Policy Papers no. 6, June 2013, http://www.oecd.org/eco/growth/Health%20FINAL.pdf.

43. Richard Cracknell, "The Ageing Population," House of Commons Library Research, http://www.parliament.uk/documents/commons/lib/research/key_issues/Key-Issues-The-ageing-population2007.pdf.

44. *Statistical Handbook of Japan 2014*, Statistics Japan website, Table 2.2, http://www.stat.go.jp/english/data/handbook/c0117.htm#c02. This table compares the proportion of population over age 65 with that of ages 15 to 64.

45. *Caring for Older Australians: Productivity Commission Inquiry Report*, June 2011, vol. 1, Chapter 5: "Assessment of the current aged care system," http://www.pc.gov .au/__data/assets/pdf_file/0004/110929/aged-care-volume1.pdf.

46. Esther Mot is at the CPB Netherlands Bureau for Economic Policy Analysis.

47. Jane Kelly, "It's Time to Admit It: The NHS Is Unable to Look after Our Elderly," the *Spectator* (London), May 18, 2013, http://www.spectator.co.uk/features/8909201 /among-the-bed-blockers.

48. Ibid.

49. "Who Needs Care?," Longtermcare.gov, http://longtermcare.gov/the-basics/ who-needs-care.

50. "Man Lay Dead for Three Years," *Stockholm News*, March 26, 2011, http:// stockholmnews.com.preview.binero.se/more.aspx?NID=6955.

51. "Stockholm Man Lay Dead in Flat for Two Years," *The Local* (Sweden), May 22, 2013, http://www.thelocal.se/20130522/48062.

52. Justin Nobel, "Japan's Lonely Deaths: A Business Opportunity," *Time*, April 6, 2010, http://www.time.com/time/world/article/0,8599,1976952,00.html?xid= rss-topstories.

53. "Current Conditions and Challenges of Japanese Senior Citizens."

54. Kleinhubbert and Windmann, "Alone by the Millions."

55. A 1994 survey claimed that one in three acknowledge feelings of "hatred," according to Hayashi, "The Care of Older People in Japan."

56. Conversation with Francesco Maietta of Censis, a socioeconomic research institute in Rome; see also Daniel González, "Italy Grants Special Treatment to Needed Immigrants," AZCentral.com, http://www.azcentral.com/news/articles/global -immigration-italy-domestic.html.

57. My informant was Francesco Maietta. The lower estimate comes from Claudia Villosio and Giulia Bizzotto, "Once There Were Wives and Daughters; Now There Are *Badanti*," WALQING Social Partnership Series, September 2011, http://www .walqing.eu/fileadmin/download/external_website/WALQING_SocialPartnership Series_2011.14_ElderlyCare_ITA.pdf. They suggest there are 684,000 immigrant caregivers.

58. "No Room for Mum and Dad: Less than 30% of Adults Would Look After Their Parents," Care U.K. website, July 30, 2014. http://www.careuk.com/news /no-room-mum-and-dad-less-30-adults-would-look-after-their-parents.

Chapter 10

1. George Orwell, *Animal Farm* (London: Secker and Warburg, 1945). *Animal Farm* was an allegory of Soviet communism. The political elite who took over the farm soon found ways to give themselves privileges.

2. "David Cameron's Speech on Public Service," *Guardian*, June 6, 2006, http:// www.guardian.co.uk/politics/2006/jun/06/publicservices.conservatives.

3. Eduardo Porter, "Health Care and Profits, a Poor Mix," *New York Times*, January 8, 2013, http://www.nytimes.com/2013/01/09/business/health-care-and -pursuit-of-profit-make-a-poor-mix.html?pagewanted=all&_r=0.

4. The description of the "rubber rooms" and the statistics are taken from Terry M. Moe, *Special Interest: Teachers Unions and America's Public Schools* (Washington, D.C.: Brookings Institution, 2011).

5. Ibid.

6. Ibid.

7. Karl Weber, "A Nation Still at Risk," in *Waiting for "Superman": How We Can Save America's Failing Public Schools*, ed. Karl Weber (New York: Public Affairs, 2010), p. 7.

8. "Michelle Apperson, Teacher of the Year, Gets Lay-Off Notice from Sacramento School District Amid Budget Cuts," *HuffPost Education*, June 15, 2012, http://www.huffingtonpost.com/2012/06/15/michelle-apperson-teacher_n_1601015.html.

9. Eric Hanushek, "The Difference is Great Teachers," in *Waiting for "Superman": How We Can Save America's Failing Public Schools*, ed. Karl Weber (New York: Public Affairs, 2010), pp. 81–100.

10. In the 1950s, teachers unions had little power. Schools were dominated by administrators. Then in the 1960s, the unions began to establish themselves. States began to adopt laws that allowed, or even promoted, collective bargaining for public employees. Teachers unions could disrupt schooling. The public schools were, in each state, a monopoly. The customers of the schools, the state and the parents, could not go elsewhere. So the unions got their way. The next stage came through the rising dues from their members. They were able to use the money to buy political influence. The teachers unions have been the biggest contributors of all to politicians in federal elections. They have bought power and used it to protect their members and, in the process, damage the education of children.

11. Moe, *Special Interest*, pp. 36, 37.

12. Ibid., pp. 282, 283.

13. The teachers unions have also opposed the creation of charter schools and schools funded by tax credits—schools that have given choice to poor people, something that was previously available only to the rich. It is easy to suspect that their motivation for doing so is not, as they claim, the well-being of students but the maintenance of their own power and income.

14. Thomas Frank, "States Expand Lucrative Pensions to More Jobs," *USA Today*, December 9, 2011, http://usatoday30.usatoday.com/news/nation/story/2011-12-08/state-pensions-workers/51750670/1?loc=interstitialskip.

15. Ibid. They rose from 48,188 to 75,135.

16. Ibid. The number of workers eligible for enhanced or early retirement rose from 59,685 to 77,394.

17. "Government Employees in Ontario Earn 14 Per Cent More Than Private-Sector Workers," Fraser Institute website, February 20, 2013, http://www.fraserinstitute.org/research-news/news/news-releases/Government-employees-in-Ontario-earn-14-per-cent-more-than-private-sector-workers. The exact figures are 97.3 percent of public sector employees and 53.5 percent of those in the private sector.

18. Ibid. In the public sector, 0.7 percent lose their jobs compared with 3.9 percent in the private sector.

19. Jason Clemens, Amela Karabegović, and Milagros Palacios, "Comparing Public and Private Sector Compensation in Ontario," Fraser Institute, February 2013, http://www.fraserinstitute.org/uploadedFiles/fraser-ca/Content/research-news/research/publications/comparing-public-and-private-sector-compensation-in-ontario.pdf.

20. Maury Gittleman and Brooks Pierce, "Compensation for State and Local Government Workers," *Journal of Economic Perspectives* 26 (2012): 217–42.

The researchers admitted that the figures are not definitive for a number of reasons, including gaps in the information they can obtain. But they added, "The data suggest that public sector workers, especially local government ones, on average, receive greater remuneration than observably similar private sector workers. Overturning this result would require, we think, strong arguments for particular model specifications, or different data."

21. Ed Holmes and Matt Oakley, "Public and Private Sector Terms, Conditions and the Issue of Fairness," Policy Exchange research note, Policy Exchange, London, May 2011, http://www.policyexchange.org.uk/images/publications/public%20 and%20private%20sector%20terms%20conditions%20and%20the%20issue%20of%20 fairness%20-%20may%2011.pdf.

22. For the purposes of this book, 1 euro = 1.10 U.S. dollars (exchange rate in March 2016).

23. Michael Lewis, "Beware of Greeks Bearing Bonds," *Vanity Fair*, October 1, 2010, http://www.vanityfair.com/business/features/2010/10/greeks-bearing-bonds-201010.

24. Colin Robinson, "Liberalisation of the Energy Market: A Favourable Supply-side Shock for the U.K. Economy?," Surrey Energy Economics Centre, June 1994, http://www.seec.surrey.ac.uk/research/SEEDS/SEEDS73.pdf. The figure of 91,500 employees was for 1986.

25. Ibid.

26. Eliana Johnson, "IRS Paying Over 200 Employees to Work Full-Time for Labor Union," *National Review*, July 8, 2014, http://www.nationalreview.com /corner/352876/irs-paying-over-200-employees-work-full-time-labor-union-eliana -johnson. In Spain, even private companies are obliged by law to pay for full-time trade union employees.

27. Adrian T. Moore, "Private Prisons: Quality Corrections at a Lower Cost," Policy Study no. 240, Reason Foundation, Los Angeles, April 1998, http://reason.org /files/d14ffa18290a9aeb969d1a6c1a9ff935.pdf.

28. Ibid., p. 18.

29. "The Life Programme," Participle website, www.participle.net. The time spent in the family home might be thought to be the most useful, but "the majority of this time was spent collecting information and data to fulfil the reporting duties."

30. "Getting IT," *The Economist*, October 17, 2002, http://www.economist.com /node/1394744.

31. Ibid.

32. For the purposes of this book, 1 pound = 1.42 U.S. dollars (exchange rate in March 2016).

33. "Getting IT," *The Economist*.

34. Ted Ritter, "Secret Papers Reveal Blair's Rushed NPfIT Plans," *Computer Weekly*.com, February 18, 2008, http://www.computerweekly.com/blogs/public -sector/2008/02/secret-papers-reveal-blairs-ru.html.

35. *Le Point* (France), June 27 2013, http://boutique.lepoint.fr/fonctionnaires -les-chouchous-du-pouvoir-596

36. Blake Hurst, "An Imaginary Dustup? The Incalculable Harm of Regulation," *The American*, January 8, 2012, http://www.american.com/archive/2012/january /an-imaginary-dustup-the-incalculable-harm-of-regulation.

37. Ibid.

38. Edward Cody, "Seven Peculiar Rules Imposed on the French," WorldViews blog, *Washington Post*, April 16, 2013, http://www.washingtonpost.com/blogs /worldviews/wp/2013/04/16/seven-peculiar-rules-imposed-on-the-french.

39. "Ces bureaucrates qui nous tyrannisent," *Le Point* (France), March 21, 2013.

40. Ibid.

41. Ibid.

42. Graham Ruddick, "U.K. Planning Laws 'A Living Nightmare,' says Red-row founder Steve Morgan," *Telegraph* (London), September 9, 2011, http://www .telegraph.co.uk/finance/newsbysector/constructionandproperty/8751013/UK -planning-laws-a-living-nightmare-says-Redrow-founder-Steve-Morgan.html.

43. David Barrett, "Police Red Tape Revealed: Reams of Paperwork to Look through a Window," *Telegraph* (London), October 16, 2010, http://www.telegraph .co.uk/news/uknews/law-and-order/8068202/Police-red-tape-revealed-reams-of -paperwork-to-look-through-a-window.html.

44. Gregory Viscusi and Mark Deen, "Why France Has So Many 49-Employee Companies," *Bloomberg Businessweek*, May 3, 2012, http://www.businessweek.com /articles/2012-05-03/why-france-has-so-many-49-employee-companies.

45. Michael Howard, "Keep the Bureaucrats' Hands off Our Hospices," *Times* (London), December 18, 2012. Lord Howard, chairman of Help the Hospices, was previously a senior government minister and then leader of the Conservative Party.

46. Ibid.

47. Edward L. Glaeser, "Growth Engines," *City Journal*, Manhattan Institute, Special Issue 2013, http://www.city-journal.org/2013/special-issue_small -businesses.html.

48. Giuseppe Nicoletti and Stefano Scarpetta, "Regulation, Productivity, and Growth: OECD evidence," World Bank Policy Research Working Papers, January 2003, http://elibrary.worldbank.org/doi/pdf/10.1596/1813-9450-2944.

49. John Dawson and John Seater, "Federal Regulation and Aggregate Economic Growth," *Journal of Economic Growth* 18 (2013): 137–77, http://www4.ncsu .edu/~jjseater/regulationandgrowth.pdf.

50. "Ease of Doing Business Index," World Bank website, http://data.worldbank .org/indicator/IC.BUS.EASE.XQ/countries/1W?display=default.

51. "Gross Domestic Product," Geostat website, http://geostat.ge/index .php?action=page&p_id=119&lang=eng.

52. "The 'Progressive' IRS," *New York Post*, June 28, 2013, http://nypost .com/2013/06/28/the-progressive-irs.

53. Quoted in "Where's the Special Prosecutor? The IRS Scandal Demands an Independent Investigation," *Chicago Tribune*, June 30, 2013, http:// articles.chicagotribune.com/2013-06-30/opinion/ct-edit-irs-20130630_1_new-irs -conservative-groups-irs-scandal.

54. Timothy Hinks and Artjoms Ivlevs, "Communist Party Membership and Bribe Paying in Transitional Economies," University of the West of England Economics Working Papers Series 1401, 2014, http://www2.uwe.ac.uk/faculties/BBS /BUS/Research/Economics%20Papers%202014/1401.pdf.

55. In Western Europe, the probability of having to pay a bribe is 0.53 percent, compared with 4.55 percent in the "transitional economies" (Ibid., Table 1).

"Communism created structural incentives for engaging in corrupt behaviors, which became such a widespread fact of life that they became rooted in the culture in these societies" Wayne Sandholtz and Rein Taagepera, "Corruption, Culture, and Communism," *International Review of Sociology* 15 (2005): 109–31. Note also a study of bribery in Uganda in which the author remarks, "Firms typically have to pay bribes when dealing with public officials whose actions directly affect the firms' business operations." Jakob Svensson, "Who Must Pay Bribes and How Much? Evidence from a Cross-section of Firms," Institute for International Economics Studies, Stockholm University, May 2012, available at http://www.diva-portal.org/smash /get/diva2:343782/FULLTEXT01.pdf.

56. Matt Chorley, "Revealed: The Health Bosses Who Ordered Cover-Up at Hospital Unit Where 16 Babies Died Are Finally Named and Shamed," *Daily Mail* (London), June 20, 2013, http://www.dailymail.co.uk/news/article-2345216 /REVEALED-The-health-bosses-ordered-cover-hospital-unit-16-babies-died-finally -named-shamed.html.

57. "Mid Staffordshire Trust Inquiry: How the Care Scandal Unfolded," *Telegraph* (London), February 6, 2013, http://www.telegraph.co.uk/health /healthnews/9851763/Mid-Staffordshire-Trust-inquiry-how-the-care-scandal -unfolded.html.

58. Andrew Gilligan, "NHS bureaucrats Care for Themselves, Not the Patients," *Telegraph* (London), April 9, 2010, http://www.telegraph.co.uk/health/7569995 /NHS-bureaucrats-care-for-themselves-not-the-patients.html. See also the official report at http://www.midstaffspublicinquiry.com/report.

59. Sebastián Galiani, Paul Gertler, and Ernesto Schargrodsky, "Water for Life: The Impact of the Privatization of Water Services on Child Mortality," *Journal of Political Economy* 113 (2005): 83–120.

60. Ibid.

61. Stuart Holder, "Privatisation and Competition: The Evidence from Utility and Infrastructure Privatisation in the U.K.," 12th plenary session of the Organisation for Economic Co-operation and Development Advisory Group on Privatisation, Helsinki, September 17–18, 1998, p. 20, http://www.oecd.org/daf/ca/corporate governanceofstate-ownedenterprises/1929658.pdf.

62. Ibid.

63. "El 82% de los funcionarios se decanta por la sanidad privada," *Libre Mercado* (Spain), February 11, 2014, http://www.libremercado.com/2014-02-11 /el-82-de-los-funcionarios-se-decanta-por-la-sanidad-privada-1276510463.

64. I gave an example of this phenomenon in *The Welfare State We're In*. A baby died unnecessarily in a private hospital. It was front-page news and was commented on extensively. However at a similar time, there were cases of several unnecessary deaths of babies in NHS hospitals that barely got into the news at all.

65. For the pensions system in Australia, see Pensionfundsonline, http://www .pensionfundsonline.co.uk/content/country-profiles/australia/80, and for Hong Kong, see Pensionfundsonline, http://www.pensionfundsonline.co.uk/content /country-profiles/hong-kong/104.

66. Karin Svanborg-Sjövall, "Privatising the Swedish Welfare State," *Economic Affairs* 34 (2014): 181–92. The article adds, "Welfare quasi-markets are increasingly subject to input-related regulation and control."

Chapter 11

1. In theory, at least, a bachelor's degree or *laurea* takes three years. Then there is a *laurea magistrale*, equivalent to a master's degree, which takes two more years, to be followed by a *dottorato di ricerca*, equivalent to a PhD, which takes another three to four years. Because secondary school continues until a person is 19, this program would easily take someone to the age of 28 or even 30, if one were allowed to progress more slowly. I am not sure how the attempt to reduce the years of study is currently working in practice, but my informants clearly thought that for many people things had not changed very much.

2. Dick M. Carpenter II, "Blooming Nonsense," *Regulation*, Spring 2011, http://object.cato.org/sites/cato.org/files/serials/files/regulation/2011/4/regv34n1-8.pdf. Carpenter is director of strategic research at the Institute for Justice and an associate professor at the University of Colorado.

3. Morris M. Kleiner and Alan B. Krueger, "Analyzing the Extent and Influence of Occupational Licensing on the Labor Market," *Journal of Labor Economics* 31 (2013): S173–S202, http://www.hhh.umn.edu/people/mkleiner/pdf/Final.occ.licensing.JOLE.pdf.

4. Adam B. Summers, "Occupational Licensing: Ranking the States and Exploring Alternatives," Policy Study 361, Reason Foundation, Los Angeles, August 2007, http://reason.org/files/762c8fe96431b6fa5e27ca64eaa1818b.pdf

5. Perdido Productions, 2013.

6. David E. Bernstein, *Only One Place of Redress: African Americans, Labor Regulations, and the Courts from Reconstruction to the New Deal* (Durham, NC: Duke University Press, 2001).

7. Ibid., p. 38.

8. Ibid.

9. David Green, *Working-Class Patients and the Medical Establishment: Self-Help in Britain from the Mid-Nineteenth Century to 1948* (Aldershot, U.K.: Gower/Maurice Temple Smith, 1985), p. 46.

10. "In 1911 and 1946 the government of the day needed professional cooperation, and paid their asking price." David Green, "Medical Care without the State," in *Re-Privatising Welfare: After the Lost Century*, ed. Arthur Seldon (London: Institute of Economic Affairs, 1996). p. 186.

11. Clayton Christensen, "The Future of Medical Education," in Clayton M. Christensen, Jerome H. Grossman, and Jason Hwang, *The Innovator's Prescription: A Disruptive Solution for Health Care* (New York: McGraw-Hill, 2009).

12. Kleiner and Krueger, "Analyzing the Extent and Influence of Occupational Licensing on the Labor Market."

13. Ibid.

14. *Report of the Mid Staffordshire NHS Foundation Trust Public Inquiry, vol. 1: Analysis of Evidence and Lessons Learned (Part 1)*, HC898-I, February 2013, p. 118, http://www.midstaffspublicinquiry.com/sites/default/files/report/Volume%201.pdf.

15. *Independent Inquiry into Care Provided by Mid Staffordshire NHS Foundation Trust January 2005–March 2009*, vol. 1, HC 375-I, February 2010, p. 57, http://webarchive.nationalarchives.gov.uk/20130107105354/http://www.dh.gov.uk/prod_consum_dh/groups/dh_digitalassets/@dh/@en/@ps/documents/digitalasset/dh_113447.pdf.

16. Ibid.

17. "Patients 'routinely neglected' at Stafford Hospital," *Telegraph* (London), February 24, 2010, http://www.telegraph.co.uk/health/healthnews/7306347/Patients -routinely-neglected-at-Stafford-Hospital.html. This newspaper report has it in indirect quotes but another report, which I now cannot find, had it in direct quotes.

18. Sophie Borland, "Trainee Nurses 'Spend Too Long in Lecture Halls and Not Enough Time with Patients,'" *Daily Mail* (London), September 23, 2011, http://www .dailymail.co.uk/health/article-2040825/Trainee-nurses-spend-time-patients.html.

19. For the purposes of this book, 1 pound = 1.42 U.S. dollars (exchange rate in March 2016).

20. "What a Waste! The NHS Spends Millions on Training, but We Are Recruiting from Overseas," *Daily Mail* online (London), January 22, 2007, http://www .dailymail.co.uk/health/article-430676/What-waste-The-NHS-spends-millions -training-recruiting-overseas.html.

21. Celia Hall, "NHS Cuts 'Leave New Nurses without Jobs,'" *Telegraph* (London), April 26, 2006.

22. Cited in Kleiner and Krueger, "Analyzing the Extent and Influence of Occupational Licensing on the Labor Market."

23. Rita Kramer, *Ed School Follies: The Miseducation of America's Teachers* (New York: Free Press, 1991).

24. Roderick Hooker, James Cawley, and David Aprey, "Economic Assessment of Physician Assistants," in *Physician Assistants: Policy and Practice*, 3rd ed. (Philadelphia: F. A. Davis, 2010).

25. James Cawley, in email to the author.

26. Victoria Stagg Elliott, "Number of Physician Assistants Doubles over Past Decade," amednews.com, American Medical Association, September 27, 2011, http://www.amednews.com/article/20110927/business/309279997/8.

27. Jacob Goldstein, "So You Think You Can Be a Hair Braider?," *New York Times Magazine*, June 12, 2012, http://www.nytimes.com/2012/06/17/magazine/so-you -think-you-can-be-a-hair-braider.html?pagewanted=all&_r=0.

28. Kleiner and Krueger, "Analyzing the Extent and Influence of Occupational Licensing on the Labor Market."

29. Union membership in the United States stood at 12 percent in 2008.

30. "Our History," ACCA website, Association of Chartered Certified Accountants, http://www.accaglobal.com/uk/en/discover/about/history.html. Also conversation with and email from Colin Davis at the ACCA.

31. Based on 1 guinea = 1.05 pounds and 1 pound = 1.42 U.S. dollars (exchange rate in March 2016).

32. "Rules for fools," *The Economist*, May 12, 2011, http://www.economist.com /node/18678963.

Chapter 12

1. Heritage History on Clodius, http://www.heritage-history.com/www /heritage.php?Dir=characters&FileName=clodius.php.

2. Ibid.

3. H. H. Scullard, *From the Gracchi to Nero: A History of Rome from 133 BC to AD 68* (Abingdon, U.K.: Routledge [1959] 2011), p. 99.

4. "Roman Society, Roman Life," Roman Empire website, http://www.roman
-empire.net/society/society.html. Bread came into general use only at the beginning
of the second century.

5. Scullard, *From the Gracchi to Nero*, p. 152.

6. Ibid., pp. 287, 152, 122.

7. Ibid, p. 287. There are some who regard the corn dole as part of the reason for
the decline of the Roman Empire: "The dole became an integral part of the whole
complex of economic causes that brought the eventual collapse of Roman civilization. It undermined the old Roman virtues of self-reliance. It schooled people to
expect something for nothing. . . . The necessity of feeding the soldiers and the idlers
in the cities led to strangling and destructive taxation. Because of the lethargy of
slaves and undernourished free workmen, industrial progress ceased.

"There were periodic exactions from the rich and frequent confiscations of property. The better-off inhabitants of the towns were forced to provide food, lodging,
and transport for the troops. Soldiers were allowed to loot the districts through
which they passed. Production was everywhere discouraged and in some places
brought to a halt. Ruinous taxation eventually destroyed the sources of revenue."
Henry Hazlitt, "Poor Relief in Ancient Rome," in Henry Hazlitt, *The Conquest of Poverty* (New Rochelle, NY: Arlington House, 1973), http://www.fee.org/the_freeman
/detail/poor-relief-in-ancient-rome.

8. The origin of this word is the tradition in the United States that neighbors who
had cut a lot of timber would find it sensible to join together to roll each other's logs,
Online Etymology Dictionary, http://www.etymonline.com/index.php?allowed_in_fr
ame=0&search=logrolling&searchmode=none.

9. The term "pork barrel" is "used in reference to the use of government
funds for projects designed to please voters or legislators and win votes. The
term, which is recorded from the early 20th century in this sense, refers to the use
of such a barrel by farmers, to keep a reserve supply of meat," Elizabeth Knowles,
ed., *Oxford Dictionary of Phrase and Fable*, 2nd ed. (Oxford: Oxford University
Press, 2005).

10. Timur Kuran, "Now out of Never: The Element of Surprise in the East European Revolution of 1989," *World Politics* 44 (1991): 7–48. This comment refers to the fall
of communism, but the same concepts apply to democratic states.

11. I first heard of "magical thinking" in conversation with Leszek Balcerowicz,
the former deputy prime minister of Poland. The phrase has different meanings
in different contexts. Its application to politics seems to me to be very useful and
identifies an important part of the psychology of government and of voting.

12. See http://thinkexist.com/quotes/plato/3.html.

13. Frédéric Bastiat, *Selected Essays on Political Economy*, tr. Seymour Cain
(Princeton, NJ: Van Nostrand, 1964).

14. Quoted in Geoffrey A. Plauché, "Idealistic Politics," *Libertarian Standard*, April
21, 2011, http://www.libertarianstandard.com/2011/04/21/idealistic-politics.

15. Frédéric Bastiat, "The State," in *"The Law," "The State," and Other Political
Writings 1843–1850* (Indianapolis: Liberty Fund, 2012), pp. 93–95.

16. The story of St. Jeanne of Jugan suggests that there was little, if any, state
support for the elderly in Bastiat's time. See "Our History," Little Sisters of the Poor
website, http://www.littlesistersofthepoor.org/ourlife/our-history. Likewise, the
history of health care was dominated by voluntary mutual benefit societies. See

Simone Sandier et al., *Health Care Systems in Transition: France* (Copenhagen: WHO Regional Office for Europe, 2004), p. 5, http://www.euro.who.int/__data/assets /pdf_file/0009/80694/E83126.pdf.

17. See usgovernmentspending website, http://www.usgovernmentspending .com/us_20th_century_chart.html. This chart shows the rise in spending. However, the precise figures for recent years are not shown. For the 2011 figure, I have used the one cited by Chris Edwards of the Cato Institute in testimony ("American Government Spending: 41% of GDP," Cato at Liberty blog, Cato Institute website, October 19, 2011, http://www.cato.org/blog/american-government-spending-41-gdp). The use of this figure was criticized as being a figure from the Organisation for Economic Co-operation and Development (OECD), but I prefer to use it because the OECD figures are more likely to be comparable internationally than are national figures. An example of the criticism is "Is Government Spending Really 41 Percent of GDP?," Off the Charts blog, Center on Budget and Policy Priorities, blog entry by Kathy Ruffing, October 18, 2011, http://www.offthechartsblog.org /is-government-spending-really-41-percent-of-gdp).

18. "Les dépenses publiques depuis un siècle," Vie Publique website, June 12, 2013, http://www.vie-publique.fr/decouverte-institutions/finances-publiques/appro fondissements/depenses-publiques-depuis-siecle.html.

19. "U.K. Public Spending as Percent of GDP," ukpublicspending website, http:// www.ukpublicspending.co.uk/total_spending_chart#copypaste.

20. "U.K. Public Spending since 1963," *The Guardian* (London), http://www .theguardian.com/news/datablog/2010/apr/25/uk-public-spending-1963#data.

21. 1900: GDP £1.885 million ($2.68 million) and defense spending £71.3 million ($101.2 million). 2010: GDP £1.458 billion ($2.07 billion) and defense spending £42.5 billion ($60.4 billion). "Total Public Spending: Expenditure—Charts—GDPDebt," ukpublicspendingwebsite,http://www.ukpublicspending.co.uk/total_spending _2010UKmn. For the purposes of this book, 1 pound = 1.42 U.S. dollars (exchange rate in March 2016).

22. Defense spending in the United States was much lower in 1900, but all government spending then was much lower at that time. 1900: GDP $20.567 million and defense spending $331.6 million. 1960: GDP $526.4 billion and defense spending $53.3 billion. 2012: GDP $15.7 trillion and defense spending $0.88 trillion. (usgovernmentspending website, http://www.usgovernmentspending.com /total_spending_1960USmn.) It is true that there has been a "peace dividend," in that governments no longer need to spend so much on defense because there appears to be no imminent threat of world war. However, it is also true that this has created extra space for welfare state spending to move into.

23. "Government Expenditure by Function," OECD.StatExtracts, http://stats .oecd.org/Index.aspx?DatasetCode=SNA_TABLE11.

24. Willem Adema, Pauline Fron, and Maxime Ladaique, "Is the European Welfare State Really More Expensive?," OECD Social, Employment and Migration Working Papers no. 124, October 2011, p. 41, http://www.oecd-ilibrary .org/docserver/download/5kg2d2d4pbf0.pdf?expires=1380823120&id=id&accname =guest&checksum=22B3FED9563363089C574081F4670D99.

25. Ibid. In 1980, the figure for "public social expenditure" was 27.2 percent, and in 1989, it was 29.3 percent. The OECD averages were 15.7 percent and 17.3 percent, respectively.

26. Goran Persson, "The Swedish Experience in Reducing Budget Deficits and Debt," *Federal Reserve Bank of Kansas City Economic Review*, Q1 (1996): 7–9, http://www.kansascityfed.org/publicat/econrev/pdf/1q96pers.pdf.

27. Government spending as a proportion of GDP reached 68 percent in 1993. This is the highest figure I remember seeing and surely is at the upper limit for a noncommunist society. The figure came down all the way to below 48 percent in 2012. See "The U.S. and Europe: Governments of Equal Size?," e21 website, Manhattan Institute, February 8, 2012, http://www.economics21.org/commentary/us-and-europe-governments-equal-size.

28. "Appenzell Innerrhoden enjoys 'pure democracy,'" *The Local* (Switzerland), May 24, 2013, http://www.thelocal.ch/20130524/appenzell-practices-democracy-in-its-purest-form.

29. The government expenditure figures are from a table of OECD figures kindly extracted and sent to me by Chris Edwards of the Cato Institute. They are marked "Annexe 25 General Government Total Outlays—Percent of Nominal GDP." The figures go up to 2013, but because those figures must be forecast ones, given that the table was published in that year, I have taken the figures for 2012. The tax statistics are OECD figures from OECD.Statextracts (http://stats.oecd.org/Index.aspx?QueryId=21699 accessed 2 December 2014). I have used the latest figure (2011) for Switzerland, but since there is no OECD figure for that year, I have taken the one for 2010.

30. There are different estimates one could use. I have used the World Bank's GDP per capita on a purchasing power parity basis for 2013 (http://data.worldbank.org/indicator/NY.GDP.PCAP.PP.CD?order=wbapi_data_value_2011%20wbapi_data_value%20wbapi_data_value-last&sort=desc). The countries ahead of Switzerland were Qatar, Macao, Luxembourg, Kuwait, Singapore, Brunei, Norway, and the United Arab Emirates. Close behind were Hong Kong and the United States.

31. Lars Feld, Justina Fischer, and Gebhard Kirchgässner, "The Effect of Direct Democracy on Income Redistribution: Evidence for Switzerland," London School of Economics and Political Science, October 2006, http://sticerd.lse.ac.uk/dps/pepp/pepp23.pdf. This paper refers in the introduction to two previous studies: C. Schaltegger, "The Effects of Federalism and Democracy on the Size of Government: Evidence from Swiss Sub-national Jurisdictions," *ifo Studien* 47 (2001): 145–62; A. Vatter and M. Freitag, "Die Janusköpfigkeit von Verhandlungsdemokratien: Zur Wirkung von Konkordanz, direkter Demokratie und dezentraler Entscheidungsstrukturen auf den öffentlichen Sektor der Schweizer Kantone," *Swiss Political Science Review* 8 (2002): 53–80.

32. Feld et al., "The Effect of Direct Democracy on Income Redistribution." See Table 2.

33. Lars P. Feld and John G. Matsuka, "Budget Referendums and Government Spending: Economic Evidence from Swiss Cantons," http://www.iandrinstitute.org/New%20IRI%20Website%20Info/I&R%20Research%20and%20History/I&R%20Studies/Feld%20and%20Matsusaka%20-%20Fiscal%20Evidence%20from%20Swiss%20Cantons%20IRI.pdf.

34. Bruno Frey, "The Role of Democracy in Securing Just and Prosperous Societies: Direct Democracy—Politico-Economic Lessons from Swiss Experience," *American Economic Review* 84 (1994): 338–42.

35. From 13.8 percent to 18.5 percent (OECD figures); see Adema et al., "Is the European Welfare State Really More Expensive?," Table A.I.1.3.

36. For the current figure, see ibid. The 1970 figure comes from *OECD Economic Surveys 1985–86: Switzerland* (Paris: OECD Publishing, 1986).

37. Patrick McGreevy and Melanie Mason, "Spending Impulse Curbed in California," *Washington Post*, September 26, 2013, http://www.washingtonpost.com /national/spending-impulse-curbed-in-california/2013/09/26/7cb43b2c-1efa-11e3 -8459-657e0c72fec8_story.html.

38. See http://en.wikipedia.org/wiki/2008%E2%80%9312_California_budget _crisis.

39. I am grateful to my friend Christian Wignall for his help with this, October 2013.

40. In my interview with economist Leszek Balcerowicz in Warsaw, he said that he introduced this limit. I see that the limit was in line with but not identical to the European Union limits on spending. But Poland is different from other EU countries by having enshrined the rule in its constitution. See also Ian Lienert, "Should Advanced Countries Adopt a Fiscal Responsibility Law?," IMF Working Paper WP/10/254, International Monetary Fund, Washington, D.C., November 2010, p. 17, http://www.imf.org/external/pubs/ft/wp/2010/wp10254.pdf.

41. See Lienert, "Should Advanced Countries Adopt a Fiscal Responsibility Law?"; Jón R. Blöndal, "Budgeting in Singapore," *OECD Journal on Budgeting* 6 (2006): 51, http://www.oecd.org/gov/budgeting/40140241.pdf.

Chapter 13

1. More of the quotation can be read here: http://www.heretical.com/British /mhistory.html.

2. Found in countries with government-operated health care, government health visitors are health care workers who visit individuals—particularly new mothers—in their homes and give advice and support about hygiene, nutrition, and so on.

3. Big Brother appears in George Orwell's novel *Nineteen Eighty-Four* (1949). He is the dictator of a totalitarian state whose citizens are under constant surveillance by the authorities.

4. "Spain's Jobless Rate Falls for First Time in Two Years," *BBC News* online, July 25, 2013, http://www.bbc.co.uk/news/business-23447087.

5. Quoted in Jonathan Haidt, *The Happiness Hypothesis: Putting Ancient Wisdom to the Test of Modern Science* (London: Arrow, 2006), p. 133.

6. Eric Klinenberg, *Going Solo: The Extraordinary Rise and Surprising Appeal of Living Alone* (New York: Penguin Press, 2012).

7. Homeschooling has been illegal in Germany since Hitler banned it in 1938. It is one of the few Nazi laws still on the books. Hitler introduced the ban to force all children to attend state-approved schools where they were to be indoctrinated with Nazi ideology. In one recent case, "the children, between 7 and 14 years old, were forcibly removed from their parents, Dirk and Petra Wunderlich, and taken into state custody at an unknown location." Peter Martino, "Europe: Treating Home-schoolers like Terrorists," Gatestone Institute website, September 10, 2013, http:// www.gatestoneinstitute.org/3969/europe-homeschoolers.

Appendix 2

1. "Labor Force Participation Rate, Male (% of Male Population Ages 15+) (Modeled ILO Estimate)," World Bank website, http://data.worldbank.org/indicator /SL.TLF.CACT.MA.ZS.

2. Sweden's functional illiteracy was worse in the 2012 Programme for International Student Assessment (PISA) than it had been in previous studies. This could be an aberration or it might reflect deterioration.

3. World Bank gross national income per capita based on purchasing power parity converted to international dollar rates, meaning the purchasing power is the same as it would be in the United States. Figures for 2013. High figures (excluding oil states and very small tax havens): Singapore $76,850, Switzerland $56,580, United States $53,960. Low figures: Portugal $25,350, Greece $25,650, Spain $31,850. See http://data.worldbank.org/indicator/NY.GNP.PCAP.PP.CD/countries.

Appendix 4

1. The phrase was popularized and perhaps invented by Gøsta Esping-Andersen in his influential book *The Three Worlds of Welfare Capitalism* (Cambridge, U.K.: Polity Press, 1989). See my blog about an extract from his book at http://www.thewelfare statewerein.com/general/2011/10/esping-andersen-and-his-three-worlds-of -welfare-capitalism.php.

2. I hope Esping-Andersen, who used the idea of "decommodification" in *The Three Worlds of Welfare Capitalism* (see Note 1), will forgive this jocular account of how the concept comes up against reality.

3. Not everyone would agree with this definition, which is probably not the original one and certainly is not the one used in insurance and finance, where "risk" is the key word.

4. Rebecca Milner, "Japan's Top Buzzwords for 2012," Japan Pulse blog, *Japan Times*, December 3, 2012, http://blog.japantimes.co.jp/japan-pulse/japans-top-10 -buzzwords-for-2012.

5. One example would be a law intended to conserve suitable habitats for endangered species by decreeing that no development should be allowed in such places. This could create an incentive for property owners to destroy anything that might be categorized as suitable for an endangered species in the fear that the possibility of development might be removed. See Sean Masaki Flynn, "In Pictures: Perverse Incentives," *Forbes*, February 19, 2009, p. 8, http://www.forbes.com/2009/02/19 /bonuses-incentives-pay-leadership-compensation_perverse_incentives_slide_8 .html.

6. Timur Kuran, "Now out of Never: The Element of Surprise in the East European Revolution of 1989," *World Politics* 44 (1991): 7–48.

7. Frédéric Bastiat, "What Is Seen and What Is Not Seen," available at Library of Economics and Liberty website, http://www.econlib.org/library/Bastiat/basEss1 .html.

Afterword

1. Peter Saunders, *When Prophecy Fails* (St. Leonards, NSW: Centre for Independent Studies, 2011), pp. 33–34.

2. Ibid., pp. 48–49.

3. Wilkinson and Pickett replied to Saunders and other critics in a revised edition of *The Spirit Level* (London: Penguin Books, 2010, pp. 273–98). They argued that there were "no hard and fast rules" about including outliers. They said that testing for third variables would have various drawbacks including creating "unnecessary noise" and they did not address the criticism that they omitted to show the R^2 figures and statistical significance or otherwise of their findings.

I asked a fellow of the Royal Statistical Society who also happens to be a qualified actuary whether these replies were satisfactory. He replied, "If you really want to draw an inference, then it would be a good idea to test robustness by removing outliers." He said that Wilkinson and Pickett's failure to address the issues of R^2 and statistical significance was itself "very significant." He also suggested that "addition of other variables does not add noise, it removes noise by providing alternative explanations and by explaining something more fully."

4. It is fair to say that there has been an active and sometimes acrimonious disagreement between Wilkinson and Saunders. I have read and made use of the critique of Wilkinson's work but only after considering the responses to it contained in the later edition of *The Spirit Level*. The responses do not include any substantive reply to the criticism that he and Pickett failed to use standard tests used by social scientists. He could well say to me that this book is full of ideas and assertions that have not been subjected to the normal tests of social science. That is wholly true. However, this book is not offered by an academic social scientist as an academic piece of work.

5. "Sweden's Gini coefficient for disposable income is now 0.24, still a lot lower than the rich-world average of 0.31 but around 25% higher than it was a generation ago." "The New Model," *The Economist*, October 11, 2012, http://www.economist.com/node/21564412. The article attributes the change to the less left-wing government and does not seem to consider the impact of immigration despite referring to it. In Malmö, in 2010, immigrants accounted for 80,000 of 300,000 inhabitants, according to the *Guardian*. Ian Traynor, "Sweden Joins Europe-Wide Backlash against Immigration," the *Guardian* (London), September 24, 2010, http://www.theguardian.com/world/2010/sep/24/sweden-immigration-far-right-asylum.

6. Japan is one of the countries that have low inequality according to the World Bank. This is the information used by Wilkinson and Pickett. But the OECD does not agree, placing it as slightly more unequal than the median. The difference is accounted for by the fact that the World Bank does not include the incomes of self-employed farmers and single-person households, but the OECD does. These people constitute 40 percent of the population in Japan. It does seem, at the least, unreliable to describe Japan as a country of low inequality. Certainly it does not have a culture of equality. But if one was going to assert confidently that it has low inequality, one should perhaps then consider to what extent this might be because Japan has had less immigration than most countries have had.

7. Michael Tanner, "The Income–Inequality Myth," *National Review* online, January 10, 2012, http://www.nationalreview.com/articles/287643/income-inequality-myth-michael-tanner. "A recent study by Mark Warshawsky of the Social Security Board suggests that nearly all of the recent increase in earnings inequality 'can be explained by the rapid increase in the cost of health insurance employee benefits, and that therefore [there] has not been as significant increase, if any, in inequality of compensation.'"

8. Ibid.

9. "First ONS Annual Experimental Subjective Well-being Results," U.K. Office for National Statistics, July 24, 2012, http://www.ons.gov.uk/ons/dcp171766_272294 .pdf.

10. Bruno S. Frey and Alois Stutzer, "The Economics of Happiness," *World Economics* 3 (2002).

11. Andrew E. Clark and Andrew J. Oswald, "Unhappiness and Unemployment," *Economic Journal* 104 (1994): 648–59.

12. David G. Blanchflower and Andrew J. Oswald, "International Happiness: A New View on the Measure of Performance," *Academy of Management Perspectives*, February 2011, pp. 6–22, http://www.dartmouth.edu/~blnchflr/papers/int% 20happiness.pdf.

13. *Men, Suicide and Society: Why Disadvantaged Men in Mid-life Die by Suicide*, Samaritans, September 2012, http://www.samaritans.org/sites/default/files/kcfinder /files/Men%20and%20Suicide%20Research%20Report%20210912.pdf.

14. "Individual level studies . . . are studies in which the units of analysis are individuals. . . . Individual level studies are most appropriate when investigators are interested in explaining variations between individuals." Anna V. Diez-Roux, "Potentialities and Limitations of Multilevel Analysis in Public Health and Epidemiology," in *Methodology and Epistemology of Multilevel Analysis: Approaches from Different Social Sciences,* ed. Daniel Courgeau (Dordrecht, the Netherlands: Kluwer, 2003). This kind of study is distinct from "ecological" studies, which have nothing to do with the environment but are those studies in which different areas, such as countries, are compared. Thus, it may be that a country with lots of unemployment does not have a high rate of suicide yet, within that country, the unemployed are nonetheless much more likely to commit suicide than are the employed. One might guess that the explanation of this difference could be that the culture of a country and other country-specific factors also affect the incidence of suicide.

15. Kouichi Yoshimasu et al., "Suicidal Risk Factors and Completed Suicide: Meta-analyses Based on Psychological Autopsy Studies," *Environmental Health and Preventive Medicine* 13 (2008): 243–56.

16. Alfonso Ceccherini-Nelli and Stefan Priebe, "Economic Factors and Suicide Rates: Associations over Time in Four Countries," *Social Psychiatry and Psychiatric Epidemiology* 46 (2011): 975–82.

17. *Men, Suicide and Society*, p. 39.

18. Admittedly it is conceivable that some Catholic countries may underreport their suicides. Cross-country comparisons unfortunately have this problem of different rates of reporting and also varying accuracy in measurement.

19. Hara Estroff Marano, "The Dangers of Loneliness," *Psychology Today*, July 1, 2003, http://www.psychologytoday.com/articles/200308/the-dangers-loneliness.

20. Louise Hawkley et al., "Loneliness Is a Unique Predictor of Age-Related Differences in Systolic Blood Pressure," *Psychology and Aging* 21 (2006): 152–64.

21. Ibid. The extent to which this is the case is not clear. At one extreme, a Swedish study found that loneliness among children ages 12–13 was associated with a three-fold increase in risk of suicide at age 24–25. Anne Lise Stranden, "Suicide Linked to Loneliness in Childhood," *ScienceNordic*, May 29, 2014, http://sciencenordic .com/suicide-linked-loneliness-childhood. At the other extreme, Cacioppo himself reported an increased risk of "premature death" of seniors of 14 percent. This would

include suicide, but would not compose suicide alone. David McNamee, "Loneliness Increases Risk of Early Death in Seniors," *MNT* (Medical News Today), February 17, 2014, http://www.medicalnewstoday.com/articles/272705.php.

22. The pattern shown in this research is very clear. There has been a big rise in the proportion of people in this age group who are living alone, because of divorce, separation, and, in some cases, never having lived with partners. Meanwhile, there has also been a (more modest) increase in the proportion of those over age 60 living alone. What is probably more significant here is that more people are living longer so the number of over-60 individuals living alone has increased significantly. This particularly affects women, who tend to outlive their husbands and partners. Among women ages 61 and above, 47.9 percent live alone—a frightening statistic. The proportion of women living alone passes 90 percent by the time they reach 85.

23. Suicide rates, like most statistics, are not always to be relied upon. The culture of one society may be such that it is particularly unwilling to admit that a person has committed suicide. There are also some strange changes in figures over time, with the rate in Denmark falling more than half in only eight years from 1990. The source for the latter is Diego De Leo and Russell Evans, *International Suicide Rates: Recent Trends and Implications for Australia,* Australian Institute for Suicide Research and Prevention, 2003.

Acknowledgments

1. It is available from the Centre for Independent Studies website: http://www.cis.org.au/publications/cis-special-publications/article/3474-when-prophecy-fails.

Index

A page reference followed by f indicates figure; t indicates table.

About the Author

James Bartholomew is a journalist and author with a wide range of international experience. After studying history at Oxford, he worked in banking briefly, before becoming a journalist, first for the *Financial Times* and then the *Far Eastern Economic Review* based in Hong Kong and then Tokyo. The rapid economic growth in Hong Kong made a strong impression on him and formed a vivid contrast with the poverty and political oppression he witnessed when travelling across communist China and the Soviet Union. After the fall of the Berlin Wall, he was an East European consultant for an investment company, travelling to most of the formerly communist countries.

When working as a writer for the *Daily Telegraph* and the *Daily Mail*, he came to believe that the British welfare state has done more harm than good. He wrote *The Welfare State We're In*, a critique of the welfare state that came to influence government reforms. It was commended by Milton Friedman and won several awards, including the Sir Anthony Fisher Memorial Award from the Atlas Foundation.

Bartholomew travelled to 11 different countries to research *The Welfare of Nations*. From charter schools in California to hospitals in Spain and from a welfare benefit office in Singapore to housing projects dominated by drug gangs in France, he has seen how welfare states work and how they are changing the nature of our civilization for the worse.

Bartholomew is a fellow of the Institute of Economic Affairs and of the Adam Smith Institute in London.

Cato Institute

Founded in 1977, the Cato Institute is a public policy research foundation dedicated to broadening the parameters of policy debate to allow consideration of more options that are consistent with the principles of limited government, individual liberty, and peace. To that end, the Institute strives to achieve greater involvement of the intelligent, concerned lay public in questions of policy and the proper role of government.

The Institute is named for Cato's Letters, libertarian pamphlets that were widely read in the American Colonies in the early 18th century and played a major role in laying the philosophical foundation for the American Revolution.

Despite the achievement of the nation's Founders, today virtually no aspect of life is free from government encroachment. A pervasive intolerance for individual rights is shown by government's arbitrary intrusions into private economic transactions and its disregard for civil liberties. And while freedom around the globe has notably increased in the past several decades, many countries have moved in the opposite direction, and most governments still do not respect or safeguard the wide range of civil and economic liberties.

To address those issues, the *Cato Institute* undertakes an extensive publications program on the complete spectrum of policy issues. Books, monographs, and shorter studies are commissioned to examine the federal budget, Social Security, regulation, military spending, international trade, and myriad other issues. Major policy conferences are held throughout the year, from which papers are published thrice yearly in the *Cato Journal*. The Institute also publishes the quarterly magazine *Regulation*.

In order to maintain its independence, the Cato Institute accepts no government funding. Contributions are received from foundations, corporations, and individuals, and other revenue is generated from the sale of publications. The Institute is a nonprofit, tax-exempt, educational foundation under Section 501(c)3 of the Internal Revenue Code.

CATO INSTITUTE
1000 Massachusetts Ave., N.W.
Washington, D.C. 20001